Clinical Updates in
Obstetrics and Gynecology

Clinical Updates in
Obstetrics and Gynecology

Editor

Usha Sharma
MBBS, MS (Obstetrics and Gynecology), DIP in Sterility, USA
Awarded Padmashri

Professor Emeritus
Obstetrics and Gynecology and Chief Hospital Administrator
Muzaffarnagar Medical College, Muzaffarnagar
Ex-Principal-cum-Professor of Gynecology and Obstetrics
LLRM Medical College, Meerut
Chief Patron, UPCOG and Meerut Obstetrics and Gynecology Society

Co-Editor

Bharti Maheshwari
MBBS, MD (Obstetrics and Gynecology), FICOG

Professor, Obstetrics and Gynecology
Muzaffarnagar Medical College, Muzaffarnagar
Joint Secretary, UPCOG
Secretary, Meerut Obstetrics and Gynecology Society

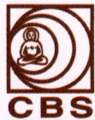

CBS Publishers & Distributors Pvt Ltd

New Delhi • Bengaluru • Chennai • Kochi • Kolkata • Mumbai
Hyderabad • Nagpur • Patna • Pune • Vijayawada

Clinical Updates in
Obstetrics and
Gynecology

ISBN: 978-93-85915-00-0

Copyright © Editors and Publisher

First Edition: 2016

Published by Satish Kumar Jain and produced by Varun Jain for
CBS Publishers & Distributors Pvt Ltd
4819/XI Prahlad Street, 24 Ansari Road, Daryaganj, New Delhi 110 002, India.
Ph: 23289259, 23266861, 23266867   Fax: 011-23243014   Website: www.cbspd.com
                                                                    e-mail: delhi@cbspd.com; cbspubs@airtelmail.in.
Corporate Office: 204 FIE, Industrial Area, Patparganj, Delhi 110 092
Ph: 4934 4934   Fax: 4934 4935   e-mail: publishing@cbspd.com; publicity@cbspd.com

Branches

- **Bengaluru:** Seema House 2975, 17th Cross, K.R. Road, Banasankari 2nd Stage, Bengaluru 560 070, Karnataka
  Ph: +91-80-26771678/79   Fax: +91-80-26771680   e-mail: bangalore@cbspd.com
- **Chennai:** No. 7, Subbaraya Street, Shenoy Nagar, Chennai 600 030, Tamil Nadu
  Ph: +91-44-26680620, 26681266   Fax: +91-44-42032115   e-mail: chennai@cbspd.com
- **Kochi:** Ashana House, 39/1904, AM Thomas Road, Valanjambalam, Ernakulam 682 016, Kochi, Kerala
  Ph: +91-484-4059061–65,67   Fax: +91-484-4059065   e-mail: kochi@cbspd.com
- **Kolkata:** No. 6/B, Ground Floor, Rameswar Shaw Road, Kolkata-700014 (West Bengal), India
  Ph: +91-33-2289-1126, 2289-1127, 2289-1128   e-mail: kolkata@cbspd.com
- **Mumbai:** 83-C, Dr E Moses Road, Worli, Mumbai-400018, Maharashtra
  Ph: +91-22-24902340/41   Fax: +91-22-24902342   e-mail: mumbai@cbspd.com

Representatives

- **Hyderabad** 0-9885175004   • **Nagpur** 0-9021734563   • **Patna**   0-9334159340
- **Pune**   0-9623451994   • **Vijayawada** 0-9000660880

Printed at Paras Offset Pvt. Ltd., New Delhi

to

---

my revered parents
Dr. Kalendri Prasad Nigam and
Dr. (Mrs.) Ram Kali Nigam
who taught me the value of hard work and
were always my inspiration and guiding light

Usha Sharma

Contributors

Abhilasha Gupta
Professor and Head
Dept of Obst and Gyne
LLRM Medical College, Meerut

Bharti Maheshwari
Professor
Dept of Obst and Gyne
Muzaffarnagar Medical College
Muzaffarnagar

Kirti Dubey
Professor
Dept of Obst and Gyne
LLRM Medical College
Meerut

Kuldeep Jain
Director
KJIVF Centre
New Delhi

Kiran Pandey
Professor and Head
Dept of Obst and Gyne
GSVM Medical College
Kanpur

Mamta Tyagi
Professor
Dept of Obst and Gyne
Subharti Medical College
Meerut

Neerja
Professor
Dept of Obst and Gyne
Muzaffarnagar Medical College
Muzaffarnagar

Nutan Jain
Director
Vardhman Hospital
Muzaffarnagar

Rukma Idnani
Ex. Professor and Head
Dept of Obst and Gyne
LLRM Medical College, Meerut
Ex. Principal, Saraswati Medical College
Hapur

Renu Misra
Senior Consultant
Endoscopic Surgery and IVF
Sitaram Bhartia Institute of
Science and Research
Miracles Medicare, Gurgaon
Former Additional Professor
All India Institute of Medical Sciences
New Delhi

Saroj Singh
Professor and Head
Dept of Obst and Gyne
SN Medical College
Agra

SK Gulati
Professor and Head
Dept of Obst and Gyne
Muzaffarnagar Medical College
Muzaffarnagar

Sushma Rastogi
Ex-Professor
Dept of Obst and Gyne
LLRM Medical College
Meerut

Usha Sharma
Professor Emeritus
Dept of Obst and Gyne
Muzaffarnagar Medical College
Muzaffarnagar

Preface

It gives me great pleasure to present this book. Many renowned authors, well known in the field, have contributed various chapters to update the present knowledge on the subject. I have tried to make this book comprehensive and easy to understand for both undergraduates and postgraduate students.

All of us very well understand that it is impossible to compete and sustain in any field of medicine today without refreshing our knowledge from time to time. There are many chapters like 'Labor', 'High Risk Pregnancy' and 'Infertility' in which challenges experienced everyday have also been taken into consideration.

Great care has been taken in the selection of topics which matter the most, not only to the students but also to one who practises the art and science of obstetrics and gynecology. Therefore, I consider that the book will not only be fruitful for the students but also for the teachers and practitioners.

I am thankful to my coeditor Dr Bharti Maheshwari who has worked very hard to help me in this endeavor. I am also obliged to all the authors who have tried to do a great job in writing their individual chapters in this book.

I believe this book shall be an immense educational resource to all concerned in the field of obstetrics and gynecology.

Usha Sharma

Contents

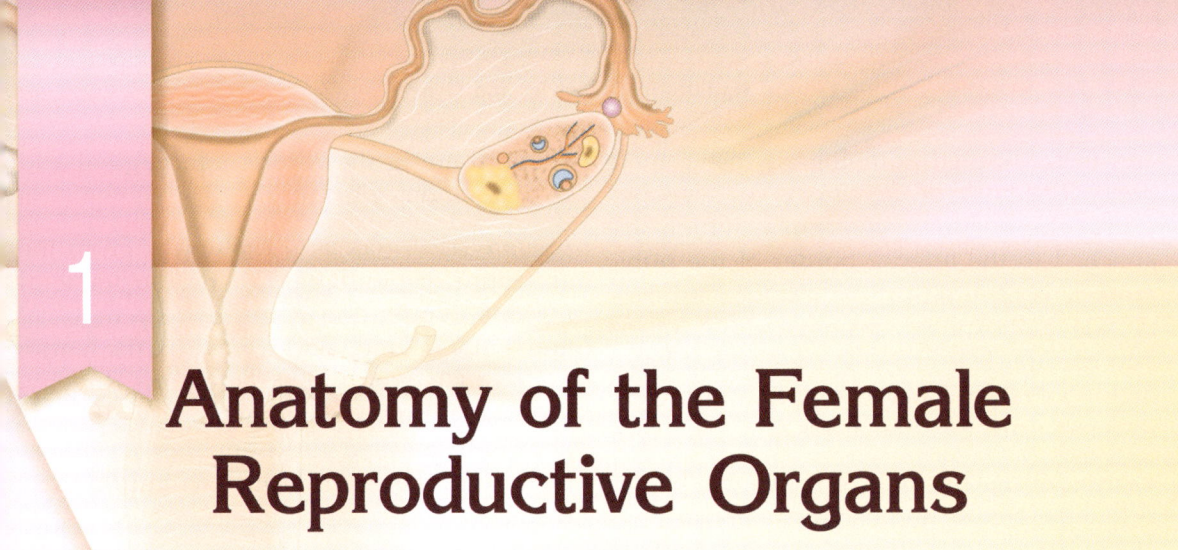

1

Anatomy of the Female Reproductive Organs

• SK Gulati

An understanding of the anatomy of the female reproductive organs are essential for obstetrical practice. The female reproductive organs are composed of external genitalia (vulva), internal genitalia like vagina, uterus, fallopian tubes and ovaries and other supportive structures like pelvic floor and perineum.

VULVA

The external female genitalia that surround the opening to the vagina; collectively consist of the labia majora, the labia minora, clitoris, vestibule of the vagina, bulb of the vestibule, and the glands of Bartholin. All of these organs are located in front of the anus and below the mons pubis (the pad of fatty tissue at the forward junction of the pelvic bones) (Fig. 1.1).

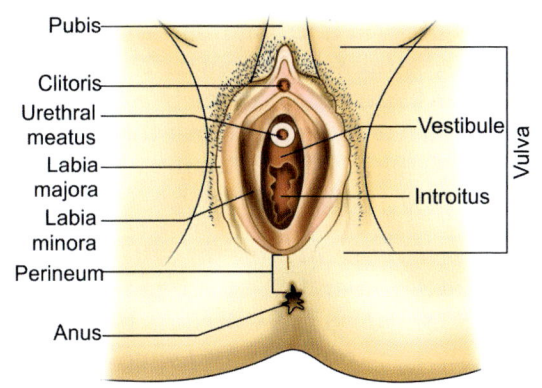

Fig. 1.1: Vulva

Mons pubis: It is composed of fibro-fatty tissue, which covers the body of the pubic bones. Inferiorly it divides to become continuous with the labium majus on each side of the vulva. In the adult, the skin that covers the mons pubis bears pubic hair, the upper limit of which is usually horizontal.

Labia majora: They are two folds of skin with underlying adipose tissue bounding either side of the vaginal opening. They contain sebaceous and sweat glands and a few specialized apocrine glands. In the deepest part of each labium is a core of fatty tissue continuous with that of the inguinal canal and the fibers of the round ligament terminate here.

Labia minora: They are two thin folds of skin that lie between the labia majora. Anteriorly they divide into two to form the prepuce and frenulum of the clitoris. Posteriorly they fuse to form a fold of skin called the fourchette. They contain sebaceous glands but have no adipose tissue and hairs. They are not well developed before puberty, and atrophy after the menopause. Their vascularity allows them to become turgid during sexual excitement.

Clitoris: It is a small erectile structure. It is capable of some enlargement caused by increased blood flow during sexual excitement and is considered homologous to the male penis. The body of the clitoris contains two crura, the corpora cavernosa, which are attached to the inferior border of the pubic rami. It is covered by the ischiocavernosus muscle; bulbospongiosus muscle and inserts into its root. It is about 1 cm long but has a highly developed nerve supply and is very sensitive during sexual arousal.

Vestibule: The vestibule of the vagina begins below the clitoris and contains the openings of the urethra, the vagina, and the ducts of the two glands of Bartholin. The urethral opening is a small slit located close to the clitoris. The vestibular bulbs are two oblong masses of erectile tissue that lie on either side of the vaginal entrance. They contain a rich plexus of veins within the bulbospongiosus muscle.

Bartholin's glands: The size of a small pea. lie at the base of each bulb and open via a 2 cm duct into the vestibule between the hymen and the labia minora. These are mucus-secreting, producing copious amounts during intercourse to act as a lubricant.

Hymen: It is a thin fold of mucous membrane across the entrance to the vagina. There are usually openings in it to allow menses to escape. It is partially ruptured during first coitus and is further disrupted during childbirth. Any tags remaining after rupture are known as carunculae myrtiformes.

Blood Supply

Arterial supply: Internal pudendal artery: The terminal branch of the anterior division of the internal iliac artery that ends as the dorsal artery of the clitoris. Branches from the femoral artery, supply the anterior part. Superficial and deep external pudendal arteries.

Venous drainage: The veins draining the vulva form a venous plexus from which veins accompany their corresponding arteries. The

veins draining the clitoris join vaginal and vesical venous plexuses.

Lymphatic drainage of the vulva: From the skin and appendages, to the superficial inguinal lymph nodes, to the deep inguinal and femoral lymph nodes of which the lymph node of Cloquet drains the clitoris directly. From the former superficial group, lymphatic channels pass to the deep pelvic nodes including; the external iliac, common iliac, then para-aortic lymph nodes.

Nerve supply of the vulva: The vulva is supplied mainly from the pudendal nerve (S2, 3 and 4). Additional sensory nerves are supplied from; the Ilioinguinal nerve (L1), the genital branch of genitofemoral nerve (L1, 2), and the posterior cutaneous nerve of the thigh.

THE INTERNAL REPRODUCTIVE ORGANS

Vagina: It is a fibromuscular canal lined with stratified squamous epithelium that leads from the uterus to the vulva forming an angle of 60° with the horizontal plane. Length: Anterior wall is 8–9 cm and posterior wall is 10–11 cm.

Vaginal fornices: The cervix projects in the upper blind end of the vagina that forms a pouch (vaginal pouch) around the cervix and is divided into four fornices: Two lateral, anterior and posterior (deeper) fornices. The vaginal walls are rugose, with transverse folds. There are no glands in the vaginal lamina propria and vaginal lubrication is provided by transudate from the blood vessels as well as by secretions of the Bartholin's and Skene's gland. The epithelium is thick and rich in glycogen, which increases in the postovulatory phase of the cycle.

Anatomical relations of the vagina: Anteriorly-upper 1/3—trigone of urinary bladder and lower 2/3—urethra. Posteriorly, upper 1/3—peritoneum of Douglas pouch, middle 1/3—ampulla of rectum and lower 1/3—the perineal body. Laterally, lower end bulbocavernosus muscle, vestibular bulb, and Bartholin's gland, 1 cm above orifice: Urogenital diaphragm, 2½ cm above the orifice: Levator ani muscle with the pelvic fascia above it. The lateral fornix gives attachment, to the lower part of the cardinal ligaments. The ureters pass through the cardinal ligaments 1 cm lateral to the vagina.

Vaginal supports: Vaginal support, as described by DeLancey in 1992, is achieved at three different levels: Level I—the uterosacral cardinal ligament complex, supports the upper vagina and the uterine cervix. Level II—the paravaginal support of the vaginal sidewalls to the arcus tendineus fasciae pelvis. Level III—the support of the distal part of the vagina to the perineum. Vaginal fascia: Connective tissue fascia that condenses anteriorly forming the vesico-vaginal fascia and posteriorly forming the rectovaginal fascia.

Histology of the vagina: The cut section of the vagina is H shaped with approximation of the anterior to the posterior vaginal walls. It is formed of three layers:
1. Mucosa, formed of squamous epithelium without glands

2. Musculosa, which is fibromuscular with some fibers from the levator ani inserted into it, and
3. Adventitia, which is connective tissue continuous with the paracolpos.

Blood Supply
Arterial supply: The vaginal artery (from internal iliac artery), additional branches from: Middle rectal artery (from internal iliac artery), inferior rectal artery (from the internal pudendal artery, the internal iliac artery).

Venous drainage: A plexus around the vagina (the vaginal plexus), drain into the internal iliac vein by veins that accompany their corresponding arteries.

Lymphatic drainage of the vagina: Lower 1/3 drains to the inguinal lymph nodes, upper 1/3 follows lymphatic drainage of the cervix, middle 1/3, drains in both upper and lower directions.

Nerve supply of the vagina: The pudendal nerve gives sensory fibers to the lower vagina (Fig. 1.2).

UTERUS
The uterus varies considerably in size, shape and weight depending on the status of

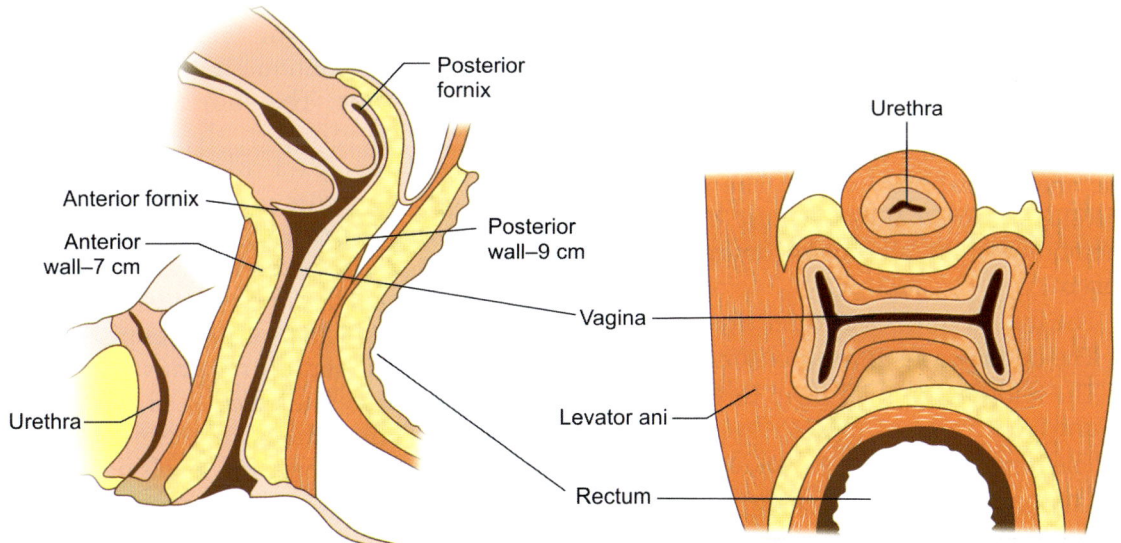

Fig. 1.2: Relations and cut section of vagina

parturition and estrogenic stimulation. The uterus is a fibromuscular organ that can be divided into the upper muscular walls. Its maximum external dimensions are approximately 7.5 cm long, 5 cm wide and 3 cm thick. An adult uterus weighs about 70 gm. The upper part is termed the body or corpus. The area of insertion of each fallopian tube is termed the cornu. The upper part of the uterus above the insertion of the fallopian tubes is called the fundus. The narrow portion situated between corpus and cervix is known as the isthmus and approximately at the level of the course of the uterine artery and the internal os of the cervix (Fig. 1.3).

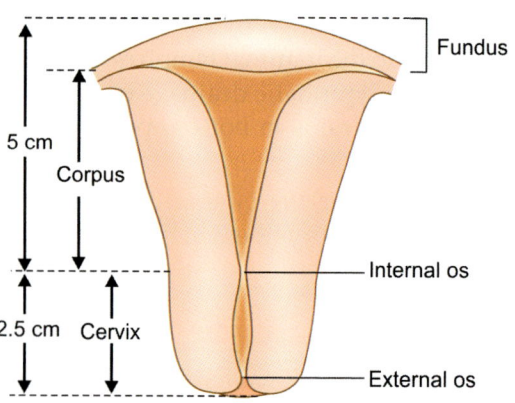

Fig. 1.3: Uterus and cervix

The cervix projects obliquely into the vagina and can be divided into vaginal and supravaginal portions. The constriction at the isthmus where the corpus joins the cervix is the anatomical internal os. The site of the histological internal os is where the mucous membrane of the isthmus becomes that of the cervix.

The uterus consists of three layers:

- The outer serous layer (peritoneum)
- The middle muscular layer (myometrium) and
- The inner mucous layer (endometrium).

The peritoneum covers the body of the uterus, and posteriorly, the supravaginal portion of the cervix. The serous coat is intimately attached to a subserous fibrous layer except laterally, where it spreads out to form the leaves of the broad ligament. The muscular myometrium forms the main bulk of the uterus and comprises interlacing smooth muscle fibers intermingling with areolar tissue, blood vessels, nerves and lymphatics. The muscular layer of the uterus has outer longitudinal layer (stratum supravasculare) continuing into the fallopian tubes and round ligaments. The vascular layer (stratum vasculare) consists of many interlacing spiral groups of smooth muscles and contains many blood vessels. An inner layer consists of muscle fibers arranged both longitudinally and obliquely. The inner endometrial layer has tubular glands that dip into the myometrium. The endometrial layer is covered by a single layer of columnar epithelium. This epithelium is mostly lost due to the effects of pregnancy and menstruation. The endometrium undergoes cyclical changes during menstruation and varies in thickness between 1 and 5 mm.

The endometrial cavity lies above the internal cervical os. It is roughly triangular in shape and measures approximately 3.5 cm in length. Ordinarily, the anterior and posterior walls of the uterus lie in apposition so that a little if any actual cavity is present. At each cornu or horn of the uterus, the cavity of the uterus becomes continuous with the lumen of a fallopian tube. The endometrium varies greatly depending on the phase of the menstrual cycle. Proliferation of the endometrium occurs under the influence of estrogen; maturation occurs under the influence of progesterone. The uterine endometrial cycle can be divided into three phases: The follicular or proliferative phase, the luteal or secretory phase, and the menstrual phase. The follicular, or proliferative phase, spans from the end of the menstruation until ovulation. Increasing levels of estrogen induce proliferation of the functionalis from stem cells of the basalis, proliferation of endometrial glands, and proliferation of stromal connective tissue. Endometrial glands are elongated with narrow lumens and their epithelial cells contain some glycogen. Glycogen, however, is not secreted during the follicular phase. Spiral arteries elongate and span the length of the endometrium.

The endometrium lines the uterine cavity and is considered to have three layers: The pars basalis, the zona spongiosa, and the superficial zona compacta. The straight branches of the radial arteries of the uterus terminate in capillaries in the basal layer, while the spiral or coiled branches penetrate to the surface epithelium, where they give rise to superficial capillaries. Sinus-like dilatations of the capillaries in the superficial layer are called "lakes". These vascular lakes and capillaries are drained by small veins.

The uterus is partially supported by three pairs of ligaments. The paired round ligaments extend from the anterosuperior surface of the uterus through the internal inguinal rings and through the inguinal canals to end in the labia majora. They are composed of muscle fibers, connective tissue, blood vessels, nerves, and lymphatics. The round ligaments stretch with relative ease, particularly in pregnancy. The uterosacral ligaments are condensations of endopelvic fascia that arise from the posterior wall of the uterus at the level of the internal cervical os. They fan out in the retroperitoneal layer and attach broadly at the second, third, and fourth segments of the sacrum. They are predominately composed of smooth muscle but also contain connective tissue, blood vessels, lymphatics, and parasympathetic nerve fibers. The paired cardinal (Mackenrodt's) or transverse cervical ligaments arise from the anterior and posterior marginal walls of the cervix and fan out laterally to insert into the fascia overlying the obturator muscles and the levator ani muscles. The cardinal ligaments form the base of the broad ligament. They are composed of perivascular connective tissue and nerves that surround the uterine artery and veins. The cardinal and uterosacral ligament complex is collectively called the parametrium.

Position of the uterus: The "positions" of the uterus are of considerable interest but of much less importance in gynecologic practice than 50 years ago. The most common position of the uterus in a nulligravid female is in moderate anteflexion or bent slightly anteriorly, and the uterus as a whole is inclined toward the symphysis in ante version against the bladder, adapting its position as the latter organ distends or empties. In a variable number of women, the uterus is retroverted or inclined posteriorly or retroflexed toward the sacrum. Quite a few disabilities were attributed to these "malpositions" in the past including dysmenorrhea, functional uterine bleeding, backache, dyspareunia, and leukorrhea. Many normal uteri are in midposition, with the axis of uterus being almost parallel to the spine.

The broad ligament is formed by folds of peritoneum covering the fallopian tubes, the infundibulopelvic vessels, and the hilus of the ovary. It contains a number of structures: fallopian tube, round ligament, ovarian ligament, uterine and ovarian blood vessels, nerves, lymphatics, and mesonephric remnants. Below the infundibulopelvic structures, the anterior and posterior leaves of peritoneum lie in apposition, leaving a clear space below the tube with its tubal branch of the uterine artery. This avascular area is useful to the surgeon in isolating the adnexal structures and in avoiding blood vessels while performing tubal ligations.

Blood Supply

The blood supply of the uterus is derived chiefly from the uterine arteries. These arise from the hypogastric artery and swing toward the uterus, which they reach at approximately the level of the internal os. Here the uterine arteries divide, the descending limb coursing downward along the cervix and lateral wall of the vagina. The ascending limb passes upward alongside the uterus and continues below the fallopian tube. Frequent anterior and posterior branches go to vagina, cervix, and uterus. The ovarian artery, which ordinarily arises from the aorta, passes along the ovary, dividing into a number of branches. At several places in the broad ligament there are anastomotic connections between the tubal branch of the uterine artery and the ovarian artery. A branch of the uterine artery nourishes the round ligament. The veins generally accompany the arteries.

Using injection and microradiographic and histologic techniques to study the vascular anatomy of the uterus. Farrer-Brown et al showed that the uterine arteries run a tortuous course between the two layers of the broad ligament along the lateral side of the uterus and turn laterally at the junction of the uterus and fallopian tube, run toward the hilum of the ovary, and terminate by joining the ovarian arteries. In the broad ligament each uterine artery supplies lateral branches that immediately enter the uterus and give off tortuous anterior and posterior arcuate divisions, which run circumferentially in the myometrium approximately at the junction of its outer and middle thirds. In the midline the terminal branches of both arcuate arteries anastomose with those of the contralateral side.

Each arcuate artery throughout its course gives off numerous branches running both centrifugally towards the serosa and centripetally towards the endometrium. The arteries to the serosa at first are directed radially and then frequently became more circumferential. There is a plexus of small arterial radicals with a radial distribution located immediately below the serosa. The inner two-thirds of the myometrium is supplied by tortuous radial branches of the arcuate arteries. They provide numerous branches terminating in a capillary network which surrounds groups of muscle fibers. An abrupt change in the density of the arterial

pattern occurs at the junction of the basal layer of the endometrium with the subjacent myometrium. The endometrial vessels are relatively sparse in comparison with those of the myometrium at all stages of the menstrual cycle.

The entire uterus has a rich lymphatic capillary bed as extensive as the blood capillary system. The lymphatic capillary bed is arranged in four zones: (1) the lower uterine segment with its rich supply of fine capillaries, (2) the subserosa of the corpus with a few lymphatics, (3) a deep subserosal network, and (4) a plentiful supply in the muscularis proper. These vessels increase greatly in number and size during pregnancy. The collecting system of the uterine lymphatics is formed from anastomoses of a lateral-uterine descending network of lymph vessels which unites with collecting vessels from the utero-ovarian pedicle and the external iliac area. Lymphatic drainage of the uterus and upper two-thirds of the vagina is primarily to the obturator and internal and external iliac nodes.

CERVIX

The cervix is narrower than the body of the uterus. Approximately 2.5 cm in length. Due to anteflexion or retroflexion, the long axis of the cervix is rarely the same as the long axis of the body of the uterus. Anterior and lateral to the supravaginal portion is cellular connective tissue, the parametrium. The posterior aspect is covered by peritoneum of the pouch of Douglas. The ureter runs about 1 cm laterally to the supravaginal cervix. The vaginal portion projects into the vagina to form the fornices. The upper part of the cervix mostly consists of involuntary muscle, whereas the lower part is mainly fibrous connective tissue. The intravaginal portion of the cervix, known as the portio vaginalis, ordinarily is covered with nonkeritinizing squamous epithelium with a number of mucus-secreting glands (see Fig. 1.2). The external os is the opening of the cervix within the vagina. Above the external os lies the fusiform endocervical canal, approximately 2 cm long and lined with columnar epithelium and endocervical glands. The intersection where the squamous epithelium of the exocervix and columnar epithelium of the endocervical canal meet, the squamocolumnar junction, is geographically variable and dependent on hormonal stimulation. It is this dynamic interface, the transformation zone, that is most vulnerable to the development of squamous neoplasia. In early childhood, during pregnancy, or with oral contraceptive use, columnar epithelium may extend from the endocervical canal onto the exocervix, a condition known as eversion or ectopy. After menopause, the transformation zone usually recedes entirely into the endocervical canal.

At the upper end of the endocervical canal at the junction with the uterine cavity is the internal os. The endocervical canal in the nullipara is lined by mucosa arranged in a series of folds. A vertical fold is present on the anterior and posterior cervical walls; from these, oblique folds radiate. These folds have been called the arbor vitae uteri or plicae palmatae. It was formerly thought that tubular glands descend vertically from the surface and divide into many branches forming compound racemose glands; however, secondary changes caused by the intense growth activity of the columnar cells result in the formation of tunnels, secondary clefts, and exophytic processes.

The Fallopian Tubes

The fallopian tubes are bilateral muscular structures of paramesonephric duct origin. They are from 7 to 12 cm in length and usually less than 1 cm in diameter. The tubes or oviducts have a lumen that varies considerably in diameter. It is extremely narrow, being less than 1 mm at its opening into the uterine cavity. It is wider in the isthmus 2.5 mm and in the ampulla is approximately 6 mm in diameter. The tube begins in the uterine cavity at the cornu and penetrates the myometrium (intramural or interstitial portion). The second portion is the relatively straight and narrow portion of the tube which emerges from the uterus posterior to and a little above the origin of the round ligament. The lumen of the narrow isthmus is relatively simple, with a few longitudinal folds. This portion of its tube is 2 or 3 cm long. There are three layers of musculature: the inner longitudinal, the middle circular layer, and the outer longitudinal layer (Fig. 1.4).

There is some evidence that the isthmus may act as a sphincter. The ampulla is the largest and longest portion of the tube, approximately 5 cm or more in length. The lumen enlarges from 1 or 2 mm near the isthmus to over a centimeter at the distal portion. The mucosa has multiple longitudinal folds. The ampulla is the portion usually involved in gonorrheal salpingitis and tubo-ovarian abscesses and is the site of most ectopic pregnancies. At the distal end of the tube is the trumpet shaped infundibulum. The tube ends in a number of fimbriae or frond-like projections; the largest of these is ordinarily in contact with the ovary and is known as the ovarian fimbria. The peritoneal cavity in the female is connected with the exterior of the body through the patent distal end of the tube by way of the uterus and vagina. The ovum must enter through the open end of a tube if fertilization is to occur in the ampullary portion, where sperm have collected by migrating "upstream" against the current. This opening is of considerable clinical importance as blood, ascending infections, or pus can pass out of the tube to invade the abdominal cavity, with resultant pain, endometriosis, or pelvic infection.

Functions of fallopian tube: Ovum pickup, provision of physical environment for conception, transport of fertilized ovum and nourishment of fertilized ovum.

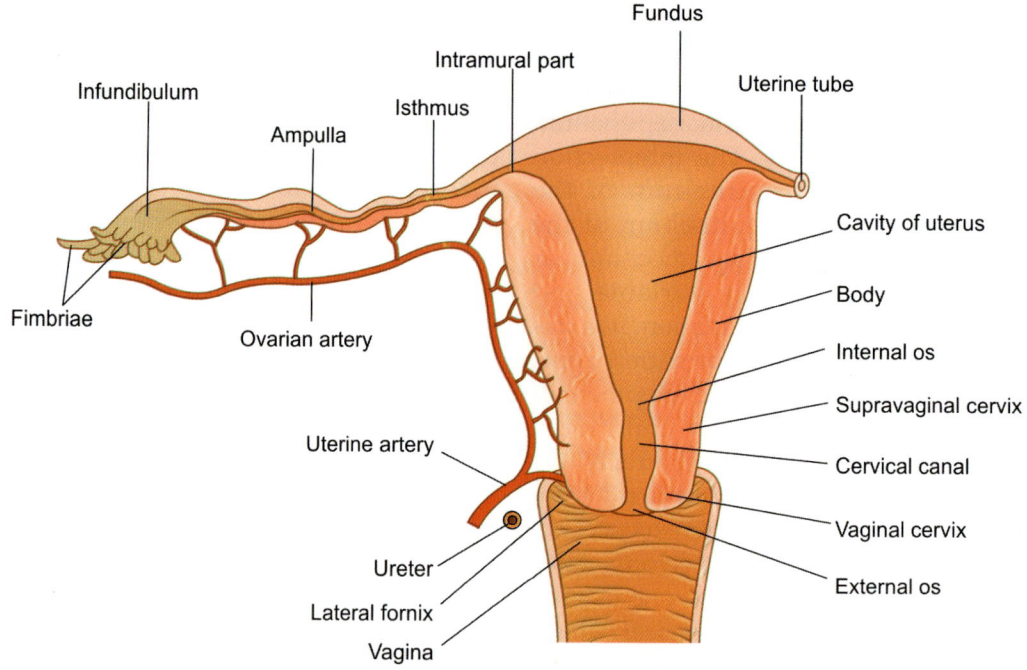

Fig. 1.4: Uterus and fallopian tube—various parts

The blood supply of the tube is from the upper end of the uterine artery, which bifurcates and sends a large branch or ramus below the tube to anastomose with the ovarian artery. The proximal two-thirds of the tube is chiefly supplied by the uterine artery. The arterial supply is quite variable and there may be three branches (medial, intermediate, and lateral) or a branch from the uterine and another from the ovarian artery. Anastomoses between uterine and ovarian arteries in the mesosalpinx are variable but always present.

The venous system accompanies the arterial distribution. Capillary networks are to be found in subserosal, muscularis, and mucosal layers. The arrangement varies in different portions of the tube, but the venous plexuses become confluent in the subserosal layer. The lymphatic drainage runs along the upper edge of the broad ligament to the lymphatic network below the hilus of the ovary. From here the flow from uterus, tube, and ovary drains to the para-aortic or lumbar nodes.

The tube is provided with both sympathetic and parasympathetic innervation. Sympathetic fibers from T10 through L2 reach the inferior mesenteric plexus. Postganglionic fibers then pass to the oviduct. The fibers from the inferior mesenteric plexus pass to the cervicovaginal plexus, which in turn, sends fibers to the isthmus and part of the ampulla. Some sympathetic fibers from T10 and T11 reach the celiac plexus and provide postganglionic fibers to the ovarian plexus, which supplies the distal ampulla and fimbriae. The parasympathetic supply is by vagal fibers from the ovarian plexus supplying the distal portion of the tube. Part of the isthmus receives its parasympathetic supply from S2, S3, and S4 via the pelvic nerve and the pelvic plexuses.

OVARY

The glistening white ovaries are generally oval in shape but may vary in size, position, and appearance, depending on the age and the

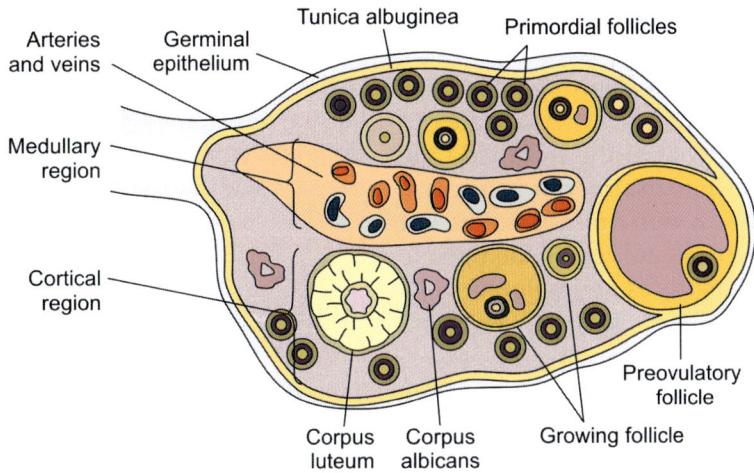

Fig. 1.5: Histology of ovary

reproductive activities of the individual (Fig. 1.5). The ovaries of a normal adult woman are 2.5–5 cm long, 1.5–3 cm thick, and 0.7–1.5 cm wide, with a weight of 3–8 g. The ovaries contain 1–2 million oocytes at birth. A woman will release up to 400 ova, on average, during her lifetime. It is the only intra-abdominal structure not to be covered by peritoneum. In the nullipara, the ovary typically lies in the ovarian fossa, a depression in the pelvic wall below the external iliac vessels and in front of the ureter. A mesovarium attaches the ovary to the posterior wall of the broad ligament, while the posterior margin is free. The peritoneum does not cover the ovary proper, which is covered by germinal epithelium. At either end the ovary is supported by ligaments. At the tubal pole the ovary is attached to the suspensory ligament, a fold of peritoneum which forms a mesentery for the ovary and contains the ovarian vessels. This suspensory ligament is often called the infundibulopelvic ligament. At the other pole is the uteroovarian ligament. Anterior to the ovary lie the fallopian tubes, the superior portion of the bladder and the uterovesical pouch. The ovary is bound behind by the ureter where it runs downwards and forwards in front of the internal iliac artery. The surface of the ovaries is covered by a single layer of cuboidal cells, the germinal epithelium. Beneath this is an ill-defined layer of condensed connective tissue, the tunica albuginea, which increases in density with age.

Histologically the ovary is divided into the outer cortex and the inner medulla. The cortex consists of a cellular connective tissue stroma in which the ovarian follicles are embedded. The medulla is composed of loose connective tissue which contains blood vessels and nerves. The cortex is surrounded by a single layer of cuboidal epithelium called the germinal epithelium.

The hilus is the base of the ovary; at this point the ovarian blood vessels enter. The ovarian arteries arise from the abdominal aorta just below the renal arteries. They pass downward across the pelvic brim, cross the external iliac artery, and traverse the infundibulopelvic fold of peritoneum. Branches go to the ureter, round ligament, and tube and anastomose with the uterine artery.

As the ovarian artery passes through the mesovarium, it separates into multiple branches that enter the ovarian hilus. Each of these arteries divides into two medullary branches which cross the ovary. Cortical branches arise from the medullary branches and supply the cortex and follicles. Two prominent veins enter the hilus and, in general, follow the arterial pattern.

At the hilus venous drainage forms a pampiniform plexus, which consolidates to form the ovarian vein. On the right side the ovarian vein drains into the inferior vena cava, while the left ovarian vein drains into the left renal vein. The ovarian as well as the uterine blood supply frequently is anomalous.

The nerve supply derives from a sympathetic plexus accompanying the vessels of the infundibulopelvic ligaments. The plexus arises at the level of the tenth thoracic segment, but fibers from renal and aortic plexuses as well as from the mesenteric and celiac ganglia are present.

VESTIGIAL STRUCTURES

Vestigial remains of the mesonephric duct and tubules are always present in young children, but are variable structures in adults. The epoophoron and the paroophoron series of parallel blind tubules, lies in the broad ligament. The duct of Gartner is a well developed caudal part of the mesonephric duct, running alongside the uterus to the internal os.

Pelvic peritoneum: The peritoneum is reflected from the lateral borders of the uterus to form, on either side, a double fold of peritoneum of the broad ligament. This is not a ligament but a peritoneal fold, and it does not support the uterus.

Ovarian ligament: It lies beneath the posterior layer of the broad ligament and passes from the medial pole of the ovary to the uterus just below the point of entry of the fallopian tube.

Round ligament: It is the continuation of the ovarian ligament and runs forwards under the anterior leaf of peritoneum to enter the inguinal canal, ending in the subcutaneous tissue of the labium majus. Together the ovarian and round ligaments are analogous to the gubernaculum in the male.

Cardinal ligaments (transverse cervical ligaments): It provides the essential support of the uterus and vaginal vault. These are two strong, fen-shaped, fibromuscular expansions that pass from the cervix and vaginal vault to the side wall of the pelvis on either side.

Uterosacral ligaments: It run from the cervix and vaginal vault to the sacrum. In the erect position they are almost vertical in direction and support the cervix.

The parametrium: It is a considerable collection of cellular tissue in the wide base of the broad ligament and at the side of the cervix and vagina.

The pelvic diaphragm: It is formed by the levator ani muscles. The two muscles, one on either side. Each is a broad, flat muscle, the fibers of which pass downwards and inwards. The muscle is described in two parts (Fig. 1.6):
1. The pubococcygeus, which arises from the pubic bone and the anterior part of the tendinous arch of the pelvic fascia (white line).
2. The iliococcygeus, which arises from the posterior part of the tendinous arch and the ischial spine. The muscle arises by a linear origin from: (i) the lower part of the body of the os pubis, (ii) the internal surface of the parietal pelvic fascia along the white line, (iii) the pelvic surface of the ischial spine. The levator ani muscles are inserted

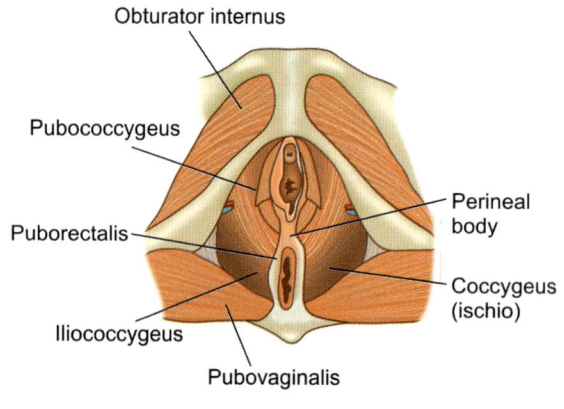

Fig. 1.6: Pelvic floor—muscles

into: (i) The pre-anal raphe and the central point of the perineum where one muscle meets the other on the opposite side, (ii) the wall of the anal canal, where the fibres blend with the deep external sphincter muscle, (iii) the postanal or anococcygeal raphe, where again one muscle meets the other on the opposite side, (iv) the lower part of the coccyx.

Urogenital diaphragm: The urogenital diaphragm (triangular ligament) lies below the levator ani muscles and consists of two layers of pelvic fascia, which fill the gap between the descending pubic rami. The deep transverse perineal muscle (compressor urethrae) lies between the two layers, and the diaphragm is pierced by the urethra and the vagina.

Perineal body: It is the perineal mass of muscular tissue that lies between the anal canal and the lower third of the vagina. The median raphe of the levator ani, between the anus and the vagina, is reinforced by the central tendon of the perineum. The bulbo-cavernosus, superficial transverse perineal, and external anal sphincter muscles also converge on the central tendon. Thus, these structures contribute to the perineal body, which provides significant perineal support. The perineal body is incised by an episiotomy incision and is torn with second-third- and fourth-degree lacerations.

Conclusion

The anatomy of the pelvic floor has been classically divided into the external and the internal genitalia. The external genital organs include the mons pubis, clitoris, urinary meatus, labia majora, labia minora, vestibule, Bartholin's glands, and periurethral glands. The internal genital organs are located in the true pelvis and include the vagina, uterus, cervix, oviducts, ovaries, and surrounding supporting structures. Pelvic organ support and continence are maintained by a complex interplay between the bony structures of the pelvis, pelvic diaphragm muscles, nerves that innervate the pelvic floor, and endopelvic fascia.

2

Fetal Growth and Development

• Neerja

Fetal growth: Fetus grows from a single cell at fertilization to about 6 billion cells at full term of pregnancy (Figs 2.1 and 2.2). There are three phases in the prenatal development.

1. *Ovular period* lasts for 2 weeks following ovulation or 4 weeks of gestational age from the last menstrual period.
2. *Embryonic period* lasts from the beginning of third week following fertilization until completion of eighth week or fifth to tenth week of gesation age. This is period of organ development (organogenesis). The average crown-rump length (CRL) of embryo is 4 mm.
3. *Fetal period* is from the beginning of 9th week to birth (post-conception) or 11th week gestation age till end of pregnancy. Organ maturation and growth occur during this period.

Normal fetal growth: There are three phases of cell growth in a normal pregnancy.

1. *First phase* (1–16 weeks of pregnancy) of cellular hyperplasia characterized by a rapid increase in cell numbers. The rate of fetal growth is 5 g/day.
2. *Second phase* (17–32 weeks) of cellular hyperplasia and hypertrophy with 15–20 g/day of fetal growth.
3. *Third phase* (33 weeks onwards) of cellular hypertrophy. Fetal growth is 30–35 g/day. Most of the fetal fat and glycogen deposition occurs during this time.

Up to 20th week the length of the fetus is measured from the vertex to the coccyx (crown-rump length) and from the vertex to the heel (crown-heel or vertex-heel length) after that. The average fetal length and weight at various gestations are shown in Table 2.1.

Haase's rule (1875): Up to 5th month, fetal length is square of lunar months in centimetres. From the 6th month, it is 5 times the number of months. However, these are rough estimates.

Estimation of fetal age (Table 2.1): Fetal gestation age is calculated from the first day of last menstrual period (LMP) and is 2 weeks more than the post-conception (fertilization) age. The fetal length is used to calculate the age of the fetus. In the first trimester, CRL (cm) + 6.5 give gestational age in weeks, e.g. if CRL is 4 cm, the gestation will be 4 + 6.5 = 10.5 weeks. Ultrasound biometry is used to accurately estimate the gestational age by measuring CRL in 1st trimester, biparietal diameter and trans-cerebellar diameter after 2nd trimester.

FACTORS AFFECTING FETAL GROWTH (BIRTH WEIGHT)

The important factors affecting fetal growth are shown in Table 2.2. Fetal genome is the main determinant of growth in early fetal life.

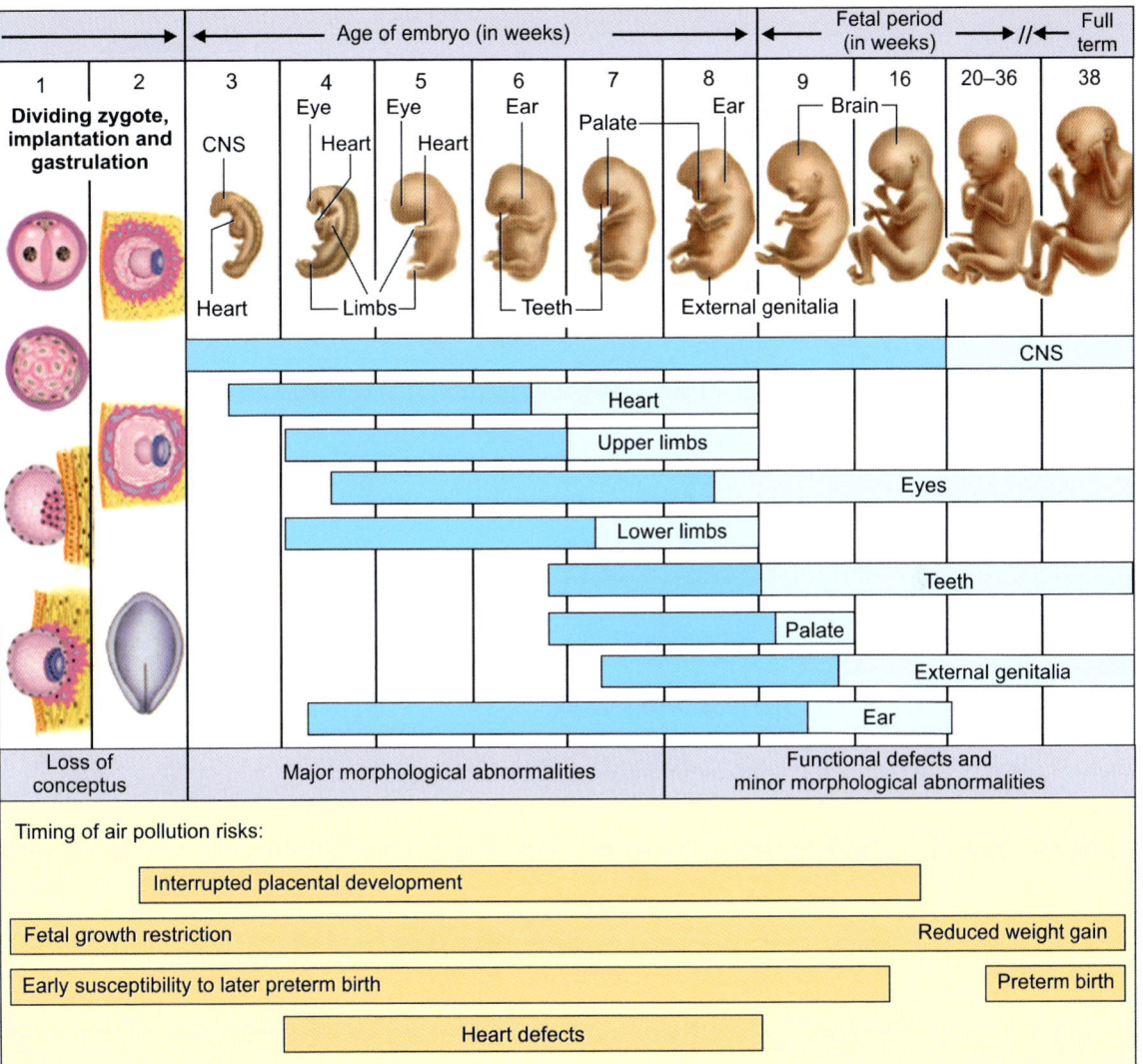

Fig. 2.1: Fetal development and growth

Environmental, nutritional and hormonal factors are more important in later pregnancy. Insulin and insulin-like growth factors (lgF I and II), obesity gene and its protein product leptin play a major role in the regulation of fetal growth and weight gain. Growth hormone is essential for postnatal growth. The fetal weight in India at term ranges from 2.5–3.5 kg with mean being 3.0 kg. The average fetal weight at various gestations is shown in Table 2.1. Various nutritional and pathological factors can adversely affect the fetal growth (Table 2.2).

FETAL PHYSIOLOGY

The various landmarks of embryonic and fetal development are shown in Table 2.3.

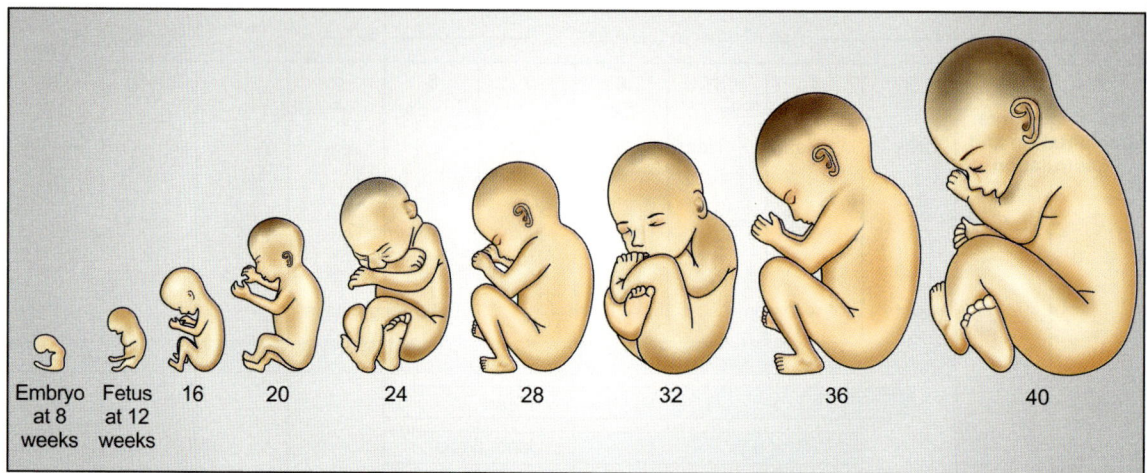

Fig. 2.2: Fetal growth from 6 to 40 weeks

Table 2.1: Average fetal length and weight at different gestations

Gestation in lunar months	In weeks	Characteristic	Average fetal length (cm)	Fetal weight (g) (approximate)
3	12	Crown-rump length	5.5	14
4	16	Crown-rump length	11.6	100
5	20	Crown-rump or vertex-heel length	16.4	300
6	24	Vertex-heel length	30	650
7	28	Vertex-heel length	37.6	1100
8	32	Vertex-heel length	42.4	1700
9	36	Vertex-heel length	47.4	2500
10	40	Vertex-heel length	51.2	3200

Table 2.2: Factors affecting fetal growth

S.No.	Factors	Effects
1.	Genetic factors, like parental height	Chromosomal abnormalities cause fetal growth restriction
2.	Fetal sex	Male fetus is 100–200 g heavier
3.	Race	Caucasian babies are heavier than Indian babies
4.	Maternal age	Mothers older than 35 years have smaller babies
5.	Socioeconomic factors	Lower socioeconomic status; poor fetal growth
6.	Nutritional factors	Malnutrition; poor fetal growth
7.	Birth order	Second- and third-order babies are heavier than first-order babies
8.	Pre pregnancy weight	Mothers weighing <40 kg have smaller babies
9.	Pregnancy weight gain	Low weight gains causes lower fetal growth
10.	Smoking and drug addiction	Poor fetal growth
11.	Maternal disease	Hypertension and anemia cause poor fetal growth. Diabetes causes excessive fetal growth
12.	Fetal factors	Fetal intrauterine infections and congenital malformations cause poor fetal growth

Table 2.3: Important landmarks of embryonic and fetal development

1.	Development of notochord and thickening of ectoderm to form neural plate and neural folds. Bilaminar embryo (ectoderm and endoderm)	14–21 days post conception
2.	Fusion of neural folds to form neural tube. Four primitive cardiac chambers. First heart beats on day 21 (7 + weeks). Trilaminar embryo (mesoderm appears)	21–28 days post conception
3.	Optic vesicles appear; complete neural tube closure (day 30). Limb buds appear. Formation of face and lens placodes	4–6 weeks post conception (4–15 mm embryo)
4.	All major structures form. Complete ventricular septum (day 46), recognition as human	6–8 weeks post conception (15–30 mm embryo)
5.	Ovaries and testes distinguishable	8 weeks
6.	External genitalia develop	8–12 weeks post conception (30–60 mm embryo)
7.	Erythropoiesis	
	i. Extraembryonic hematopoiesis in yolk sac	10–14 days of gestation
	ii. In liver	6 weeks
	iii. In bone marrow	16 weeks
8.	Lymphocytes development	
	i. In thymus	9 weeks
	ii. In lymph nodes	10 weeks
9.	Swallowing	13–14 weeks
10.	Breathing movements start	11–12 weeks
11.	Secretion of urine	End of first trimester (10–12 weeks)
12.	Fetal skeleton seen on radiology	12–16 weeks
13.	Swallowing reflex is present	16 weeks
14.	Quickening felt by mother. Fetal heart heard on auscultation	16–20 weeks
15.	Grasp reflex appears	17 weeks
16.	Skin is covered with lanugo. Vernix caseosa is present	20 weeks
17.	Appearance of meconium	20 weeks
18.	Tests descend to the internal inguinal ring	24 weeks
19.	Baby is viable	24–28 weeks (24 weeks in western countries)
20.	Eyes open, turns head down	26–28 weeks
21.	One testicle usually descends into the scrotum. Lanugo tends to disappear. Ear cartilage develops. Plantar crease is visible	32–36 weeks
22.	Fetus becomes fully mature with firm skull. Both the testicles descend into the scrotum. Nails project beyond the finger tips. Closure of posterior fontanelle	40 weeks

Nutrition: There are three phases of fetal nutrition following fertilization:

1. *Absorption:* Post-fertilization, the developing zygote is nourished by the nutrients stored in cellular cytoplasm, secretions of the fallopian tube and interstitial fluid of endometrium.

2. *Histotrophic transfer:* After implantation but before establishment of uteroplacental circulation, nutrition is derived from the decidual cells and surrounding maternal tissues.

3. *Hematotrophic:* After 3rd week, fetal circulation is established which leads to active and

passive transfer of nutrients from mother to fetus.

About 65% of calcium, 75% of proteins and 80% of the total iron in fetus are obtained from mother in the last trimester. This is the reason for poor stores of essential nutrients in preterm babies.

Fetal hematopoiesis: It is demonstrable in the yolk sac by 14th day which produces macrocytic nucleated red cells. The liver becomes the next major site of erythropoiesis between 6 and 10 weeks. Hematopoiesis starts in bone marrow (15–16 weeks) and in spleen (19–20 weeks). In 3rd trimester, the thymus and lymph nodes can be the additional sites of hemopoiesis. At term, the bone marrow is the chief site of red cell production producing normoblastic cells. At 40 weeks the fetal RBC count is 5–6 million per cu mm; Hb is 16–18 g/dl and packed cell volume is 40%.

In early gestation, the embryo forms some rare hemoglobins in yolk sac. From 24 weeks onwards when bone marrow takes over the hemopoiesis, adult type of hemoglogin (HbA) with alpha and beta chains appears. At 40 weeks, about 75–80% of the total hemoglobin is of fetal type (HbF), 20% if HbA and 5–10% is HbA2 with alpha and delta chains. Between 6–12 months after birth, the fetal hemoglobin is totally replaced by adult hemoglobin and is <10%. The change from fetal to adult Hb is mediated by glucocorticoids and is irreversible. The fetal hemoglobin has much higher affinity for oxygen due to less binding of 2, 3-diphosphoglycerate as compared with HbA. This gives an advantage anabling fetal Hb to bind with O_2 even at lower pressure of oxygen as is present in umbilical blood. Fetal hemoglobin (HbF) is more resistant to denaturation by alkaline reagents than adult hemoglobin. This quality is used in the detection of fetal blood in antepartum hemorrhage is vasa previa (Apt's test). Fetal hemoglobin is also more resistant to acid elution than adult Hb and is used for the determination of the presence of fetal RBCs

in maternal circulation to see quantity of feto-maternal hemorrhage (Kleihauer-Betke test). Total fetoplacental blood volume at term is about 400–600 ml. The red cells develop their ABO group antigen and Rh factor by 38 days. The lifespan of the fetal RBC is about 80 days.

Leukocytes first appear at 8 weeks of gestation. B lymphocytes appear in fetal liver by 9 weeks and in blood and spleen by 12 weeks. T lymphocytes start to leave thymus at about 14 weeks. Inspite of this, newborns respond poorly to immunization possibly due to deficient response of B cells. The leukocyte count at term is 14,000–18,000/cu mm. Magakaryocytes appear as early as 5 weeks with platelet counts equal to adult at term. Maternal immunoglobulins IgG (but not IgM) are passed from mother to fetus from 12 weeks onwards giving passive immunity to fetus.

Urinary system: Fetal kidneys start producing urine at 12 weeks, produce 15 ml/day at 18 weeks which increases to 650 ml/day at term. They help in the control of composition and volume of liquor amnii. Chronic anuria causes oligohydramnios and pulmonary hypoplasia.

Gastrointestinal tract: The fetal swallowing of amniotic fluid begins at 10–12 weeks increasing to 250 ml/day at term. Intestinal glands and villi develop in the first trimester with digestive enzymes being present by 16–18 weeks. Fetal bowel contains intestinal secretions, desquamated fetal cells, lanugo, scalp hair, vernix and undigested debris from swallowed amniotic fluid. Its dark green black color is from beliverdin secreted from liver. Meconium may be passed at term by normal bowel peristalsis but often occurs due to fetal hypoxia causing relaxation of anal sphincter due to vagal stimulation.

Respiratory system: Lung development occurs in three stages.

1. The pseudoglandular stage includes growth of intersegmental bronchial tree

between 5th and 17th weeks of gestation when lungs are solid.

2. The canalicular stage is between 16 and 25 weeks when terminal bronchioles give rise to several respiratory bronchioles which divide into multiple saccular ducts.

3. Terminal sac stage begins after 25 week when alveoli form pulmonary alveoli.

Surfactant production: Surfactant is produced by type II pneumocytes that line the alveoli. The main active component of surfactant is a lecithin; dipalmitoyl phosphatidyl choline (DPPC) followed by other lecithins, phosphatidyl glycerol (PG) and phosphatidyl inositol.

At birth, with the first breath, an air to tissue interface is produced in the lung alveoli. Surfactant spreads to line the fetal alveoli to prevent their collapse during expiration.

Fetal cortisol is the natural trigger for surfactant production. Maternal administration of betamethasone or dexamethasone can accelerate fetal lung maturity in preterm labors by stimulating surfactant production.

The fetal breathing and chest movements appear by 11 weeks and become established by 20 weeks leading onto movement of amniotic fluid in and out of respiratory tract.

Fetal endocrinology: Thyroid is the first endocrine gland to develop in fetus around the 4th post-conception week and is able to secrete thyroid hormones by 11 weeks. Fetal thyroid hormones play an important role in normal development of most fetal tissues especially the brain. The pancreas develops as an outgrowth of the duodenal endoderm and insulin secretion is observed by the 12th week.

Pituitary gland: Adrenocorticotrophic hormone (ACTH) is first observed in fetal pituitary at 7 weeks while growth hormones and luteinizing hormone are identified by 12 week. By 18th week, the fetal pituitary is capable of synthesizing all pituitary hormones. It also secretes endorphin and lipotropin. The posterior pituitary gland is well developed by 10–12 weeks with demonstration of oxytocin and arginine vasopressin. Intermediate pituitary gland is also well developed in fetus (disappears at term) and secretes melanocyte-stimulating hormone and endorphin.

Adrenal glands: The relatives size of fetal adrenal gland is much bigger as compared to adults. The main bulk is made by the inner (reticular) or fetal zone of adrenal cortex which involutes after birth. It secretes precursor of estriol and cortisol. Fetal ovaries usually are inactive; fetal testes are active helping in the development of male reproductive organs.

Skin: The thin fine hairs called lanugo are seen at 16 weeks of gestation disappearing by term. Sebaceous glands are present at 20th week and secrete vernix-caseosa, the thick white secretion of the sebaceous glands mixed with the exfoliated epidermal cells. Prior to keratinization of the skin before the 20th week, the fetal skin allows transudation of fluid into the liquor amnii adding to its quantity. Sweat glands appear late.

Fetal circulation (Fig. 2.3): The embryo develops separate fetal circulation from the 16th post-fertilization day with the fetal heart starting to beat from 21st day of fertilization. The single umbilical vein containing well-oxygenated blood (about 80% oxygen) and nutrients required for fetal growth and maturation from the placenta enters the fetus at the umbilicus. It runs beneath the anterior abdominal wall to reach the liver where it divides into ductus venosus and portal sinus.

The ductus venosus is the large branch which bypasses (first bypass) the liver to enter inferior vena cava mixing with venous blood from lower extremity. It then enters the right atrium of heart with 75% oxygen saturation. The smaller branch, the portal sinus, joins with portal vein. It then goes to liver where from hepatic veins drain into inferior vena cava carrying relatively deoxygenated blood.

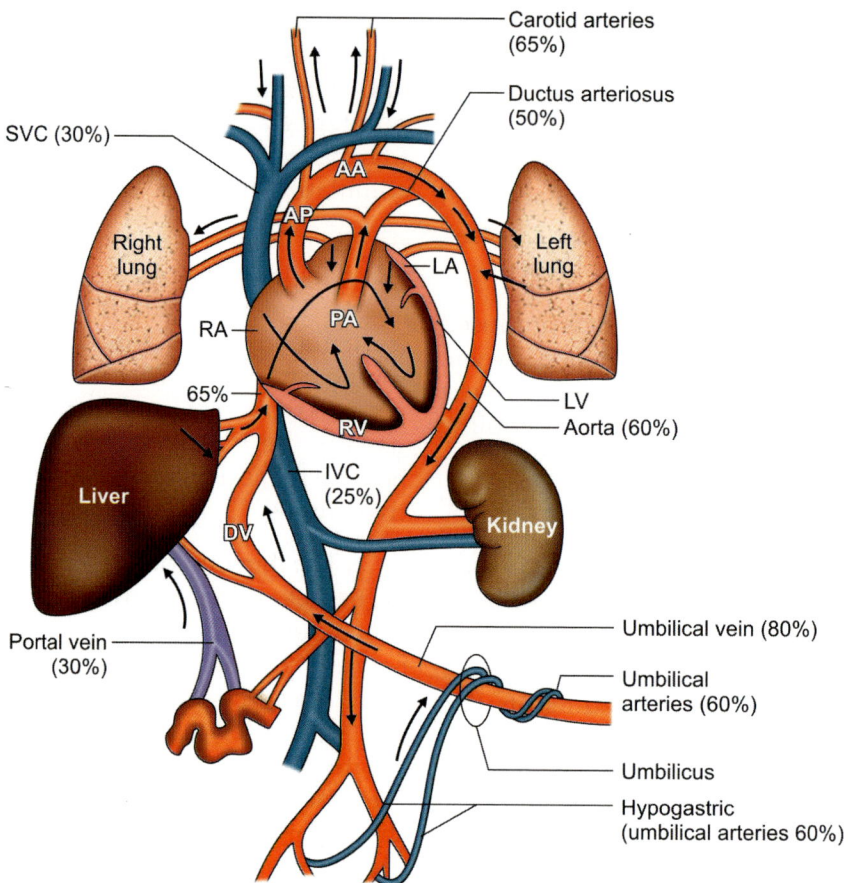

Fig. 2.3: Fetal circulation

Two separate circulations are maintained by the right atrium depending upon its oxygen content which is aided by the pattern of blood flow in inferior vena cava. The well-oxygenated blood courses along the medial aspect of the inferior vena cava while the less oxygenated blood stays along its lateral wall. When the blood reaches the rights atrium, the configuration of the upper interatrial septum—the crista dividens is such that it preferentially shunts the well-oxygenated blood from the medial side of inferior vena cava and ductus venousus through the foramen ovale into the left atrium (second bypass). The left ventricular blood with high oxygen saturation is pumped into the ascending part and arch of aorta to supply to the head, neck, brain, heart and arms through its branches.

The remaining right atrium blood coming through superior vena cava and lateral part of inferior vena cava (carrying less oxygenated blood) passes through the tricuspid valve into the right ventricle. Blood from coronary sinus also returns via this pathway.

The right ventricular blood with low oxygen saturation passes into the pulmonary trunk. Due to very high pulmonary vascular resistance and comparatively lower resistance in the ductus arteriosus during fetal life, about 90% of blood exiting the right ventricle passes directly through the ductus arteriosus into the descending aorta bypassing the lungs (third bypass). The mixed blood is distributed by the descending aorta to the rest of the fetal body. In fetus, only 8–10% of the total cardiac output (15% of right ventricle output) goes directly to the lungs and returns to the left atrium via the pulmonary veins. Only one-third of the blood passing through the ductus arteriosus is delivered to the body. The remaining two-thirds of right ventricle output returns to the placenta through two hypogastric arteries which distally become umbilical arteries. They reach the placenta carrying deoxygenated blood where the blood gets oxygen and nutrients for recirculation through the umbilical vein and the cycle is repeated. The fetal cardiac output is quite high being about 300–350 ml per kg per minute.

The fetal circulation differs from adult circulation as the chambers of the fetal heart work in parallel in contrast to series in adults. So, the brain and the heart get more oxygenated blood than the rest of the body.

Changes in fetal circulation at birth (Fig. 2.4): The fetal circulation undergoes great changes within a few minutes after cord clamping and first breath due to: (1) Stoppage of the placental blood flow with massive reduction in venous return to the right heart and (2) onset of respiration. The following changes occur in the circulation.

1. *Closure of the foramen ovale:* With the first breath, alveolar expansion and increase in alveolar capillary oxygen tension cause marked decrease in pulmonary vascular resistance. It causes marked accompanying decrease in right atrial afterload and right atrial pressure. Clamping of umbilical cord reduces venous return to right atrium reducing its pressure significantly. Secondly, the increase in pulmonary flow increases venous return into the left atrium and therefore the left atrial pressure. The combined effect of the two events is to increase the left atrial pressure above right atrial pressure and provide a physiological closure of foramen ovale which occurs soon after birth but anatomical closure may take up to one year. The closure is reversible in early neonatal life as cyanosis may develop during crying due to shunting of blood from right atrium to left atrium.

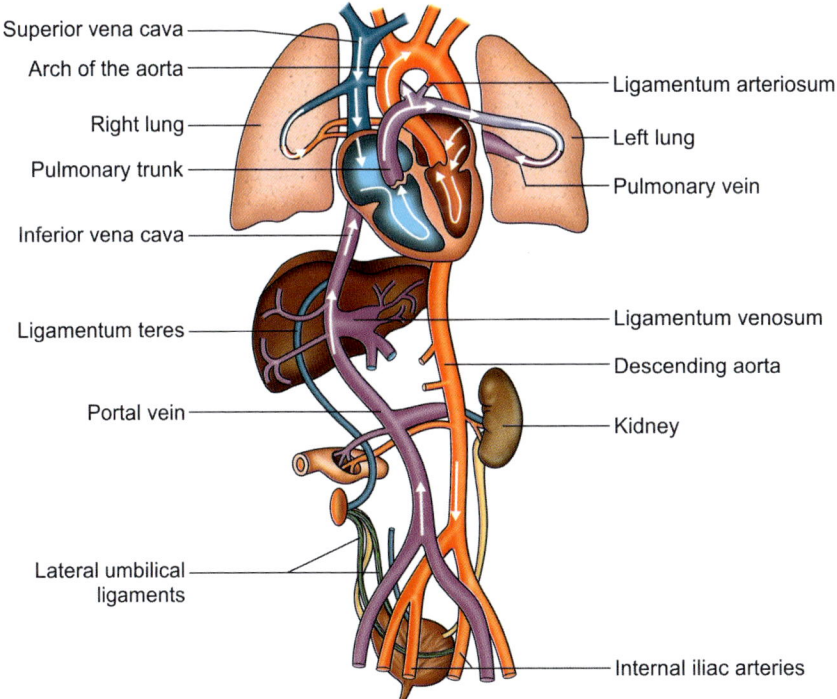

Fig. 2.4: Changes in the fetal circulation at birth

2. *Closure of the ductus arterious:* The functional closure of the ductus arteriosus usually occurs soon after the establishment of pulmonary circulation due to local increase in ductus arteriosus oxygen tension which alters the ductus response to prostaglandins and causes a marked localized vaso-constriction. Prostaglandin synthetase inhibitor (e.g. indomethacin) given to mother may cause premature closure of ductus arteriosus while prostaglandins may delay the closure. Immediately the ventricles start working in series as opposed to in parallel in fetal life. The anatomical closure from fibrosis takes 2–3 months and it forms ligamentum arteriosum in adults.

3. *Closure of the umbilical arteries:* There is immediate functional closure to prevent any fetal blood loss. Umbilical arteries undergo atrophy and obliteration within 3–4 days after birth. The proximal parts of umbilical arteries remain open as superior vesical arteries. The distal parts become the lateral umbilical ligaments.

4. *Closure of the umbilical vein:* The closure of umbilical vein occurs shortly after the umbilical arteries to enable transfer of about 80–100 ml of placental blood to the fetus. After closure, the remnant of the umbilical vein forms the ligamentum teres.

5. *Closure of ductus venosus.* The ductus venosus constricts functionally by 12–96 hours after birth and closes anatomically by 2–3 weeks to form ligamentum venosum.

The neonatal cardiac output is about 450–500 ml per minute and the heart rate is about 110–140 beats per minute.

Bibliography

1. Human Embryology, Inderbir Singh & GPPa, 10th Edition l.
2. Langman's Medical Embryology, TW sadler, 11th Edition.
3. Turnbull Obstetrics, 3rd Edition, Edited by Geoffrey Chamberlain & Philip Steer.
4. Williams Obstetrics, Cunningham, Levend, Bloom, Hauth, Rouse 7 Spong, 24th Edition.

3

Antenatal Care

• Kirti Dubey

- Systematic supervision (examination and advice) of a woman during pregnancy is called antenatal (prenatal) care.
- Should be regular and periodic nature according to the need of individual.

AIM OF ANTENATAL CARE

1. To screen high risk cases.
2. To prevent and detect and treat at the earliest any complications.
3. To educate mother about physiology of pregnancy, labor (mother craft classes).
4. To discuss about place, time, mode of delivery and motivate for family planning.

Initial Prenatal Evaluation

- Ideally, the first appointment needs to be earlier in pregnancy (prior to 12 weeks).
- Detail history with special concern for
  - Menstrual history (estimation of EDD by Naegele's rule)
  - Obstetric history
  - Medical and surgical disorder (hypertension, diabetes, epilepsy, tuberculosis)
  - Personal history (history of steroidal contraceptive use, smoking, alcohol habits, drug allergy, immunization)
  - Family history (hypertension, diabetes, tuberculosis, blood dyspraxia, twinning, known hereditary disease).

- Physical examination including detail general examination, breast examination, systemic examination and bimanual pelvic examination.
- Routine investigations including hemoglobin, ABO-Rh grouping, VDRL, hepatitis B, hepatitis C serology, HIV after counseling, Pap smear and urine RIM should be done in every patient.
  - Glucose challenge test and TSH to be done in selected patient.
  - High risk women should be screened for syphilis, hepatitis B in third trimester again. (High risk women are unmarried, recent change in sexual partners, multiple concurrent partner and history or presence of STD.)
- *Ultrasound:* First trimester scan helps to detect
  - Early pregnancy
  - Accurate dating
  - Number of fetuses. Scan at 18–20 weeks tells detailed fetal anatomy and detects structural
  - Abnormality
- Identify women who needs additional care
  - Underweight (BMI18 or less at first contact)
  - Obesity (BMI 35 or more at first contact)
  - Extremes of age

- Anemia
- Cardiac disease
- Hypertension (essential as well as pregnancy induced)
- Renal disease
- Thyroid, diabetes and other endocrine disorders
- Epilepsy requiring anticonvulsant drugs
- Asthma and other respiratory disorders
- Hematological disorder
- HIV or HBV infected
- Drug use such as heroin, cocaine
- Autoimmune disorders
- Psychiatric disorders
- Women who have experienced any of the following in previous pregnancies
  - Recurrent pregnancy loss
  - Preterm birth
  - Severe pre-eclampsia, HELLP syndrome or eclampsia
  - Rhesus isoimmunization or other significant blood group antibodies
  - Uterine surgery including cesarean section, myomectomy or cone biopsy
  - Antepartum or postpartum hemorrhage
  - Previous MRP
  - Puerperal psychosis
  - Grand multiparity (more than five pregnancies)
  - A stillbirth or neonatal death
  - A baby with a congenital anomaly (structural or chromosomal).

Subsequent Prenatal Visit

- Subsequent visits are planned at 4-week intervals until 28 weeks, then every 2 weeks until 36 weeks, weekly thereafter.
- Women with complicated pregnancies require return visits at 1- to 2-week intervals.
- WHO recommends at least 4 visits, first around 12 weeks, second between 24 and 28 weeks, third visit at 32 weeks and the fourth visit at 36 weeks.

- History taking (appearance of any new symptom like headache, dysuria), general examination (weight, pallor edema, leg, blood pressure), abdominal examination (fundal height, fetal lie, presentation, position, fetal heart rate, liquor volume, abdominal girth) should be done in each visit.
- Hemoglobin estimation is repeated at zs" and ss" week and urine RIM should be done at every antenatal visit.

ANTENATAL FETAL ASSESSMENT

Aim: To ensure satisfactory fetal growth and well-being of fetus and screen out high risk factor that affects growth of fetus.

Indications

- Pregnancy with obstetric complications, e.g. IUGR, multiple pregnancies, poly-hydramnios or oligohydramnios.
- Pregnancy with medical complications, e.g. diabetes mellitus, hypertension, epilepsy, renal or cardiac disease.
- Other indications are advanced maternal age >35 yrs, previous stillbirth or recurrent pregnancy loss, previous baby with structural or chromosomal anomaly.

Clinical Method

- *Weight gain:* During second half of pregnancy, the average weight gain is 1 kg a fortnight.
- *Blood pressure:* Hypertension, pre-existing or pregnancy induced may impair the fetal growth.
- *Symphysio-fundal height and abdominal girth:* After 24 weeks of pregnancy SFH measured in cm corresponds to POG in weeks. After 30 weeks of pregnancy AG measured in inches corresponds to POG weeks, measured at lower border of umbilicus.
- *Clinical assessment of liquor:* Scanty liquor may indicate placental insufficiency.

Biochemical Method

- *Maternal serum alpha fetoprotein test (MSAFP)* in done between 15 and 20 weeks. High levels are seen in open neural tube defect, wrong gestational age, anterior abdominal wall defect, Intrauterine fetal death (IUFD) while low levels are seen in trisomy, gestational trophoblastic disease.
- *Dual test:* It includes free β-hCG and PAPP-A, done between 10 and 14 weeks, NT + NB + dual test has detection rate of 97% in fetus with Down syndrome.
- *Triple test* is done between 15 and 18 weeks. It includes MSAFP, hCG, unconjugated estradiol (UE3). It can detect trisomy 21 in 70% of affected pregnancy with false positive rate as 5%.
- *Quadruple test* includes MSAFP, hCG, UE3 and inhibin. It can detect trisomy in 80% of affected pregnancy and false positive rate is 7%.

Cytogenetic Test

- *Amniocentesis:* Performed between 14 and 16 weeks under USG guidance. It can detect chromosomal anomalies (trisomy 21, monosomy), single gene disorder (cystic fibrosis, Tay-Sachs disease). Risks are fetal loss (0.5%) and amniotic fluid leakage.
- *Chorionic villus biopsy:* It is carried out transcervically between 10 and 12 weeks and transabdominally from 10 weeks to term. False positive results are 2–3% and may need amniocentesis for confirmation. Complications are fetal loss (0.5–1%), oromandibular limb deformity.
- *Cordocentesis:* Done under LA from 18 weeks onwards, and gives all information obtained from amniocentesis and CVS. It can also detect fetal anemia, bleeding disorder, hemoglobinopathies, fetal infections, and fetal blood acid–base status and also useful for fetal therapy ego blood transfusion, drug therapy. Overall fetal loss is 1–4%.

Biophysical Method

1. Fetal Movement Count

- *Cardif 'count 10':* Patient counts fetal movements starting at 9 am. The counting comes to the end as soon as 10 movements are perceived.
- *Daily fetal movement count:* Three counts each of one hour duration (morning, noon and evening) are recommended. The total counts multiplied by four gives daily (12 hours) fetal movement count.
- If count is <10 in 12 hours, it suggest fetal compromise. Count should be performed daily starting at 28 weeks of pregnancy.

2. Non-stress Test

Testing should be started after 30 weeks of pregnancy. The test looks for presence of temporary accelerations of fetal heart rate with fetal movement. NST is reactive if there are >2 accelerations of >15 beats lasting longer than 15 seconds in 20 minutes observation. Test has false negative rate of <0.5% and false positive rate of 50%. Vibroacoustic stimulation—reactive NST after VAS indicate a reactive fetus.

3. Contraction Stress Test

It is an indicator of uteroplacental function. False negative rate of CST is 0.4 per 1000.

Biophysical Profile

- It includes NST, fetal breathing movement, gross body movement, fetal muscle tone and amniotic fluid with score of 2 for each.
- BPP score 8–10 suggest no fetal asphyxia, a score of 6 is equivocal and requires further testing to verify fetal well-being, score <4 indicate asphyxia and urgent delivery is required regardless of gestational age.
- False negative rate of BPP is 0.7 per 1000 while false positive rate is 30%.
- Modified BPP consists of NST and AFI. It is considered abnormal if NST is non-reactive and AFI is <5.1. It has false positive rate of only 0.05%.

Ultrasonography

- In early pregnancy (11–14 weeks) increased *Nuchal translucency* (NT) >3 mm IS associated with aneuploidy, triploidy, congenital heart disease, diaphragmatic hernia.
- If NT >4 mm, incidence of aneuploidy is so significant that it is appropriate to perform CVS without testing for biochemical analysis.
- *Absent nasal bone (NB)* is associated with fetal Down's syndrome. When NB and NT were combined, detection rate of trisomy 21 was 90% with a false positive rate of 3.5%.
- With NT alone, detection rate is 75%. In genetic sonogram of fetus affected with aneuploidy, one may see absent NB, NT >3 mm, cardiac anomaly, echogenic bowel, short digits, short humerus, short femur, hydronephrosis, echogenic focus. Detection rate for aneuploidy is 59%. In late pregnancy IUGR can be diagnosed accurately with serial measurement of BPD, AC, FL, HC and amniotic fluid volume. AC is single measurement which best reflects fetal nutrition. When the HC/AC ratio is elevated (>1.0) after 34 weeks, IUGR is suspected.
- *Doppler ultrasound velocimetry:* Arterial Doppler waveforms are helpful to assess the downstream vascular resistance. In normal pregnancy the SID ratio, pulsatility index, resistance index decreases as pregnancy advances. Higher values >2 SDs above POG indicate reduced diastolic flow and increased placental vascular resistance. Venous Doppler parameter provides information about cardiac forward function. Fetus with abnormal cardiac function shows pulsatile flow in the umbilical vein.

ANTENATAL ADVICE

- Rest and sleep—patient should be in bed for 10 hours especially in last 6 weeks.

- *Nutritional supplements*
  - Folic acid supplementation: The recommended dose is 400 micrograms per day.
  - Iron (40 mg daily-needed 16 weeks onwards), protein (60 gm daily, preferably animal source) and calcium (at least 1 litre of milk daily) supplementation should be offered routinely to all pregnant women.
  - The increased calorie requirement is to extent of 300 calories more over non-pregnant state during 2nd half of pregnancy. Women with normal BMI should gain 11–12 kg weight while women with BMI 26–29 should limit weight gain to 7 kg and obese women with BMI >29 should gain less weight.
- *Exercise in pregnancy:* A moderate course of exercise during pregnancy is not associated with adverse outcomes.
- *Coitus:* Pregnant woman should be informed that sexual intercourse in pregnancy is not known to be associated with any adverse outcome. Women with increased risk of miscarriage or preterm labor should avoid coitus, if they feel uterine activity.
- *Alcohol and smoking in pregnancy:* Due to increased fetal risks, it is suggested that women should avoid alcohol consumption when pregnant. Pregnant women should be informed about the specific risks of smoking/tobacco use during pregnancy (low birth weight, IUGR and preterm).
- *Travel during pregnancy:* Travel is safe. However, patient should be counseled regarding risks of long distance travel, especially the risk of DVT with long flight.
- *Immunization:* Live virus vaccine (MMR, yellow fever, polio, varicella) should be avoided. Tetanus toxoid is given IM at 6 weeks interval for 2 such, the first one to be given between 16 and 24 weeks.

MANAGEMENT OF COMMON SYMPTOMS OF PREGNANCY

- *Nausea and vomiting in early pregnancy:* Women should be informed that most cases of nausea and vomiting in pregnancy will resolve spontaneously by end of first trimester. Non-pharmacological agents or safe antiemetic can be prescribed.
- *Heartburn:* Manage by lifestyle and diet modification. Antacids may be offered to women whose heartburn remains troublesome despite lifestyle and diet modification.
- *Constipation:* Pregnant woman should be advised regarding diet modification and medication, if needed.
- *Hemorrhoids:* Topically applied anesthetics, stool softening agents can be used. Surgical treatment is better to be avoided.
- *Varicose veins:* Women should be informed that varicose veins are a common symptom of pregnancy that will not cause harm and that compression stockings can improve the symptoms.
- *Vaginal discharge:* Assurance and local cleanliness are advised. If this is associated with itch, soreness, offensive smell or pain on passing urine there may be an infective cause. In these cases, evaluation and treatment should be considered.
- *Backache:* Massage therapy, analgesic and rest relieve the pain due to muscle spasm.

PRECONCEPTION COUNSELING

Objective is to ensure that a woman enters pregnancy with an optimal state of health which would be safe both to herself and the fetus. Preconception counseling is a part of preventive medicine. It includes risk assessment and education.

- Identification of high risk factors by detailed evaluation of obstetric, medical, family and personal history and examination.
- Base level health status including blood pressure is recorded.
- Routine testing for rubella IgG antibodies prior to planning pregnancy is recommended. All susceptible patients should be immunized and advised against attempting pregnancy for subsequent 3 months.
- Use of iodized salt and practice of screening all patients for thyroid disorder are recommended.
- Folic acid supplementation (4 mg a day) starting 4 weeks prior to conception up to 12 weeks of pregnancy is advised. This reduces the incidence of neural tube defects.
- Maternal health is optimized preconceptionally. Pre-existing chronic disease (hypertension, diabetes, epilepsy) are stabilized in optimal state by intervention.
- Woman should be urged to stop smoking, taking alcohol and abusing drugs.
- Inheritable genetic diseases (thalassemia, Sickle cell disease) are screened before conception and risk of passing the condition to offspring is discussed.
- Couple with history of recurrent pregnancy loss or with family history of congenital abnormality are investigated and counseled properly.

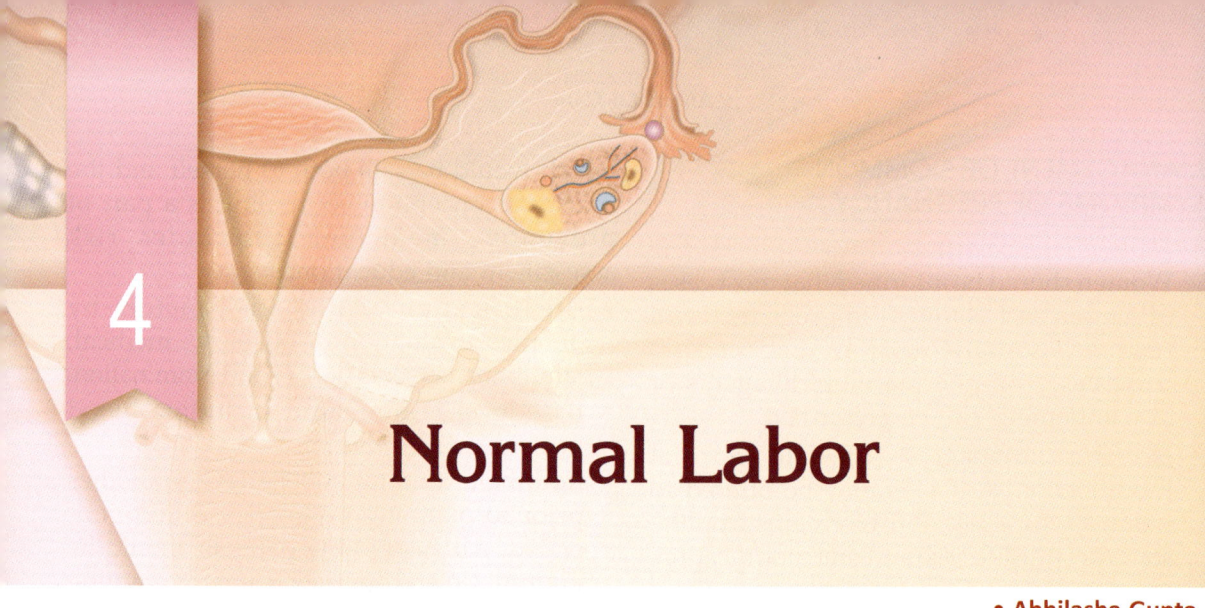

Normal Labor

• **Abhilasha Gupta**

Labor by definition is the process of expulsion of products of conception after the fetus attains viability. In the developed world a fetus is considered viable after 22 wks of gestation or with a weight of ≥ 500 gm but that is because of advanced neonatal resuscitation facilities. In India, this is not available at most places hence this cut off period practically remains 28 weeks of gestation. Normal labor (eutocia) is one where labor:

- Starts spontaneously
- Starts at term
- Presentation is vertex
- Without undue prolongation
- Without any harm to mother and baby
- Delivery occurs per vaginum without any artificial aids (episiotomy is not considered artificial aid)
- Any deviation from this is considered abnormal labor (dystocia).

ONSET OF LABOR

After so many years of research, what exactly triggers labor is still not fully known. Many theories have been postulated. It appears that multiple factors are involved including role of:

1. Prostaglandins
2. Oxytocin
3. Estrogen and progesterone
4. Inflammatory mediators
5. Mechanical factors
6. The fetus itself through its hypothalamo-pituitary adrenal axis.

During pregnancy, the progesterone levels are very high and dominate over estrogen levels. Near term, there is dramatic fall in progesterone, so there is relative rise in estrogen levels leading to destabilization of lysosomes. This liberates prostaglandins which play a role in initiation of labor. Oxytocin does not appear to have a role in initiation of labor but has its main role in final expulsive stages of labor. Inflammatory mediators (cytokines, platelet activating factor, endothelins) also appear to play a role via synthesis of prostaglandins. Fetal cortisol inhibits progesterone synthesis thus contributing to prostaglandin synthesis. Overstretching of uterus as in polyhydramnios and multiple pregnancies may increase muscle excitability and thus may initiate labor.

Facilitators of prostaglandin synthesis

- Estrogen
- Oxytocin
- Inflammatory mediators

Inhibitor of prostaglandin synthesis

- Progesterone

Identification of labor: During labor the Braxton-Hick's contractions of pregnancy become contractions of labor. The difference between the two is retraction, i.e. permanent shortening. It is not present in Braxton-Hick's whereas, it is the feature of true labor pains. Although differentiation between true and false labor is sometimes difficult, the associated features of labor like cervical dilatation, show and formation of bag of waters can help in diagnosis. In the absence of ruptured membranes or bleeding, uterine contractions every 5 mins for 1 hour, i.e. ≥12 contractions per hour may signify onset of labor.

FETUS *IN UTERO*

The fetus *in utero* must be in a position to be comfortable enough in that limited space of amniotic sac and also its position should be suitable for its journey through the birth canal.

Lie: The relation of long axis of the fetus to that of the mother. Commonest and most favorable lie is longitudinal (99.5%). It could be transverse or oblique lie. The latter being unstable and converts to longitudinal or transverse lie during labor (Fig. 4.1).

Presentation and presenting part: That part of fetus which presents at the pelvic inlet is presentation and that part of presentation which overlies the internal os is presenting part. In cephalic presentation, the presenting part can be vertex (occiput), brow or face depending on the degree of flexion or extension of head (Fig. 4.2). The terms presentation and presenting part are often used synonymously.

Attitude: A general disposition of fetus in uterus is known as attitude. Normally fetus is in flexed attitude where body, neck and limbs are all flexed. In breech presentation sometimes the legs may be extended.

Denominator: It is an arbitrarily chosen fixed point on the presenting part.

Position: It is the relation of denominator to the different quadrants of pelvis. Pelvis is divided into four equal quadrants—right and left anterior, and right and left posterior. So various positions of vertex presentation are: Left occipitoanterior (LOA), right occipito-anterior (ROA), right occipitoposterior (ROP) and left occipitoposterior (LOP). Often the head is lying in transverse position when it is

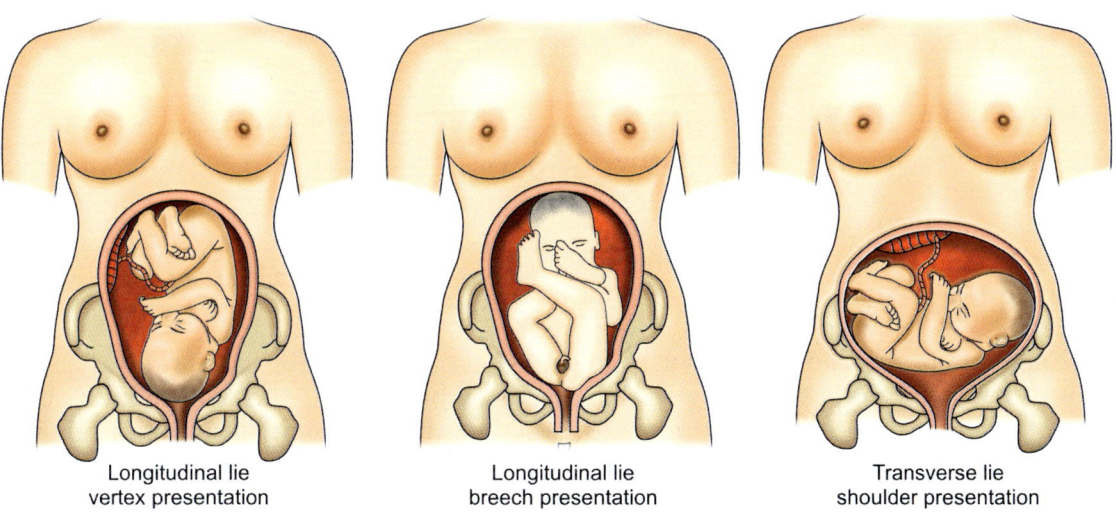

| Longitudinal lie vertex presentation | Longitudinal lie breech presentation | Transverse lie shoulder presentation |

Fig. 4.1: Longitudinal and transverse lie

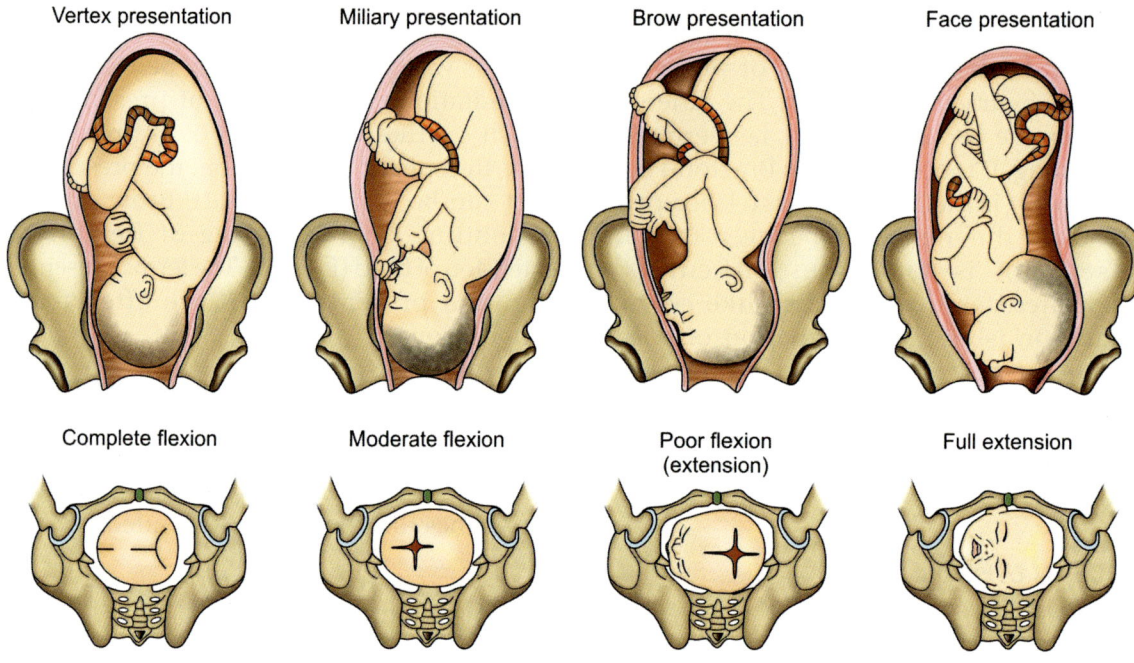

Fig. 4.2: Various presentations of head

known as occipito transverse (LOT or ROT) (Fig. 4.3).

Commonest presentation is cephalic because head is heavier and smaller as compared to podalic extremity and adapts lower pole better. The left positions are commoner due to dextrorotation of uterus. Left anterior positions are commoner as the left posterior quadrant is occupied by sigmoid colon.

MECHANISM OF LABOR

Mechanism of labor is defined as the series of movements undertaken by the fetal head in the process of adaptation during its journey through the curved pelvic cavity. Although principally the movements take place in the head, the rest of the fetal trunk also participates in the mechanism of labor. In the majority of women, the position of head at the onset of labor is left occipitoanterior (LOA) or occipitotransverse (LOT). These movements occur as a continuous process but can be described as:

1. Flexion

Although some degree of flexion is seen at the beginning of labor, full flexion is achievable after the head meets the resistance of birth canal during descent.

Flexion is essential in keeping smaller diameter of fetal head entering the pelvis.

2. Descent

The various forces helping in descent (Fig. 4.4) are:
1. Pressure of the amniotic fluids
2. Direct pressure of the fundus upon the breech.
3. Maternal bearing down efforts.
4. Extension and straightening of the fetal body.

Asynclitism: While the fetal head is descending, the sagittal suture may not be midway between symphysis pubis and sacral promontory. It is frequently deviated towards either of them. If it is closer to pubic symphysis, it is posterior parietal bone presentation or

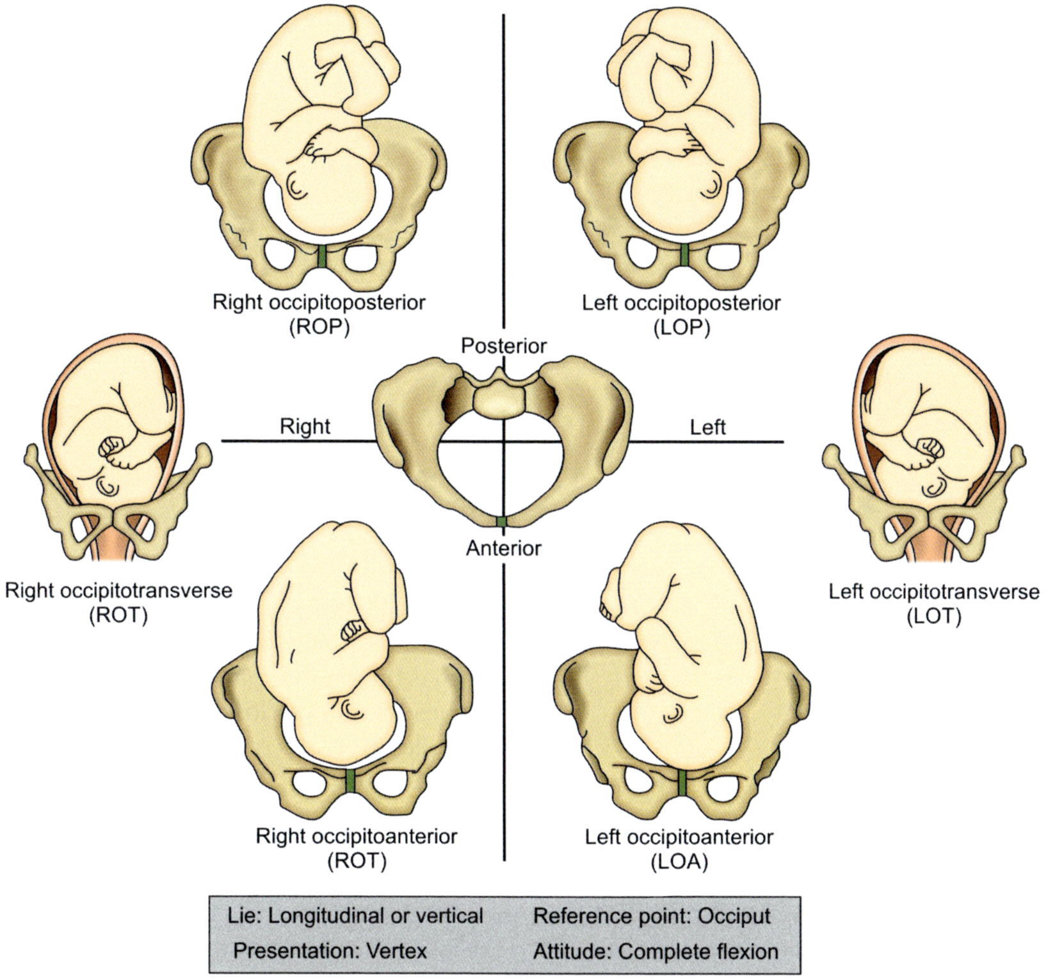

Right occipitoposterior
(ROP)

Left occipitoposterior
(LOP)

Posterior

Right

Left

Anterior

Right occipitotransverse
(ROT)

Left occipitotransverse
(LOT)

Right occipitoanterior
(ROT)

Left occipitoanterior
(LOA)

Lie: Longitudinal or vertical	Reference point: Occiput
Presentation: Vertex	Attitude: Complete flexion

Fig. 4.3: Various positions of vertex

posterior asynclitism. If it is closer to sacral promontory, it is anterior parietal bone presentation or anterior asynclitism. Moderate degree of asynclitism is the rule in normal labor. Successive shifting from posterior to anterior asynclitism aids descent. Severe persistent asynclitism indicates cephalopelvic disproportion (Fig. 4.5).

3. Engagement

Engagement is when biparietal diameter, the greatest transverse diameter of the fetal head, passes through the pelvic inlet (Fig. 4.6).

In primigravida, it often occurs in last few weeks of pregnancy and in multipara, it occurs during labor. However, delivery

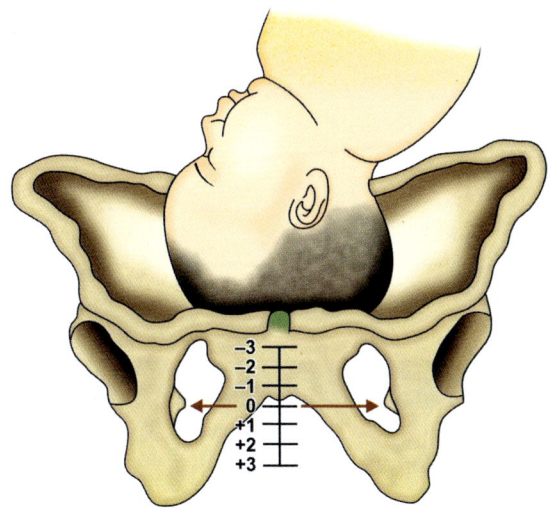

Fig. 4.4: Descent of fetal head in relation to ischial spine

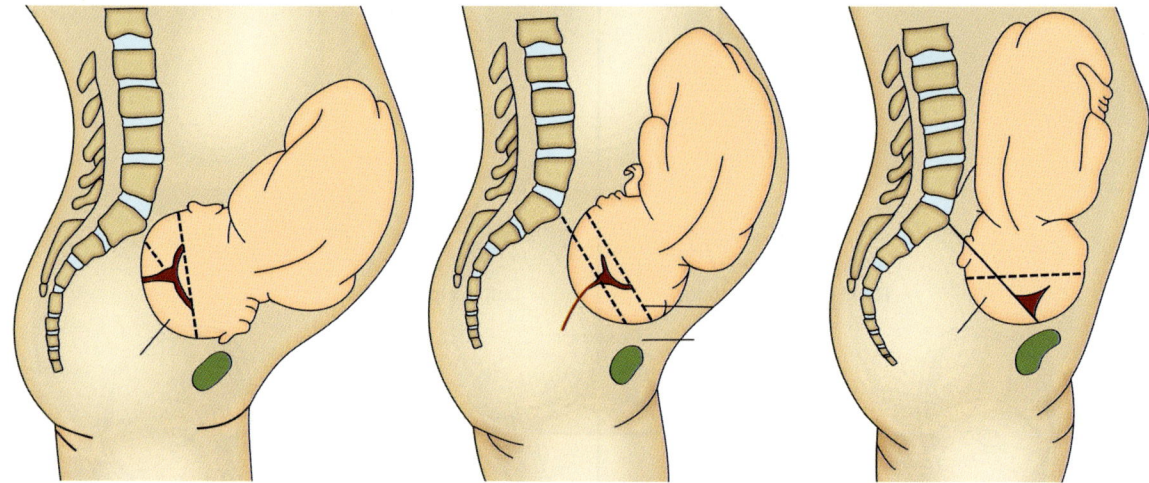

Fig. 4.5: Anterior, normal and posterior asynclitism

outcome is not influenced by the engagement of head at the time of labor, spontaneous or induced.

4. Internal Rotation

The internal rotation takes place at the level of ischial spines and the pelvic floor when the head reaches and meets with resistance. Fetal head enters the inlet in transverse diameter and rotates internally into the anteroposterior diameter as it reaches the outlet, for normal birth to take place. Hence, internal rotation is absolutely necessary. When the occiput, which is the leading part in a well-flexed head, touches the pelvic floor, there is elastic recoil of the levator ani muscles. This causes the head to rotate 45° to the midline in occipito-anterior positions and 90° in occipitotransverse positions, thereby bringing the occiput to lie near the pubic symphysis. Internal rotation is brought about by following mechanisms:

- Elastic recoil of levator ani

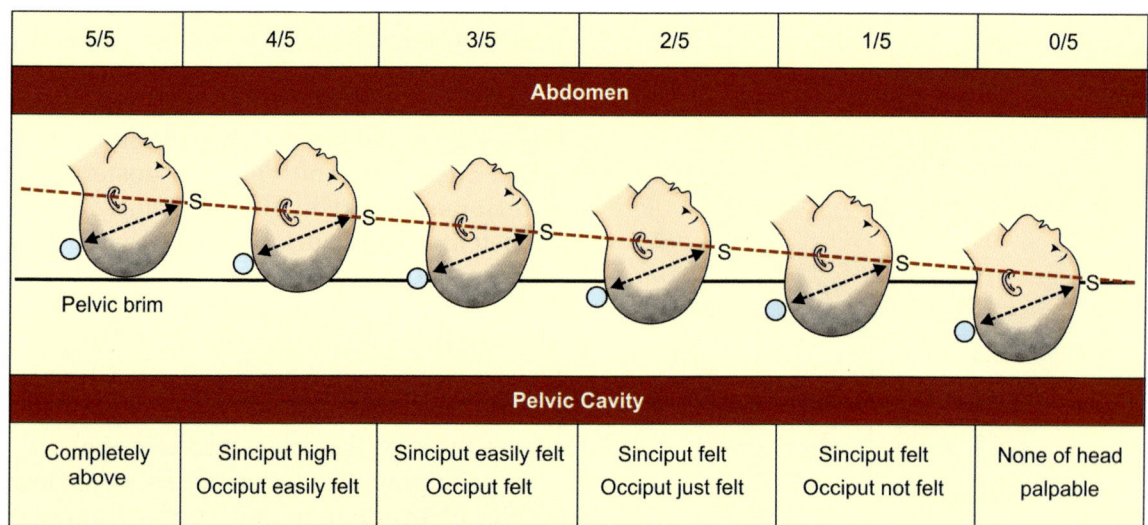

5/5	4/5	3/5	2/5	1/5	0/5
Abdomen					
Pelvic Cavity					
Completely above	Sinciput high Occiput easily felt	Sinciput easily felt Occiput felt	Sinciput felt Occiput just felt	Sinciput felt Occiput not felt	None of head palpable

Fig. 4.6: Descent and engagement of head

- Gutter like shape of the pelvic floor formed by two levator ani
- Favorable shape of the pelvis
- Well-flexed head
- Efficient uterine contractions

5. Extension

Delivery of head occurs by extension. The driving forces push the head downwards and the pelvic resistance pushes it upwards. As the anterior wall is deficient (pubic symphysis being smaller), the head is pushed anteriorly to be born by extension. The vertex, brow and face are born successively.

Restitution: Once the head is born, the neck untwists and the head rotates back by 45° and gains its original position. The occiput thus turns towards the mother's left thigh in LOA position and towards the right thigh in ROA position. This movement is called restitution.

6. External Rotation

This movement is brought as the outward manifestation of the internal rotation of the shoulders. Thus, the head, which had already restituted by 45°, now rotates another 45° to maintain its normal relation to shoulders.

7. Lateral Flexion and Delivery of Shoulders

First the anterior shoulder then the posterior shoulder followed by the trunk are delivered by lateral flexion. The shoulders engage with the bisacromial diameter in the oblique diameter of the pelvis, opposite to that of head. The anterior shoulder reaches the pelvic floor first and undergoes internal rotation into the anteroposterior diameter. This rotation obviously is in a direction opposite to the direction of rotation of head. The anterior shoulder is born under pubic symphysis and pivots there. Then by the process of lateral flexion, posterior shoulder slides over the perineum and is born.

FETAL HEAD SHAPE CHANGES DURING LABOR

Caput succedaneum: In vertex presentations, labor forces alter fetal head shape. In prolonged labor before complete cervical dilatation, the portion of fetal scalp immediately over the cervical os becomes edematous this swelling is known as caput succedaneum and is usually only a few millimeters thick. But in prolonged labor it may be so thick as to interfere with examination of various sutures and fontanels (Fig. 4.7). More commonly it forms when a rigid vaginal outlet offers resistance. Because it

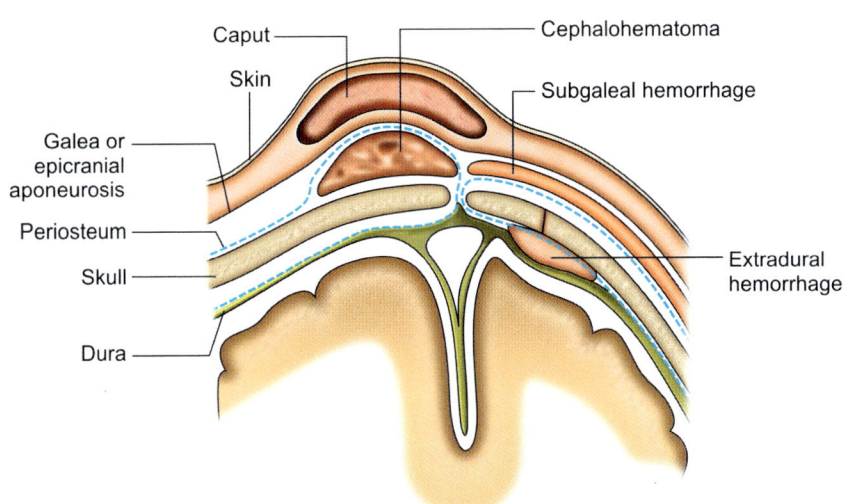

Fig. 4.7: Sites of caput, cephalohematoma and subgaleal and subdural hemorrhage

develops over most dependent area of head, one can deduce the original fetal head position by noting the location of caput succedaneum.

Molding: The bony fetal head shape is also altered by compressive forces of labor referred as molding. Some molding can occur even before labor, possibly due to Braxton Hick's contractions. There is seldom overlapping of parietal bones due to locking mechanism at anterior and posterior fontanels. The frontal and occipital bones slip under parietal bones resulting in some shortening of suboccipito-bregmatic diameter and corresponding lengthening of mentovertical diameter. This can be of a great significance in cases of mildly contracted pelvis. Excessive molding to overcome severely contracted pelvis is dangerous to baby (Fig. 4.8).

STAGES OF LABOR

Prelabor or preparatory phase: Prelabor occurs as a preparation to actual labor. During this oxytocin receptors on myometrium increase. The lower segment becomes well-formed leading to changes:

- *Lightening:* As the lower segment is formed, there is descent of the presenting part into the pelvis resulting in decrease in fundal height thus bringing a sense of relief in the mother.

- *Cervical ripening:* Under the effects of prostaglandins, there is relative decrease in collagen and dermatan sulfate and increase in hyaluronic acid, the net result being cervical ripening or softening and relaxation. A ripe cervix is short, soft and dilatable cervix.

- *False labor pains:* Irregular contractions not accompanied by cervical dilatation. They may be due to bowel problems.

Labor: Even though a continuous process, for the sake of description, labor is divided into three stages (Table 4.1).

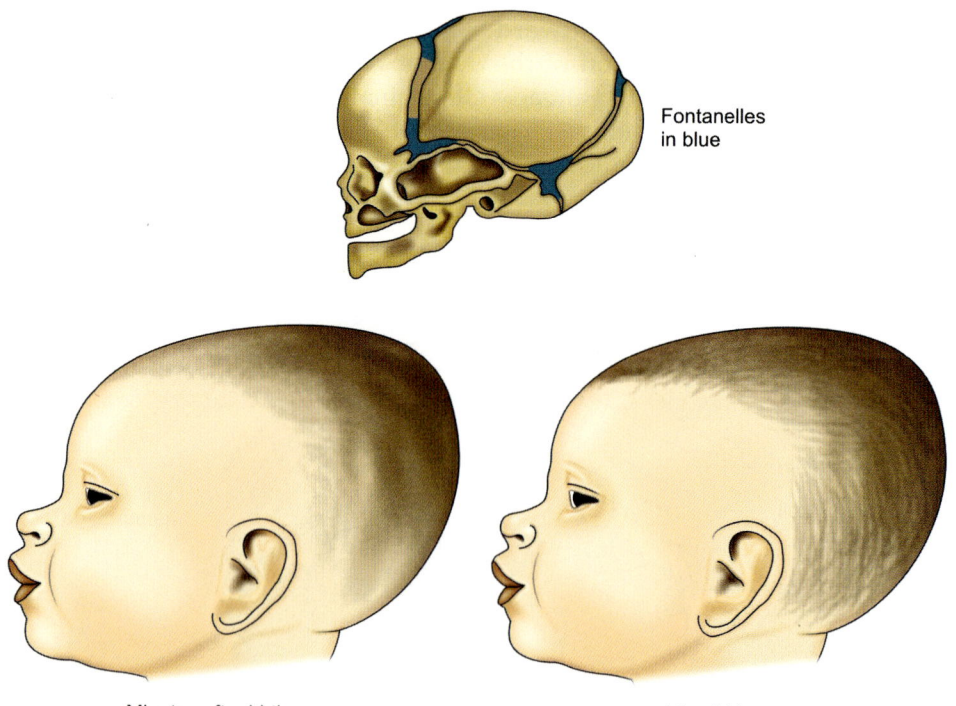

Fontanelles in blue

Minutes after birth   After 24 hours

Fig. 4.8: Molding which quickly disappears within a few hours

Table 4.1: Stages of labor	
First stage	Onset of true labor pains to complete cervical dilatation
Second stage	Complete cervical dilatation to delivery of the fetus or fetuses
Third stage	Separation and expulsion of the placenta and the membranes

First Stage

The stage of opening of the passages marked by cervical effacement and dilatation. In primigravida, effacement occurs first followed by dilatation. In multigravida, both effacement and dilatation occur simultaneously. The first stage is divided into two phases:

1. Latent phase: Mainly involves cervical dilatation up to 3–4 cm. It lasts for about 6–8 hrs in nullipara and 4–6 hrs in multipara.

2. Active phase: Extends from 4 cm of dilatation (WHO) to complete cervical dilatation. The average duration is about 5 hrs in nullipara and 3 hrs in multipara. The mean rate of cervical dilatation is 1.2 cm/hr in nullipara and 1.5 cm/hr in multipara, minimal acceptable progress rate is 1 cm/hr. The pattern of cervical dilatation is a sigmoid curve and that of fetal descent is a hyperbolic curve (Fig. 4.9).

The first stage is also divided into the following phases:
1. Acceleration phase (3–4 cm of cervical dilatation)
2. Phase of maximum slope (4–9 cm of cervical dilatation)
3. Deceleration phase (9–10 cm of cervical dilatation)

First stage is charactertized by
1. *Uterine contractions:* Contractions of labor are regular and increase in duration and frequency. In active labor, these contractions last for 30–90 sec and the frequency is at least 3 in 10 mins. These contractions have a fundal dominance along with a rise in intra-amniotic pressure. In the first stage of labor, the peak intrauterine pressure is 40–50 mm Hg and in the second stage it is 80–100 mm Hg (resting tone is about 6–10 mm Hg).

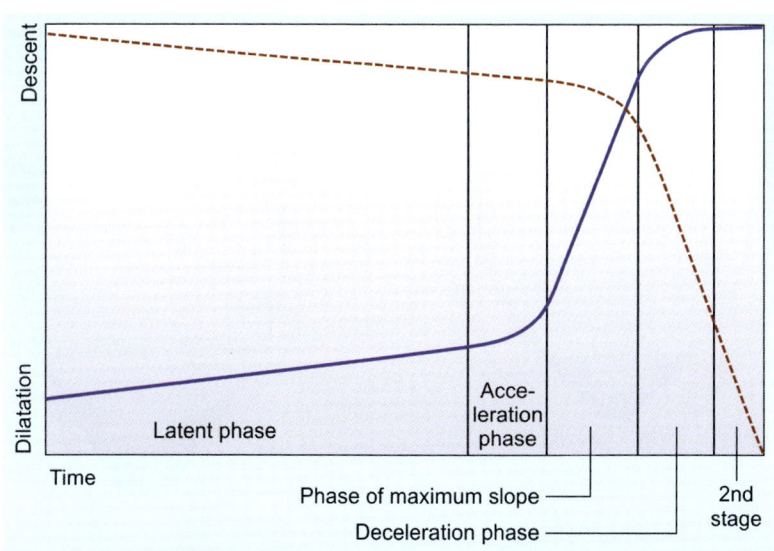

Fig. 4.9: Phases of labor and descent of head

2. *Cervical changes (effacement and dilatation):* Effacement is taking up of cervix or shortening of cervical canal to a circular opening with paper thin edges, cervix is being incorporated into lower uterine segment. Uterine contractions exert a hydrostatic pressure through the intact membranes, which dilates the cervix. When the membranes rupture, the presenting part is forced directly against the cervix and the lower segment. Mechanical dilatation of the cervix enhances uterine activity known as Ferguson reflex, probably mediated through prostaglandins.

3. *Show:* Cervical mucus plug mixed with blood is called show.

Formation of lower uterine segment: The lower segment is the part of the uterus below the uterovesical fold of peritoneum where the peritoneum is loosely attached. It is around 7–10 cm in length and is derived from isthmus and cervix. During labor, after effacement and dilatation, cervix is also incorporated in the LUS. Following successive uterine contractions, the upper segment becomes thicker and thicker because of progressive shortening and the lower segment becomes thinner and thinner because of progressive lengthening of muscle fibers. However, in normal labor this junction between upper and lower segments is not visible per abdomen. In obstructed labor when this phenomenon becomes exaggerated, the junction becomes visible per abdomen in the form of an oblique groove, known as the retraction ring or Bandl's ring.

4. *Descent of fetus:* Descent mainly begins with the phase of maximal slope, but is maximal in the deceleration phase and in the second stage. Once descent begins, it should be progressive.

5. *Formation of bag of water* and finally rupture of membranes due to stretching of the lower uterine segment, membranes detach from their loose attachment to deciduas and bulge into the cervical canal as it dilates (Fig. 4.10). When the uterus contract, this bag of water become tense and exerts hydrostatic pressure, which in turn dilates the cervix like a wedge. Finally, towards the end of first stage, the membranes rupture as the lower part of the uterus becomes unsupported.

Second Stage

This is the stage of expulsion of the fetus. The average duration is 1 hour in nullipara and half an hour in multipara. It is mainly concerned with the descent of the fetus. It is considered to have two phases (Fig. 4.11):

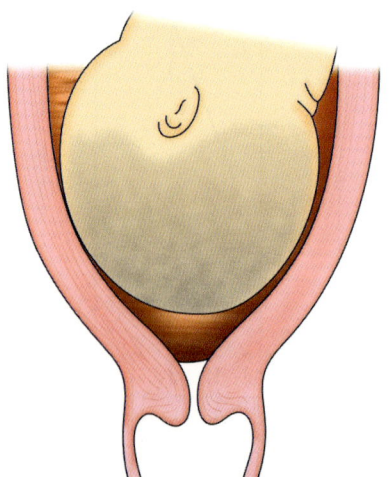
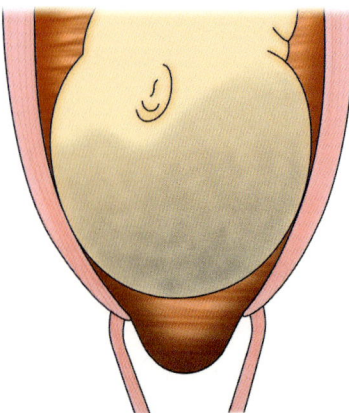

Fig. 4.10: Cervical effacement, dilatation and formation of bag of water

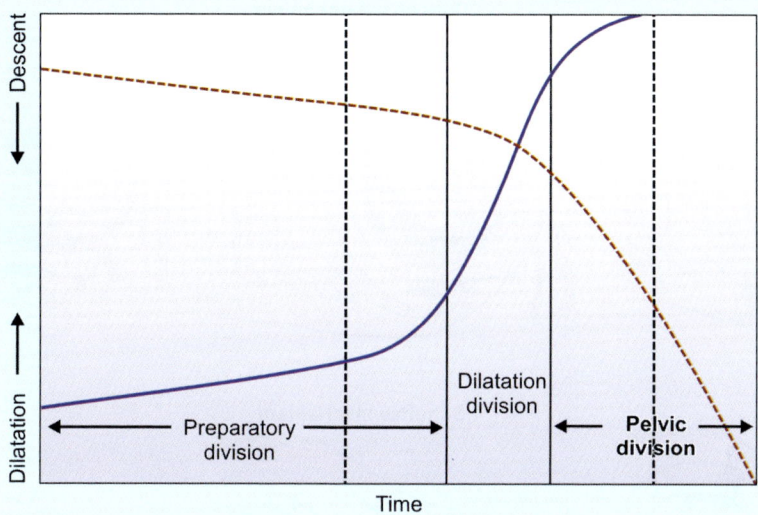

Fig. 4.11: Phases of labor and descent of head

Phase 1/passive phase/pelvic phase/phase of descent

This phase is from complete cervical dilatation until the head reaches the pelvic floor. Physiologically, it is more like an extension of the first stage.

Phase 2/active phase/perineal phase/phase of expulsion

This active phase is marked by bearing down efforts. Instrumental delivery if indicated should be undertaken in this stage.

A second stage can be considered within normal limits in nullipara for up to 3 hrs when regional anesthesia is used and up to 2 hrs when it is not. The comparable values in multipara are 2 hrs, and 1 hr, respectively.

Second stage is characterized by:

1. *Descent of the head:* Assessed by abdominal palpation and vaginal examination.

2. Bearing down pains

3. *Crowning:* The head is said to crown when its maximum diameter (biparietal) stretches the vulval outlet and does not recede in between contractions.

4. Expulsion of the fetus

Clinically one can identify second stage by noting

- A change in the character of pains (bearing down type).
- Gaping of introitus and anus during pains due to pressure of head on the levator ani muscle.
- The cervical rim cannot be felt as the uterus, cervix and vagina become one single birth canal.

Third Stage

This is the stage of placental separation and expulsion and the mean duration is about 15 mins. Immediately after the baby is born, the uterus contracts and retracts and thus decreases markedly in size. As a result, there is a decrease in area of the implantation site, which causes the placenta to buckle. This leads to placental separation at decidua spongiosa, the weakest layer of placental attachment.

There are two methods of placental separation.

1. Central Separation or Schultze Method

Here, a retroplacental hematoma is formed and the placenta separates like an inverted

Duncan's mechanism

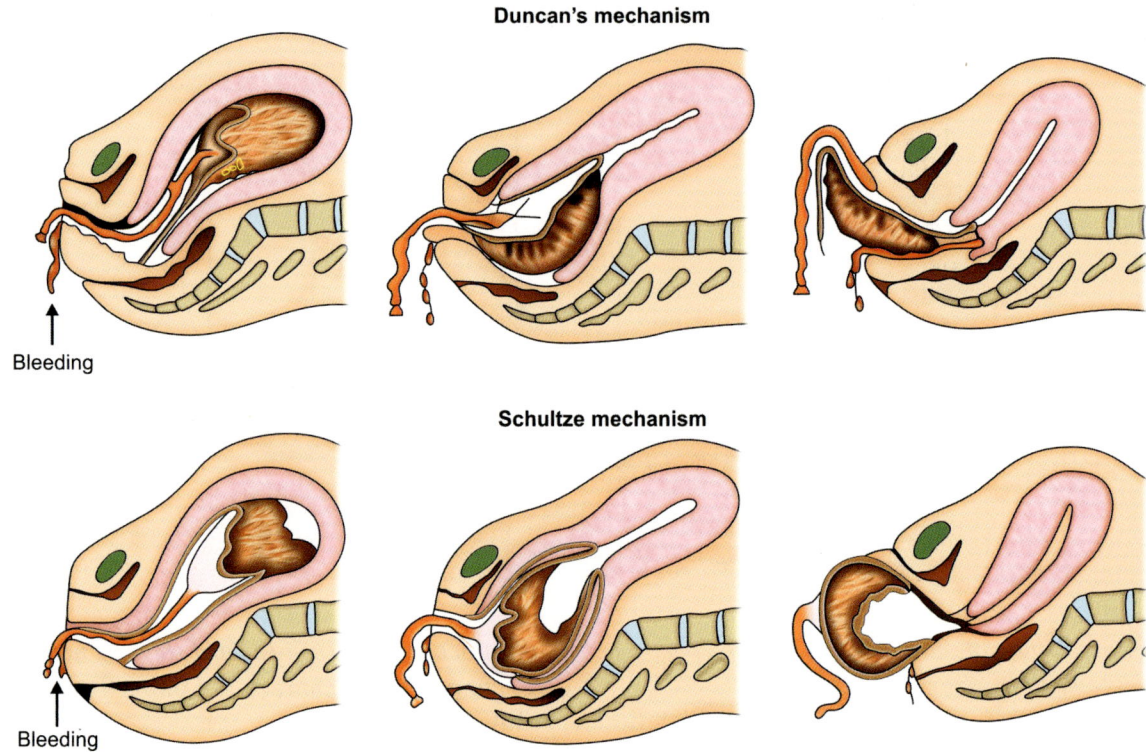

Bleeding

Schultze mechanism

Bleeding

Fig. 4.12: Central and marginal separation of placenta

umbrella. Blood is usually collected behind the placenta in the membranes.

2. Marginal Separation or Mathew Duncan's Method

Separation begins at the periphery, blood escapes into the vagina between the membranes and the uterine wall, the placenta descends sideways and the maternal surface appears first at vulva (Fig. 4.12).

After separation, the placenta is usually expelled by controlled cord traction. There is an inevitable amount of blood loss, which should not normally exceed 300 ml. This is followed by contraction and retraction of the uterine muscle fibers around the uterine vessels forming living ligatures and thus the vessels are occluded preventing further blood loss.

The signs of separation of placenta are: The uterine fundus becomes well contracted, smaller, fundal height rises somewhat with a suprapubic bulge as the placenta shifts in the lower segment, apparent lengthening of cord and a small gush of blood.

Bibliography

1. Adams SS, Eberhard-Gran M, Eskild A. Fear of childbirth and duration of labour: a study of 2206 women with intended vaginal delivery. BJOG 2012;119(10):1238.

2. Alexander JM, Sharma SK, McIntire DD, et al. Epidural analgesia lengthens the Friedman active phase of labor. Obstet Gynecol 2002;100:46.

3. Caldwell WE, Moloy HC, D'Esopo DA. A roentgenologic study of the mechanism of engagement of the fetal head. Am J Obstet Gynecol 1934;28:824.

4. Calkins LA. The etiology of occiput presentations. Am J Obstet Gynecol 1939;37:618.

5. Carlan SJ, Wyble L, Lense J, et al. Fetal head molding: diagnosis by ultrasound and a review of the literature. J Perinatol 1991;11:105.

6. Carollo TC, Reuter JM, Galan HL, et al. Defining fetal station. Am J Obstet Gynecol 2004; 191: 1793.

7. Dupuis O, Silveira R, Zentner A, et al. Birth simulator: Reliability of transvaginal assessment of fetal head station as defined by the American College of Obstetricians and Gynecologists classification. Am J Obstet Gynecol 2005; 192: 868.

8. Kilpatrick SJ, Laros RK Jr. Characteristics of normal labor. Obstet Gynecol 1989;74:85.

9. Pates JA, McIntire DD, Leveno KJ. Uterine contractions preceding labor. Obstet Gynecol 2007;110:566.

10. Segel SY, Carreno CA, Weiner MS, et al: Relationship between fetal station and successful vaginal delivery in nulliparous women. Am J Perinatol 2012;29:723.

5

Abnormal Uterine Action

• Saroj Singh

Over last quarter of century the incidence of cesarean section due to dystocia has increased. Abnormal uterine actions are one of the important causes of dystocia.[1] Overall labor abnormalities occur in about 25% of nulliparous women and 10% of multiparous women.

PHYSIOLOGY OF NORMAL UTERINE CONTRACTIONS

The pacemaker of uterine contractions lies in the cornua of uterus near fallopian tubes with left being dominant and leads to commencement of waves of uterine contractions and retractions, that passes downwards towards the lower segment and become progressively less intense. Though the lower segment needs to be passive and relaxed in order to efface and dilate to facilitate normal labor (Fig. 5.1).

- During normal labor the uterus contracts every 3–4 minutes and each contraction increase the intrauterine.
- Pressure 25–75 mm Hg above a baseline of 5–20 mm Hg.
- Interval gradually shortens and intensity increases.
- Associated with cervical dilatation
- Associated with discomfort in back and abdomen not relived by sedation.

In contrast, Braxton Hicks contractions, are contractions that may start around 26 weeks gestation and are sometimes called "false labor", should be infrequent, irregular and involve only mild cramping.[2]

In the second stage of labor the uterine work is complmented by maternal expulsive efforts that become an important part of the power required to achieve vaginal delivery.

Any deviation of normal uterine contraction and or coupled with inadequate cervical dilatation and descent of presenting fetal part affecting the course and outcome of labor is defined as abnormal uterine action.

Dystocia literally means difficult labor and is characterized by abnormally slow labor progress. It may be a result of abnormal uterine action.[3]

Classification

1. *Over-efficient uterine action*
   - *Precipitate labor:* In absence of obstruction
   - *Excessive contraction and retraction:* In presence of obstruction.
2. *Ineffient uterine action*
   - Hypotonic inertia
   - Hypertonic inertia
     - Colicky uterus
     - Hyperactive lower uterine segment
     - Constriction (contraction) ring

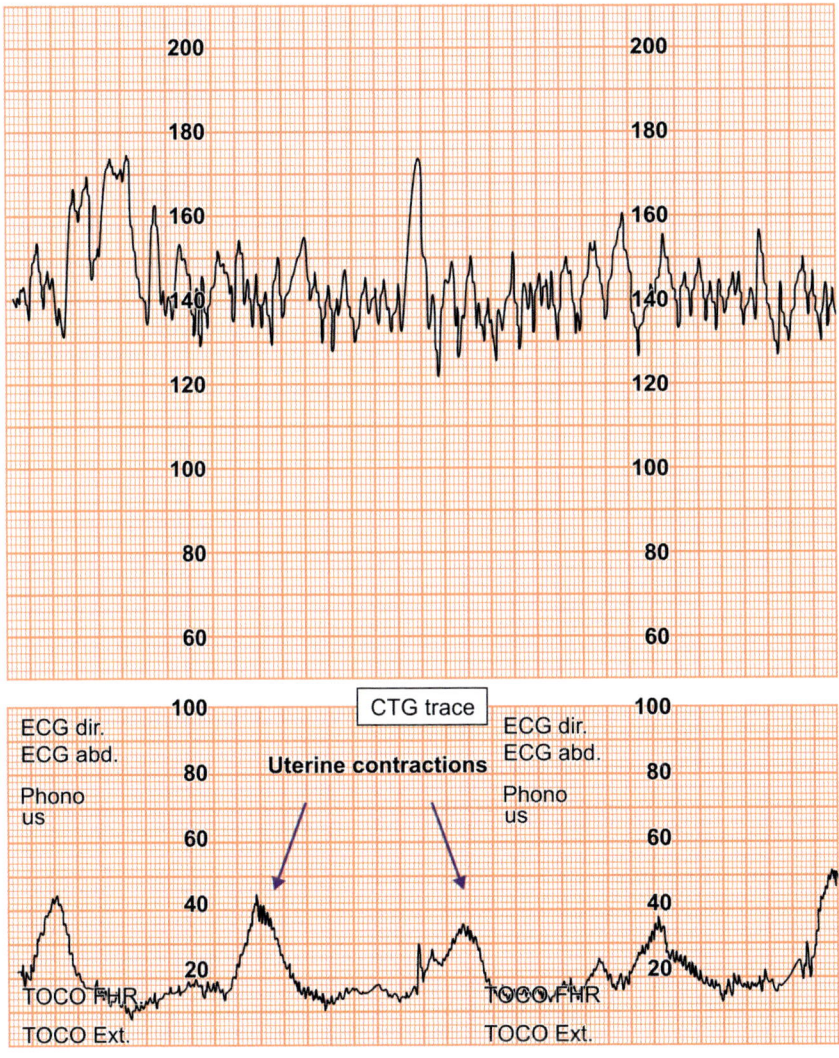

Fig. 5.1: Uterine tracings of normal labor

3. *Cervical dystocia*

Dystocia usually arises from four distinct abnormalities that may exist singly or in combination:

1. Abnormalities of the expulsive forces.
2. Abnormalities of presentation, position, or development of the fetus.
3. Abnormalities of the maternal bony pelvis.
4. Abnormalities of soft tissues of the reproductive tract that forms an obstacle to fetal descent.

It may be simplified as abnormalities of the powers—uterine contractility, the passenger—the fetus, and the passage—the pelvis.[4]

1. Overefficient Uterine Action

Precipitate Labor

Precipitous labor is extremely rapid labor and delivery.

According to Hughes (1972), precipitous labor terminates in expulsion of the fetus in less than 3 hours. It is more common in multiparous.[5]

Etiology: The etiology is not clear; it may result from following predisposing factors:

a. Abnormally low resistance of soft parts of the birth canal.

b. Abnormally strong uterine contractions.

c. *Rarely* from the absence of painful sensations.

Maternal effects: Only seldom precipitous labor is accompanied by serious maternal outcomes if cervix, vagina and perineum are effaced, compliant, stretched and compliant. Conversely, vigorous uterine contractions coupled with noncompliant birth canal may lead to following consequences:

- Extensive lacerations of the cervix, vagina, vulva or perineum.
- Uterine rupture.
- Postpartum hemorrhage.
- Amniotic fluid embolism.

Fetal and neonatal efects

- Fetal asphyxia due to vigorous uterine contractions.
- Intracranial trauma.
- Due to rapid birth, baby may fall to the floor and may suffer from head injury.
- Due to unattended birth, baby may not receive timely resuscitation.
- Erb's or Duchenne's brachial palsy may be associated in one-third of cases.

Management

- In women with such previous history, timely admission should be advised.
- Supervised and controlled induction of labor may be performed.
- Role of tocolytic agents and analgesia is unproven.
- Any oxytocic agent is contraindicated.
- Prophylactic episiotomy may be given.
- As the delivery is quite rapid, the patient should be carefully examined to exclude any cervical, vaginal and perineal tear.

Excessive Uterine Contraction and Retraction

It generally develops in presence of obstruction.

Prior to the onset labor, the junction between the lower and upper uterine segments is a slightly thickened ring which is termed as normal physiological retraction ring. In abnormal and obstructed, after the cervix is fully dilated further contractions cause the upper uterine segment muscle fibers myometrium to shorten, so that the actively contracting upper segment becomes thicker and shorter and on other hand the lower segment becomes stretched and thinner. The demarcation between the two segments become prominent and it takes the form of a well-defined ridge/ring, which may be seen and felt abdominally, is a warning of impending uterine rupture. Also called Bandl's ring or retraction ring (Fig. 5.2).[6]

Etiology

Unknown but predisposing factors are as follows:

- It is more common in primigravidas.
- Malpresentations and malpositions.
- Clumsy intrauterine manipulations.
- Improper use of oxytocin.

Clinical picture: It simulates that of obstructed labor. Patient is usually dehydrated and may present with rupture of lower uterine segment.

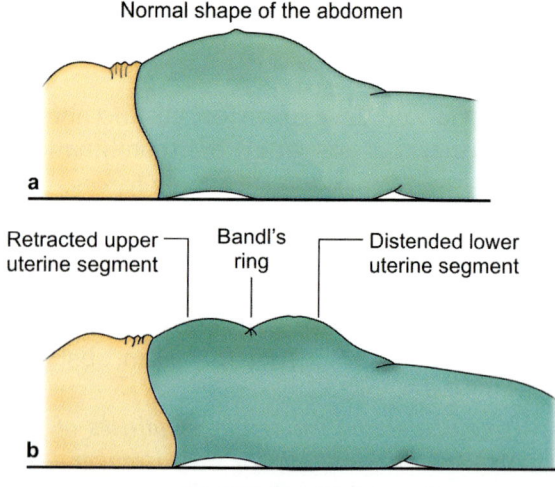

Fig. 5.2: Bandl's ring

(bucket handle tear) due to continuous pressure of the head.

Management

- If cervix is not favorable, cesarean section is treatment of choice.
- However, if fetal head is low down in birth canal with only a rim of cervix well applied on fetal head ventouse delivery can be tried.
- Duhrssen's incisions can be given at 2 and 10 o'clock positions of the cervix, an additional incision if required may be given at 6 o'clock position. These incisions are stitched after delivery using vicryl no. 1-0 suture.[10]

Summary

1. Dystocia means difficult labor.

2. Abnormal uterine action is an important cause of abnormal labor patterns and inefficient uterine contractions, excessive contractions and retractions and cervical dystocia.

3. Hypotonic uterine action is the most common cause of uterine dysfunction.

4. Hypertonic dysfunction is characterized by frequent, intense and painful contractions having no effect on cervical dilatation.

5. Bandl's ring is formed in obstructed labor at the junction of upper and lower uterine segment. It is felt per abdominally.

6. Constriction ring is formed at the junction of upper and lower segment of uterus. It is felt from inside on vaginal examination.

7. Duhressen's incision is given at 2 and 10 o'clock positions in cases of cervical dystocia for delivery of fetus.

Bibliography

1. Bakker JJ, Jansen PF, Van Halem K, et al. Internal versus external tocodynamometry during induced or augmented labor. Cochrane Database Syst. Rev, 2013; 8.

2. Cronje HS, Poor progress in labor, In.Cronje HS, Cilliers JBF, Pretorious MS, Clinical Obstetrics-a south African prespective. 3rd edition, Pretoria, SA 2011; 314–327.

3. Cunningham FG, Lenevo KJ, Bloom SL, et al. Abnormal Labor-Labor and Delivery, Williams Obstetrics, 23rd edition, 2010; 464–489.

4. Gibbons L, Belizan JM, Lauer JA, et al. The global numbers and costs of additionally needed and unnecessary cesarean section performed per year: overuse as a barrier to universal coverage. World Health Report (2010), Background paper, 30. WHO, Geneva.

5. Hinshaw K, Kenyon S, Abnormal labor, Bhide A, Arulkumaran S, Damania KR, et al. Aria's Practical guide to high risk pregnancy and delivery, 4th edn, Haryana, Elsevier, 2015; 333–345.

6. Hugh R Arthur, Cervical dystocia, BJOG: An International Journal of Obstetrics and Gynaecology, August 2005;56(6):983–993.

7. Leah Hennen, Murray, Linda, Jim Scott. *The Baby Center Essential Guide to Pregnancy and Birth: Expert Advice and Real-World Wisdom from the top Pregnancy and Parenting Resource* Emmaus, Pa: Rodale Books 2005; 293–295.

8. Thomson A. Precipitate labor and slow labor: In Magowan B, Owen P, Clinical Obstetrics and Gynaecology, 2nd edn. Edinburgh, UK: Saunders Elsevier, 2009; 355–364.

9. Turrentine MA, Andres RL. "Recurrent Bandl's ring as an etiology for failed vaginal birth after cesarean section". *Amer J Perinatol,* Jan 1994;11(1):65–66.

10. Pandey K, Arya S, Pandey S. Pregnancy with uterine prolapse: Duhressn's incison still valid in today's scenario; Int J Reprod Contracep Obstetrics and Gynaecolgy, 2013;2(4):586–590.

6

Hypertensive Disorders in Pregnancy

• Usha Sharma

Hypertension is one of the common complication in pregnancy and important cause of maternal morbidity and mortality. Pregnancy may induce hypertension in women who are normotensive and may aggravate hypertension in those who are hypertensive before pregnancy. It is difficult to differentiate between pregnancy induced hypertension with hypertension independent of pregnancy so dangerous delay in treatment may occur.

Definitions (According to American College of Obstetricians and gynecologist (ACOG))

Diagnosis of hypertension in pregnancy is made by one of the following criteria:

1. A rise of 30 mm Hg or more in systolic BP.
2. A rise of 15 mm Hg or more in diastolic BP.
3. A systolic BP of 140 mm Hg or more.
4. A diastolic BP of 90 mm Hg or more.

Blood pressure should be observed on at least 2 different occasions at 6 hrs apart.

Hypertension in pregnancy is classified in to following groups:

1. Pregnancy induced hypertension
   a. Pre-eclampsia
   b. Eclampsia
2. Chronic hypertension independent of pregnancy.

3. Pre-eclampsia/eclampsia—superimposed on chronic hypertension
4. Transient hypertension.
5. Unclassified hypertensive disorders.

According to ACOG each form is defined as follows:

Pre-eclampsia

1. Hypertensive with proteinuria greater than 0.3 g/L in 24 hr urine or >1 gm/L in random sample.
2. Generalized edema after 24 hrs of rest in bed.
3. Weight gain of 5 lb or more in 1 week. after 20 wks of gestation.

Eclampsia: Convulsion in patients with pre-eclampsia.

Chronic hypertension: Presence of sustained blood pressure of 140/90 mm Hg or more before pregnancy or before 20 wks of gestation.

Pre-eclampsia/eclampsia superimposed on chronic hypertension: Rise of 30 mm Hg or more in diastolic BP associated with proteinuria, generalized edema or both.

Transient hypertension: The development of hypertension during pregnancy or in early puerperium in a previous normotensive woman whose BP normalizes within 10 days postpartum. There must be no evidence of pre-eclampsia.

UNCLASSIFIED HYPERTENSIVE DISORDERS

Cases who do not have enough informations for classifications.

Etiology

Hypertensive disorders due to pregnancy are more likely to devlop in women who:

1. Are exposed to chorionic villi for the first time.
2. Are exposed to excessive chorionic villi, as in twins or hydatidiform mole.
3. Have preexisting vascular disease.
4. Generally predisposed to hypertension developing during pregnancy.

According to Sibai (2003), currently plausible potential causes include the following:

1. Abnormal trophoblastic invasion of uterine vessels.
2. Immunological intolerance between maternal and fetoplacental tissues.
3. Maternal maladaptation to cardiovascular or inflammatory changes of normal pregnancy.
4. Dietary deficiencies.
5. Genetic influence.

1. *Abnormal trophoblastic invasion:* In pre-eclampsia there is incomplete trophobslastic invasion. Early pre-eclamptic changes include endothelial damage, exudation of plasma constituents into vessel wall, proliferation of myometrial cells, medial necrosis, lipid accumulation in myometrial cells and macrophages termed 'Atherosis'. Obstruction of spiral arteriolar lumen by atherosis impair placental blood flow. These changes cause diminished placental perfusion leading to "pre-clampsia syndrome".

2. *Immunological factors:* There are strong evidences to support the theory that pre-eclampsia is immune mediated. Risk of pre-eclampsia is enhanced in circumstances where formation of blocking antibody to placental antigenic sites might be impaired as in first pregnancy where effective immunization by previous pregnancy is lacking or number of antigenic sites provided by placenta is more than antibodies as in multiple pregnancies.

In early 2nd trimester, women destined to develop PET have lower proportion of helper T cell. These helper T lymphocytes secreate specific cytokines that promote implantation and their dysfunction may favor pre-eclampsia. In women with anticardiolipin antibodies placental abnormalities and pre-eclampsia develop more commonly.

3. *The vasculopathy and inflammatory changes:* Pre-eclampsia is considered a disease due to an extreme state of activated leukocyte in maternal circulation. Cytokine such as tumor necrosis factor (TNF) and interleukins may contribute to oxidative stress associated with PET. Oxidative stress is characterized by reactive oxygen species and free radicals the lead to formation of self propagating lipid peroxides. These in turn, generate highly toxic radicals that injure endothelial cells, modify their nitric oxide production and interfere with prostaglandin balance. Other consequences of oxidative stress include production of lipid laden macrophage foam cell seen in atherosis. Activation of microvascular coagulation seen as thrombocytopenia and increased capillary permeability seen as edema and proteinuria.

4. *Nutritional factors:* A number of dietary deficiencies or excess have been blamed as the cause of eclampsia. Blood pressure in women is affected by a number of dietary influences including minerals and vitamins. Various elements such as zinc, magnesium and calcium are found to be useful in prevention of pre-eclampsia in some studies. Some studies proved that diet rich

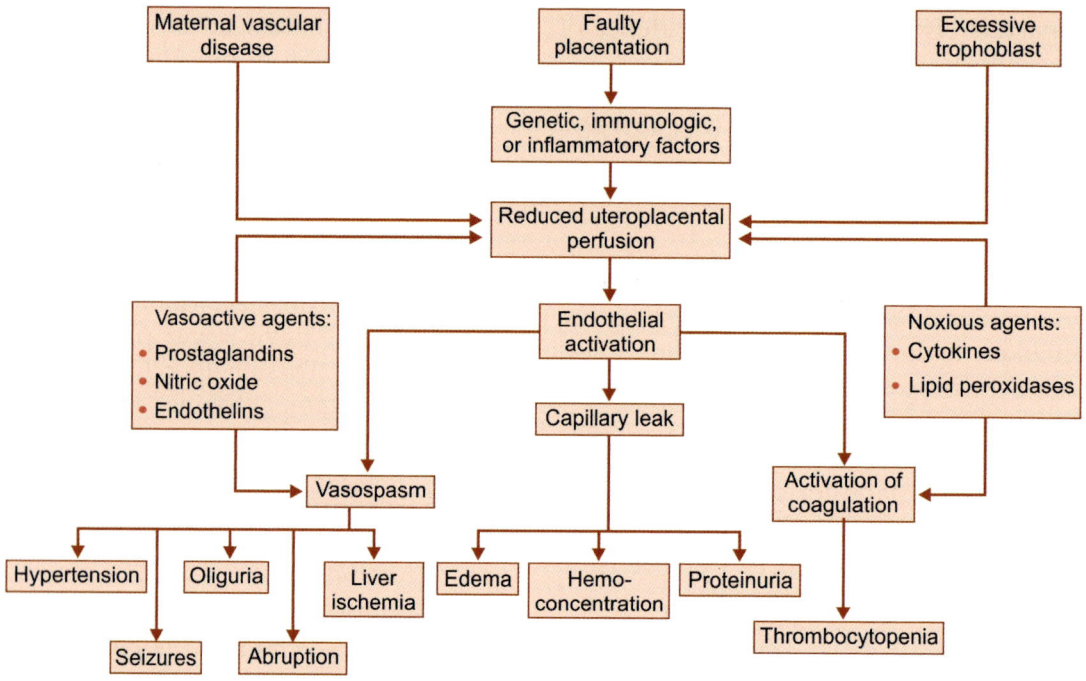

Fig. 6.1: Pathophysiology of pre-eclampsia

in fruits and vegetables that have antioxidant activity is associated with decreased blood pressure. Low intake of ascorbic acid (<85 mg/day) is associated with double fold increase in incidence of pre-eclampsia. Obesity is a potent risk factor for hypertension in nonpregnant women which causes endothelial activation and systemic inflammatory response associated with atherosclerosis. C-reactive protein, an inflammatory marker was shown to be increased in obesity, which in turn, was associated with PET.

5. *Genetic factors:* Predisposition to hereditary hypertension undoubtedly is linked to tendency for PET and eclampsia. Association between HLA-DR-4 and proteinuric hypertension is documented by Haryward and co-workers (1992). Number of single gene mutations have been studied in women with PET. Zhang (2003) and their associates reported that women heterozygous for angiotensinogen gene variant T-235 had a higher incidence of PET and

fetal growth restriction. Some of inherited thrombophilias predispose some women to PET. Polymorphisms of gene for TNF, lymphotoxins and interleukin-1 have been studied with varying results.

Pathophysiology

Several important pathophysiological changes in pre-eclampsia (Fig. 6.1) are:

Hyperdynamic circulation: Present studies suggest that the increase in cardiac output rather than the increased peripheral vascular resistance, is the most common feature of PET.

Cardiac output values are significantly higher in pre-eclamptic patients than in normotensive gravidas. This elevation of cardiac output is already apparent at 11 wks and continues in puerperium despite resolution of hypertension. Systemic vascular resistance of PET patients was always less than that of normotensive patients.

These findings of hyperdynamic left ventricular function and decreased peripheral vascular resistance in PET give important guidance for selecting best antihypertensive drugs. Beta-adrenergic blockers are drug of choice rather than vasodilators.

Changes in intravascular volume: Increase in intravascular volume that normally occur in pregnancy is minimal or completely absent in patients with pre-eclampsia due to generalized constriction of the capacitance vessels. The reduced volume is predominantly of plasma, and as a result, hemoconcentration occurs as the diseases progresses. After delivery plasma volume increase leads to decrease in hemoglobin and hematocrit values.

Loss of resistance to angiotensin II and catecholamines: Patients destined to develop pre-eclampsia show a progressive loss of resistance to pressure effect of catecholamines and angiotensin II in contrast women who remain normotensive during pregnancy. Loss of resistance is also found in patients with pre-eclampsia superimposed on hypertension.

Coagulation abnormalities: Coagulation abnormalities exist in only a minority of patients with severe pre-eclampsia. The most serious hematologic complication of PET is HELLP (hemolytic anemia, elevated liver enzyme, low platelet count) syndrome. The prognosis of this complicated form of PET is guarded and would be best cared in tertiary centre. There is decreased in platelet, fibrinogen, antithrombin III, plasminogen level in blood.

Morphological Changes

Kidney

Kidney is most studied organ in women with PET distinctive lesion in PET is—"Glomerular endotheliosis". Capillary lumen is narrowed due to deposits of osmophilic material between the basal membrane and endothelial cell. There is no change in epithelial cells or foot processes, no prolferation of inter-capillary cells and no alteration in architecture of renal medulla.

With the development of PET, number of reversible changes occurs. Renal perfusion and glomerular filtration is reduced. Plasma uric acid level is typically increased especially in severe disease. There is diminished urinary excretion of calcium due to increased tubular reabsorption, mild to moderately diminished glomerular filtration and severe intrarenal vasospasm leads to increase in plasma creatinine level several times—2–3 mg/L in severe pre-eclampsia. Oliguria develop despite normal ventricular filling pressure, urinary sodium is also increased in most of the women. Urine osmolarity, urine plasma creatinine ratio and fractional excretion of sodium are indicative of involvement of prerenal mechanism.

Liver

Characteristic lesions commonly found are periportal hemorrhage at liver periphery. Bleeding from these lesions may cause hepatic rupture which may extend beneath the hepatic capsule and form subcapsular hematoma. There is elevation of hepatic transaminase level. They are more common in women with HELLP syndrome. Mostly conservative treatment is preferred in hematoma but in some cases surgery may be required.

HELLP syndrome: This is hemolysis (H), elevated liver (EL) enzymes, low platelets (LP) syndrome. It is rare complication of PIH (10–15%). It can be associated even with mild PIH and proteinuria.

Symptom: Nausea, vomiting, epigastric pain. Parenchymal necrosis of liver causes increased level of hepatic enzymes (AST and ALT—>70 µu/l, LDH >600 µu/L). There may be subcapsular hematoma or liver may rupture and causes sudden hypotension due to hemoperitoneum.

Management: Anticonvulsant treatment with magnesium sulphate is started. Termination of pregnancy is recommended. Corticosteroids is given to improve pulmonary maturity of fetus and it also increases platelet counts and urinary output. Epidural anesthesia is usually used safely. Platelet transfusion is indicated if platelet count is <50,000/mm³. Recurrence risk of HELLP syndrome is 3–10%.

Patients should be managed in ICU:
1. Bed rest
2. Plasma volume expanders (5–25% albumin infusion)
3. Dipyridamole (antithrombotic agents)
4. Steroids
5. Others—fresh frozen plasma

Maternal mortality—up to 25%, perinatal mortality—5–60%.

Brain

There are two distinct types of cerebral pathology
1. *Cerebral hemorrhage:* Caused by severe hypertension. More common in women with chronic hypertension, may be fatal.
2. *Focal lesion:* Mainly demonstrated with pre-eclampsia and in eclampsia, rarely fatal.

The principal features are edema, hyperemia, ischemia, thrombosis and hemorrhage ranges from petechiae to gross bleeding. With use of CT and MRI, it is reported that nearly all women with eclmapsia have abnormal brain findings. Most commonly seen with CT is hyperdense area in cortex and infarction. Extent and location of ischemic lesions influence the severity of disease and neurological complications occur ranging from blindness to coma.

Cerebral Blood Flow

Pre-eclampsia is associated with increased cerebral perfusion pressure counterbalanced by increased carebrovascular resistance with no net change in cerebral blood flow.

Blindness

It is rare with pre-eclampsia alone. It follows eclamptic convulsion in up to 10% of women.

Blindness may develop up to a week or more following delivery. The condition is also called amaurosis and affected women have extensive occipital lobe vasogenic edema on CT and MRI. Blindness can lasts from four hours to eight days but usually completely resolves in all cases.

Rarely permanent visual defects may be caused by cerebral infarction or by retinal artery ischemia and infarction.

Retinal Detachment

Usually it is one-sided and seldom causes total vision loss. Sometimes it occurs with cortical edema and visual defects. Surgical treatment is seldom indicated. Vision usually returns to normal within a week.

Cerebral Edema

Symptomatic cerebral edema is rare. It is usually associated with severe PET. Symptoms ranged from lethargy, confusion, blurred vision to coma. Careful blood pressure control is essential. Mannitol and dexamethasone can be useful.

Uteroplacental Perfusion

Compromised uteroplacental perfusion from vasospasm is important contributing factor for perinatal morbidity and mortality associated with pre-eclampsia. It is assessed by Doppler velocimetry of uterine and umbilical arteries by measuring mean resistance which is higher in all women of pre-eclampsia compared to normotensive women.

Clinical Types

Clinical classification depends on degree of blood pressure elevation and proteinuria.

Mild

Sustained rise of blood pressure of more than 140/90 mm of Hg but less than 160/110 without significant proteinuria.

Severe

1. Persistent rise of systolic blood pressure of >160 mm of Hg and diastolic blood pressure >110 mm.

2. Epigastric pain, visual disturbances, oliguria.

3. Protein excertion of more than 5 gm/day.

4. Platelet count <1,00,00/mm³.

5. HELLP syndrome.

6. Retinal hemorrhages.

7. IUGR.

8. Pulmonary edema.

From prognostic point of view diastolic blood pressure is more important. Serious complications or convulsions may occur even with moderate rise of blood pressure.

Clinical Features

Pre-eclampsia is common in primigravida (70%). Other high risk cases are pregnancy with polyhydramnios, pre-existing hypertension, diabetes, multiple pregnancy, etc. Usually symptoms appear after 20th weeks of gestation.

Symptoms

a. *Mild:* Swelling initially over the ankle, gradually extends to the face, abdominal wall, vulva and whole body.

b. *Alarming symptoms:* Usually associated with acute onset of syndrome and are mainly confined to:

   a. *Headache:* Occipital or frontal region.

   b. *Eye symptoms:* Most common visual symptom in patients going to develop PET is scotoma, i.e. transient perception of bright or black contrast. Blurring of vision or complete blindness are due to spasm of retinal vessels, occipital lobe damage and retinal detachment. Vision is usually regained within 4–6 weeks following delivery due to reattachment of retina following subsidence of edema and normalization of blood pressure.

   c. *Epigastric pain:* Acute pain in epigastric region associated with vomiting sometimes coffee color is due to hemorrhagic gastritis or subcapsular hemorrhage in the liver usually accompanied by marked alteration in AST, ALT and LDH values.

   d. Decreased urinary output, i.e. less than 400 ml/24 hr is ominous sign.

Signs

1. *Blood pressure elevation:* Hypertension is the most important sign of PET especially diastolic blood pressure because it reflects the severity of disease. Following precautious should be taken to avoid error:

   1. BP should be always measured in same position preferably in sitting position with hand at heart level.

   2. In obese patient it should be measured by large cuff as regular size cuff gives higher reading.

   3. Diastolic blood pressure should be noted at Korotkoff V sound.

   Rise of BP should be evident at least on 2 occasions at 6 hrs apart. An absolute rise of BP of at least 140/90 mm Hg. If BP is not known then rise of at least 30 mm Hg in systolic and 15 mm Hg in diastolic blood pressure.

2. *Abnormal weight gain:* More that 5 lb/month or 1 lb/week in later months of pregnancy is significant.

3. *Edema:* Visible edema over ankle in the morning on rising from the bed is pathological. Sudden and generalized edema may indicate imminent eclampsia.

4. *Abdominal examination:* Evidence of chronic placental insufficiency like amount of liquor, fetal growth retardation should be seen.

5. *Proteinuria:* Extremely valuable as a prognostic sign in PET. It may be in traces to copious so that urine becomes solid on boiling (10–15 gm/L). 24 hrs of urine collection for proteinuria measurement is

ideal. Presence of total protein in 24 hrs urine of more than 0.3 gm or >2 + (1 gm/L) on at least 2 random clean catch urine samples tested >4 hrs apart in absence of urinary tract infection is significant.

Test for proteinuria by strips:

Trace = 0.1 gm/L, 1 + = 0.3 gm/L, 2 + = 1 gm/L, 3 + = 3 gm/L, 4 + = 5–10 gm/L

Investigations (Lab Findings)

Altered renal function: In severe pre-eclampsia, there is elevation of serum creatinine, blood urea nitrogen (BUN), uric acid as well as decrease in creatinine clearance, proteinuria and change in urinary sediments. Serum uric acid level of >4.5 mg/dl indicate presence of PET. Serum creatinines may be more than 1 mg/dl. Blood urea is usually normal or slightly raised.

Changes in liver function test: AST, ALT and LDH are raised in severe pre-eclampsia. After delivery AST and ALT levels rapidly decrease and reach at normal level by 5th postpartum day.

Hematological abnormalities: Only hematological change found in patients with mild pre-eclampsia is an elevation of hemoglobin and hematocrit. In more severe disease thrombocytopenia may be present. Plasma fibrinogen is usually slightly increased or normal and it is unusual to find plasma fibrinogen <200 mg/L unless clinical course is complicated by placental abruption. Thrombin time is prolonged in about 50% of patients of severe pre-eclampsia. Level of D-dimer a peptide derived from degradation of fibrin more than 5 mg/L suggest more severe form of disease.

Abnormal fetoplacental function: Common finding in women with moderate to severe PET is intrauterine growth retardation. Head to abdomen and femur to abdomen ratio are abnormally elevated in these cases. The non-stress test (NST) and Doppler waveform analysis may be helpful in assessing the progress of disease.

PREDICTION AND PREVENTION

Prediction

Several test have been proposed to identify women at risk of developing pre-eclampsia.

1. *Angiotensin sensitivity test:* Abnormal vascular reactivity of patients destined to develop pre-eclampsia may be detected several week before development of clinical signs and symptoms, the degree of sensitivity of angiotensin II may be used as screening test to identify patients at risk for the disease. Unfortunately this test has high false positive and negative results and angiotensin II preparation is not available for use, so not practically useful test.

   Test: At 26–30 weeks women requiring angiotensin II <8 ng/kg/mm infusion to raise BP >20 mm Hg are called test positive.

2. *Roll over test:* It was originally described as noninvasive office procedure having excellent correlation with angiotensin sensitivity test and excellent predictor of development of pre-eclampsia but test has poor sensitivity and specificity and is of limited clinical value.

   Positive test: This test is done between 28 and 32 wks. Elevation of 20 mm Hg or more in blood pressure when patient rolls over from lateral decubitus to supine position. About 30–35% of women with positive roll over test developed hypertension later. Negative test is significant.

   Second trimester mean arterial pressure: Mean arterial pressure during 2nd trimester is a predictor. Average mean arterial pressure >90 mm Hg in 2nd trimester may predict onset of pre-eclampsia.

3. *Urinary calcium:* Several recent studies suggest association of PET with hypocalciuria. A urinary calcium concentration equal to or less than 12 mg/dl in 24 hrs

collection has positive and negative predictive value of 85% and 91% respectively. Determination of calcium/creatinine ratio is also very significant.

4. *Fibronectin:* Patients with pre-eclampsia have elevated level of fibronectin by 12 weeks. Fibronectin is a glycoprotein having important role in cellular adhesions. Positive predictive value is only 29% and negative predictive value is around 98%.

5. *Doppler ultrasound:* (At 20–24 wks)
   1. Presence of diastolic notch at 24 weeks gestation in uterine artery can predict development of PET.
   2. Absence of diastolic blood flow or reverse diastolic blood flow in umbilical artery usually indicates poor perinatal outcome.

Unfortunately abnormal Doppler waveforms at 20–24 wks of gestational age have a low sensitivity and low positive predictive value.

PREVENTION OF PRE-ECLAMPSIA

1. *Regular antenatal checking:* For early detection of rapid weight gain, edema, tendency of rising diastolic blood pressure or serum uric acid test.

2. *Antithrombotic agents:* Low dose asprin 60 mg daily may be useful in high risk group, if started from early in pregnancy. Asprin reduces platelet thromboxane production and in low doses it inhibit cyclooxygenase in platelets so preventing the formation of thromboxane A2 without interfering with prostacyline generation. Most of trails demonstrated that low dose asprin reduces risks of PET and results in longer gestational age, increased birth weight without major side effects.

3. *Calcium supplementation:* Literature suggest that dietary calcium supplementation is effective in preventing the development of PET. Normal pregnant women receiving 2 gm calcium/day after 15 wks of gestation had significantly lowered blood pressure.

4. *Antioxidants:* Vitamin E, vitamin C taking from 16 to 22 weeks onward reduce the risk of pre-eclampsia. Women should be provided well-balanced diet-rich in protein.

Nutritional supplementation: With magnesium, zinc, fish oil, high protein diet have been tried with limited advantages.

Management

Objective

1. To correct/stabilize altered physiology.
2. Prevention of complication.
3. Prevention of seizures.
4. Delivery of healthy baby in optimal time with minimum maternal morbidity.

Treatment

1. Ideally all patients should be admitted.
2. Rest is advocated preferably in left lateral position to decrease the effect of vena caval compression.

Rest is helpful in

1. Increasing renal blood flow.
2. Increasing uterine blood flow.
3. Improving the placental perfusion.
4. Reducing the blood pressure.

Diet

1. Diet should contain adequate amount of protein, i.e. about 100 gm/day.
2. Total caloric requirement is 1600 cal/day.
3. Usually salt and fluid intake is not restricted.

Sedative: To relieve anxiety 2.5–5 mg diazepam at bed time may be given.

Diuretic: Usually diuretics are not indicated as they decrease placental perfusion and cause electrolyte imbalance which is harmful for the fetus. The indication for its use are:

1. Pulmonary edema.

2. Cardiac failure.
3. Massive edema not relieved by rest and producing discomfort to patient.

Antihypertensives: The use of antihypertensive drugs is to prolong pregnancy or modify perinatal outcomes in pregnancies complicated by various types and severities of hypertensive disorder has been of considerable interest. The objective of antihypertensive treatment is to prevent intracranial bleeding and left ventricular failure. Some investigators believe that antihypertensive treatment is useful in avoiding selective cerebral arterial vasospasm that causes eclamptic seizure. Anti-hypertensive has limited value in controlling BP due to pre-eclampsia.

The unavoidable indication for its use:

1. Persistent rise of blood pressure especially when diastolic pressure is >110 mm Hg and associated with protenuria.
2. In severe pre-eclampsia to bring down the blood pressure during continued pregnancy or during induction of labor.

The commonly used oral drugs are:

a. *Methyl dopa:* Central peripheral anti-adrenergic action dose—250–500 TDS/QID.
b. *Labetalol:* α and β blocker (adrenoceptor blocker) dose—250 mg TDS/QID.
c. *Nifedipine:* Calcium channel blocker dose—10–20 mg BD.
d. *Hydralazine:* Vascular, smooth muscle relaxant—10–25 mg BD.

In hypertensive crisis: Any of the following drug can be used till blood pressure comes down to <110 mm Hg.

1. *Labetalol:* 200 mg in 200 ml of normal saline at the rate of 20 mg/hr to be doubled every ½ hr.
2. *Hydralazine:* 5 mg IV bolus to be followed by infusion of 25 mg in 200 ml normal saline, rate is 2.5 mg/hr to be doubled every 30 min.

3. *Nitroglycerin:* 5 µg/min IV or sodium nitroprusside—0.25–5 µg/kg/min

Once the blood pressure is under control, oral therapy can be continued.

Monitoring of patient: The effect of treatment is evaluated by recording:

• *Blood pressure:* At least every 6 hourly.
• Daily observation of weight gain and edema.
• Fluid intake and urinary output charting.
• Daily urinary protein estimation.
• Once a week blood examination for:
  – Hematocrit, platelet count.
  – Serum uric acid estimation.
  – Creatinine level.
  – Liver function test.
• *Ophthalmoscopic examination:* On admission and if necessary repeated.
• Fetal well-being assessment

Definitive treatment of pre-eclampsia is termination of pregnancy. The role of antihypertensive drugs is only to continue pregnancy, if possible without affecting the maternal prognosis till fetal maturity.

Criteria for Delivering Patients with Severe Pre-eclampsia

1. Blood pressure persistently 160/100 or greater despite treatment.
2. Urine output <400 ml/24 hr.
3. Platelet counts <50,000/mm³
4. Progressive increase in serum creatinine.
5. LDH >1000 IV/L.
6. Repetitive late deceleration with poor variability.
7. Severe IUGR with oligohydramnios
8. Decreased fetal movement.
9. Reversed umbilical diastolic blood flow.

Method of Termination of Pregnancy

1. Induction of labor.
2. Cesarean section.

1. Induction of Labor

Indication

a. Aggravation of the pre-eclamptic features in spite of medical treatment.
b. Hypertension persists inspite of medical treatment and pregnancy completed 37 weeks or more.
c. Acute fulminating pre-eclampsia.

Method

If cervix is ripe, surgical induction by low rupture of membrane and oxytocin infusion. If cervix is unripe and termination is not an urgent one, prostaglandin gel should be inserted to make the cervix ripe. In severe pre-eclampsia, antihypertensive drugs should be used during induction.

2. Cesarean Section

Indication of cesarean section:
1. When urgent termination is indicated in unfavorable cervix.
2. Severe pre-eclampsia with a tendency to prolong induction delivery interval.
3. Associated complicating factors such as elderly primi, contracted pelvis or mal-presentation.
   Epidural anesthesia is preferred and operation should be done by an experienced surgeon with the help of an expert anesthetist.

Management during Labor

1. Labor duration is cut short by low rupture of membrane in first stage and forcep/ventouse in 2nd stage.
2. Intravenous ergometrine should be withheld as it may cause increase in blood pressure though intramuscular ergometrine can be given.
3. Patient should be sedated immediately following delivery to prevent postpartum eclampsia.

Puerperium

1. Patient should be monitored closely for at least 48 hrs.

2. Hypotensive drug should be continued if diastolic blood pressure is raised beyond 100 mm Hg.
3. Patient is to be kept in hospital till BP is brought down to safe level and disappearance of proteinuria.

ACUTE FULMITANT PRE-ECLAMPSIA (EMINENT ECLAMPSIA)

Onset of pre-eclamptic manifestation is acute with rapid deterioration over a short period of time. There are very high chances of convulsion or coma.

Management

Sedation: By diazepam 10 mg IM if detected at home and immediate shifting to the hospital is advocated. In hospital patient should be admitted and prophylactic anticonvulsant should be given urgently. Blood pressure should be stabilized by giving antihypertensive drug parenteraly. Response to treatment should be watched by careful monitoring of blood pressure, urinary output, proteinuria and hematological values.

Termination of pregnancy should be done urgently if pregnancy is >37 weeks or irrespective of gestational age if the condition fails to improve inspite of treatment. Corticosteroid should be given if pregnancy is <34 weeks.

ECLAMPSIA

Pre-eclampsia when complicated with convulsion/coma is called eclampsia. It is more common in primigravida (75%), twins and in late pregnancy (after 36 wks).
Incidence in India ranges from 1:500 to 1:50

Causes of Convulsions

Convulsions occur due to cerebral irritation which can be provoked by:
a. Cerebral anoxia
b. Cerebral edema
c. Cerebral dysrhythmia

Usually fits occur in late trimester but it can occur in early months also as in cases of hyatidiform mole.

Following are the types of eclampsia according to period of gestation.

Antepartum: Incidence is 50%, usually fits occur before onset of labor.

Intrapartum: Incidence is 30% usually fits occur fist time during labor.

Postpartum: Incidence is 20% usually fits occurs for the first time in puerperium with in 48 hrs of delivery. Fits occurring after 7 days of delivery rules out eclampsia.

Differential Diagnosis

1. Epilepsy
2. Hysteria
3. Meningitis
4. Puerperal cerebral thrombosis
5. Poisoning
6. Encephalitis
7. Cerebral malaria
8. Intracranial tumor

Features Favoring Eclampsia

1. No past history of convulsion.
2. Presence of edema, hypertension and proteinuria.

Maternal prognosis depends on various factors and ominous features are:
1. Late referral
2. Number of fits more than 10
3. Coma in between fits
4. Temperature over 102°f with P/R >120/min
5. BP—more than 200 mm Hg systolic
6. Oliguria (<400 ml urinary output in 24 hrs)
7. Nonresponse to treatment
8. Jaundice

Maternal mortality due to eclampsia in India varies from 2 to 30% however, it can be reduced to <2%, if treated early and adequately.

Causes of Maternal Death

1. Cardiac failure
2. Pulmonary edema
3. Aspiration
4. Cerebral hemorrhage
5. Anuria
6. Pulmonary embolism
7. Sepsis and shock

Causes of Fetal Death

Perinatal mortality is 30–50% due to prematurity, intrauterine asphyxia and trauma.

Management

The principles of management
1. Resuscitation
2. Oxygen
3. Arrest convulsion
4. Hemodynamic stabilization (BP control)
5. Delivery within 6–8 hrs
6. Postpartum care

General Management

1. Patient should be kept in isolated room at tertiary hospital.
2. Detailed history from the relatives should be taken.
3. Catheterization should be done and urine is tested for protein in unconscious patient.
4. ½ hrly pulse, BP, respiration rate should be recorded. Hourly urine output should be noted.
5. *Fluid:* Crystalloid solution (RL) is first choice. Total fluid should not be given more than previous 24 hrs urine output plus 1000 ml.
6. Antibiotic should be given to prevent infection.

Specific Management

Magnesium sulfate: It is drug of choice literature suggest that it is ideal anticonvulsant in pre-eclampsia. It blocks neuromuscular transmission by decreasing acetylcholine release in response to nerve action potentials. An intravenous dose of 4 gm of magnesium sulfate causes an immediate elevation of normal Mg^{++} level 1.6–2.1 mEq/L to 7–9 mEq/L. Intracellular transfer of ion and elimination through kidney cause drop in plasma concentration to 4–5 mEq/L 1 hr after injection.

It is necessary to monitor those patients receiving magnesium sulfate to prevent serious side effects. The clinical variables to monitor are urinary output, patellar reflex and respiratory rate. Urine production is decreased in pre-eclamptic patients which may lead to abnormally high Mg^{++} level resulting in respiratory or cardiac arrest. A urinary output of at least 30 mg/hr is necessary for continuous administration of magnesium sulphate.

Disappearance of patellar reflex is important because it is the first sign of impending toxicity. The patellar reflex is usually lost when plasma Mg^{++} concentration reaches 8–10 mEq/L. In these cases drug must be discontinued until reflex returns. If plasma level will continue to increase and reaches more than 12 mEq/L than respiratory depression may occur. If respiratory depression occurs, intravenous calcium gluconate 10 ml of 10% solution given over 3 min. Magnesium sulfate may be harmful to fetus, respiratory depression and hyporeflexia may be observed in newborn delivered to mother undergoing intravenous magnesium sulfate therapy. This problem is less frequent with the drug given intramuscularly.

Magnesium sulfate acts synergistically with the muscle relaxant used for general anesthesia so obstetrical anesthetist should give smaller dosage of such medicine when giving GA to patients on magnesium sulphate therapy.

In nutshell magnesium sulphate is drug of choice. It blocks neuronal calcium influx also. It induces cerebral vasodilatation, dilates uterine arteries, increases endothelial prostacycline and inhibit platelet activation. It has no detrimental effects on neonate within therapeutic level (4–7 mEq/L). It has got excellent result with maternal mortality of 0.4%.

Regime of $MgSO_4$ for management of severe pre-eclampsia and eclampsia.

Regime

a. *Intramuscular* (Pritchard)
  a. *Loading dose:* 4 gm IV over 3–5 min followed by 10 gm deep IM (5 gm in each buttock).
  b. *Maintenance dose:* 5 gm IM–4 hrly in alternate buttock.
b. *Intravenous (Zuspan or Sibai)*
  a. *Loading dose:* 4–6 gm IV over 15–20 mins.
  b. *Maintenance dose:* 1–2 gm/hr IV infusion.

Repeat injection should be given only when urine output exceeds 30 ml/hr, respiration rate is more than 12/min and knee jerks are present. It should be continued for 24 hr after the last fits. If fits recur, further 2 gm IV bolus is given over 5 mins in the above regimens. In eminent eclampsia only maintains dose can be used for prophylactic purpose.

Lytic cocktail regime: Menon (1961) suggested this regime using chlorpromazine, phenergan and pethidine and got satisfactory result with mortality to 2.2%.

Protocol

a. Chlorpromazine (25 mg) and pethidine (100 mg) in 20 ml of 5% dextrose are given intravenously along with intramuscular 50 mg chlorpromazine and 25 mg promethazine IM.
b. Subsequently give promethazine (25 mg) and chlorpromazine (50 mg) IM at 4 hrs interval for a period up to 24 hrs following last fits.
c. IV 500 ml of 10 dextrose drip is started with 100 mg pethidine with drip rate 20–30 drops/min. Pethidine drip should be continued up to 24 hrs following last fit.

Diazepam therapy (lean): Initially given as 40 mg intravenously further 40 mg in 500 ml of 5% dextrose is infused at 30 drops/min or adjusted per need. Maternal mortality rate—0.5%.

Phenytoin therapy: Given by slow intravenous route—10 mg/kg followed by 5 mg/kg two hrs later.

Role of antihypertensive and diuretics: If BP >160/100 mm Hg, inspite of anticonvulsants anal sedatives than antihypertensive should be added. Parentral antihypertensive like labetalol, hydralazine or nitroglycerin can be given. Diuretic is indicated in presence of pulmonary edema, 20–40 mg frusemide can be given.

Management during Fits

1. Patient's head is to be turned to one side and pillow is taken off.
2. Mouth gag should be placed in between teeth to prevent tongue bite in clonic phase.
3. Air passage is to be cleared off the mucus with suction.
4. Oxygen should be given till cyanosis disappears.

Status epilepticus: Thiopentone sodium (0.5 gm) dissolves in 20 ml of 5% dextrose is given IV very slowly under supervision of anesthetist in unresponsive cases. Complete anesthesia, muscle relaxant and assisted ventilation can be employed. Cesarean section at tertiary centre may be life saving attempt.

Treatment of Complications

Pulmonary edema: Frusemide 40 mg IV followed by 20 gm of mannitol IV reduces the pulmonary edema and prevents adults respiratory distress syndrome. Aspiration of mucus from tracheobronchial tree should be done by suction apparatus.

Prophylactic use of antibiotics markedly reduced the complications like pulmonary and puerperal infection.

Heart failure: Oxygen inhalation, parenteral lasix and digitalis are used.

Hyperpyrexia: Cold sponging and antipyretics may be tried.

Psychosis: Trifluoperazine is effective.

Role of intensive care monitoring: Patient with multiple medical problems should be admitted in intensive care unit (ICU) under supervision of obstetrician, physician and anesthetist. Use of blood gas analyzer (to detect hypoxia and acidosis) pulse oximeter and central venous pressure monitor should be done. A deeply unconscious patient with raised intracranial pressure may need steroid and diuretics. CT or MRI may be needed for the diagnosis.

Obstetric management: Usually labor starts soon after convulsion but when labor fails to start the management depends on:
1. Whether the fits are controlled or not.
2. Gestational age
    1. *If fits controlled and baby mature:* Termination of pregnancy is indicated. Route of delivery is decided according to cervical condition. No contraindication for vaginal delivery. If cervix is unfavorable or contraindication for vaginal delivery—cesarean section is preferable.
    2. *Baby premature:* Continuation of pregnancy for a few more weeks should be weighed against risk involved in such a procedure. The underlying disease may flare up at any moment and risk of the baby dying *in utero* may be increased so only in selected cases, one may continue pregnancy at tertiary centre with close supervision.

Baby dead: Usually pre-eclampsia process gradually subsides and eventually expulsion of fetus occur.

Fits not controlled: If fits not controlled, termination of pregnancy should be done irrespective of fetal maturity, if vaginal examination indicates quick response to indication, low rupture of membranes is done, oxytocin infusion may be added. In presences of unfavorable factors, cesarean section gives a quick results.

Management during Labor

2nd stage of labor should be curtailed by forceps or ventouse. Prophylactic intravenous ergometrine following delivery of anterior shoulder is withheld. Intramuscular ergometrine is not contraindicated.

Indication of Cesarean Section

1. Uncontrolled fits inspite of therapy
2. Unconscious patient and poor prospects of vaginal delivery
3. Malpresentation

Follow-up and Prognosis

Patient should be followed up for 6 wks. Persistence of hypertension proteinuria and abnormal blood chemistry needs further investigation. Recurrence risk varies between 2–25%.

Pre-eclampsia is multisystem disorder usually manifest clinically as hypertension, proteinuria and placental insufficiency. Management at present focuses on controlling blood pressure and monitoring mother and fetus to optimise the timing and mode of delivery. However, there is no established prophylactic therapy, although several areas including antioxidant, vitamin supplementation are under investigation, much research is required to further unravel the enigma of pre-eclampsia. There is need for further coordination to make the best use of resources and improve the rate of progress to protect our patients from continued threat of pre-eclampsia.

Bibliography

1. Abdul-Karim R, Assali NS. Pressure response to angiotensis in pregnant and nonpregnant women, Am J Obstet Gynecol 1961;82:246.
2. Alexander JM, Bloom SL, McIntire DD, et al. Severe pre-eclampsia and the very low birth weight infant: Is induction of labor harmful? Obstet Gynecol 1999;93:485.
3. Barron WM, Hackerling P, Hibbard JU, et al. Reducing unnecessary coagulation testing in hypertensive disorders of pregnancy Obstet Gynecol 1999;94:364.
4. Belfort MA, Taskin O, Buhur A, et al. Intravenous nimodipine in the controlled clinical trial. Am J Obstet Gynecol 1996;174:451.
5. Berg CJ, Chang J, Callaghan WM, et al. Pregnancy-related mortality in the United States 1991-1997. Obstet Gynecol 2003;101:289.
6. Borghi C, Esposti DD, Immordino V, et al. Relationship of systemic hemodynamics, left ventricular structure and function and plasma natriuretic peptide concentration during pregnancy complicated by preeclampsia. Am J Obstet Gynecol 2000;183:140.
7. Brown MA, Zammit VC, Lowe SA. Capillary permeability and extracellular fluid volumes in pregnancy-induced hypertension. Clin Sci. 1989; 77:599.
8. Bush KD, O' Brien JM, Barton JR. The utility of umbilical artery Doppler investigation in women with HELLP (hemolysis, elevated liver enzymes, and low platelet count) syndrome. Am J Obstet Gynecol 2001;184:1087.
9. Chadwock HS, Easterling T. Anesthetic concerns in the patients with pre-eclampsia. Semin Perinatol 1991;15:397.
10. Chang CH, Chang FM, Chen CP, et al. Antithrombin III activity in normal and toxemic pregnancies. J formos Med Assoc 1992;91:680.
11. Cigarette smoke protect women from pre-eclampsia: The specific roles of carbon monoxide and antioxidant systems in the placenta. Med Hypotheses 2005;64:17.
12. Clark BA, Halvorson L, Sachs B, et al: Plasma endothelin levels in pre-eclampsia: Elecation and correlation with uric acid levels and renal impairment. Am J Obstet Gynecol 1992;166:962.
13. Coetzee EJ, Dommisse J, Anthony J. A randomized controlled trial of intravenous magnesium sulphate versus placebo in the management women with severe pre-eclampsia. Br J Obstet Gynaecol 1998;105:300.
14. Cotton DB, Janusz CA, Berman RF. Anti-convulsant effects of magnesium sulfate on hippocampal seizures: Therapeutic implications in pre-eclampsia–eclampsia. Am j Obstet Gynecol 1992;166:1127.

15. Crowther CA, Hilles JE, Doyle LW, et al. Effect of magnesium sulfate given for neuroprotection before birth: A randomized controlled trial, JAMA 2003;290:2669.

16. Cunningham FG, Lindheimer MD: Hypertension in pregnancy. Current concepts N Engl J Med 1992;326:927.

17. Douglas KA, Redman CWG. Eclampsia in the United Kingdom. BMJ 1994;309:1395.

18. Dyer RA, Els I, Farbas J, et al. Prospective, randomized trial comparing general with spinal anesthesia for cesarean delivery in pre-eclamptic patients with a nonreassuring fetal heart trace. Anesthesiology 2003;99:561.

19. Easterling TR, Benedetti TJ, Schmucker BC, et al. Maternal hemodynamics in normal and pre-eclamptic pregnancies: A longitudinal stud. Obstet Gynecol 1990;76:1061.

20. Eastman NS, Hellman LM. Tozemias of pregnancy. Williams Obstetrics, 12th ed. New York, Appleton-Century-Crofts, Inc., 1961; p 756.

21. Florio P, Ries FM, Pezzani I, et al. The addition of activin A and inhibin A measurement to uterine artery Doppler velocimetry to improve the early prediction of pre-eclampsia. Ultrasound Obstet Gynecol 2003;21:165.

22. Forster JG, Peltonen S, Kaaja R, et al. Plasma exchange in severe postpartum HELLP syndrome. Acta Anaesthesiol Scand 2002;46:955.

23. Gilbert WM, Towner DR, Field NT, et al. The safety and utility of pulmonary artery catheterization in severe pre-eclampsia and eclmapsia. Am J Obstet Gynecol 2000;182:1397.

24. Hall DR, Odendaal HJ, Steyn DW, et al. Expectant management of early onset, severe pre-eclampsia: Maternal outcome. Br J obstet Gynecol 2000b; 107:1252.

25. Halligan A, Bonnar J, Sheppard B, et al. Haemostatic, fibrinolytic and endothelial variables in normal pregnancies and pre-eclampsia. Br J Obstet Gyanecol 1994;101:488.

26. Hauth J, Sibai B, Caritis S, et al. Maternal serum thombozane B_2 concentrations do not predict improved outomes in thigh risk pregnancies in a low-dose aspirin trial. Am J Obstet Gynaecol 179:1993, 1998.

27. Lara-Torre E, Lee MS, Wolf MA, et al. Bilateral retinal occlusion progressing to long-lasting blindness in severe pre-eclampsia. Obstet Gynaecol 2002;100:940.

28. Livingston JC, Livingston LW, Ramsey R, et al. Magnesium sulfate in women with mild pre-eclampsia: A randomized controlled trial. Obstet Gynecol 2003;101:217.

29. Lucas MJ, Sharma S, McIntire DD, et al. A randomized trial of the effects of epidural analgesia on pregnancy-induced hypertension. Am J Obstet Gynecol 2001;185:970.

30. Martin JA, Hamilton BE, Ventura SS, et al. Births: Final data for 2001. National Vital Statistics Report, Vol. 51. No. 2. Hyattsville, Md, National Centre for Health Statistics, 2002.

31. Matthys LA, Coppage KH, Lambers DS, et al. Delayed postpartum pre-eclampsia: an experience of 151 cases. Am J Obstet Gynecol 2004;190:1464.

32. O'Brien JM, Shumate SA, Satchwell SL, et al. Maternal benefit of corticosteroid therapy in patients with HELLP (hemolysis elevated liver enzymes, and low platelet count) syndrome. Impact on the rate of regional anesthesia. Am J obstet Gynecol 2002;186:475.

33. Powers RW, Dunbar MS, Gallaher MJ, et al. The 677 C-T methylenetetrahydrofolate reductase mutation does not predict increased maternal homocysteine during pregnancy. Obstet Gynecol 2003;101:762.

34. Redman CWG, Sacks GP, Sargent IL: Pre-eclampsia: An excessive maternal inflammatory response to pregnancy. Am J Obstet Gynecol 1999;180:499.

35. Roberts JM. Preeclampsia: What we know and what we do not know? Semin Perinatol 2000; 24:24.

36. Sibai BM, Hauth J, Caritis S, et al. Hypertensive disorders in twin versus singleton gestations. Am J Obstet Gynecol 2000;182:938.

37. Somjen G, Hilmy M, Stephen CR: Failure to anesthetize human subjects by intravenous administration of magnesium sulfate. J Pahrmacol ExpTher 1966;154:652.

38. Trogstad L, Skrondal A, Stoltenberg C, et al. Recurrence risk of pre-eclampsia in twin and singleton pregnancies. Am J Med Genet 2004; 126A:41.

39. Young P, Johanson R. Haemodynamic, invasive and echocardiographic monitoring in the hypertensive parturient. Best Pract Res Clin Obstet Gynaecol 2001;15:605.

40. Zeeman GG, Flackenstein JL, Twickler DM, et al. Cerebral infarction in eclampsia. Am J Obstet Gynecol 2004a;190:714.

41. Zhang XQ, Varner M, Dizon-Townson D, et al. A molecular variant of angiotensinogen is associated with idiopathic intrauterine growth restriction. Obstet Gynecol 2003;101:237.

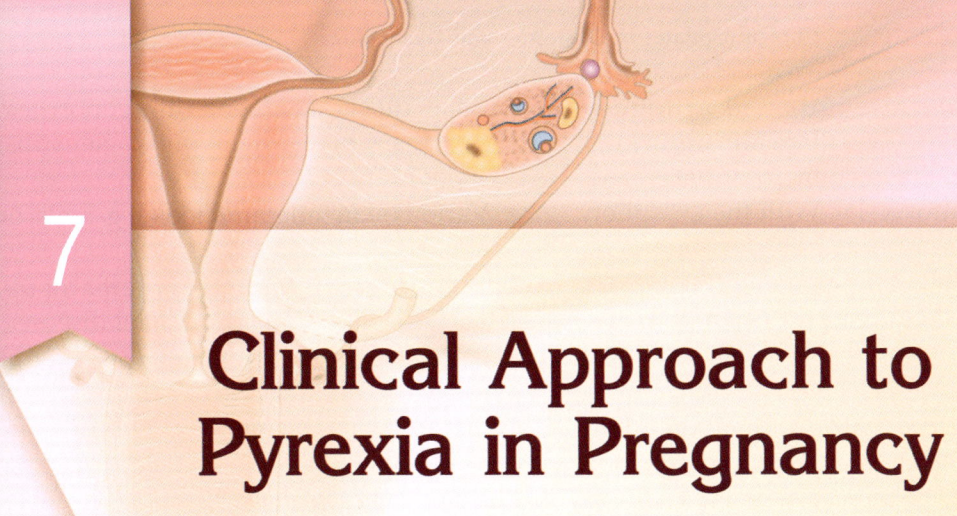

7

Clinical Approach to Pyrexia in Pregnancy

• Bharti Maheshwari

Temperature is ultimately regulated in the hypothalamus. A trigger of the fever, called a pyrogen, causes a release of prostaglandin E2 (PGE2) which acts on the hypothalamus to generates a systemic response back to the rest of the body, causing heat-creating effects to match a new temperature level.

In many respect hypothalamus works like a thermostat. When the set point is raised, the body increases its temperature through both active generation of heat and retaining heat.

Increased temperature in humans can be defined as:

PYREXIA, HYPERPYREXIA AND HYPERTHERMIA

Pyrexia

It s one of the most common *medical sign* and is characterized by an elevation of body temperature above the normal range of 36.5–37.5°C (97.7–99.5°F) due to an increase in the temperature regulatory set point: Harrison's textbook of internal medicine defines a fever as a morning temperature of >37.2°C (>98.9°F) or an evening temperature of >37.7°C (>99.9°F) while the normal daily temperature variation is typically 0.5°C (0.9°F) (Box 7.1).

Hyperpyrexia

Hyperpyrexia is a fever with an extreme elevation of body temperature greater than or

Box 7.1: Ranges of normal temperature at different sites

- Temperature in the anus (rectum/rectal) is at or over 37.5–38.3°C (99.5–100.9°F)
- Temperature in the mouth (oral) is at or over 37.7°C (99.9°F)
- Temperature under the arm (axillary) or in the ear (otic) is at or over 37.2°C (99.0°F)

equal to 41.5°C (106.7°F). Such a high temperature is considered a medical emergency as it may indicate a serious underlying condition or lead to significant side effects. The most common cause is an intracranial hemorrhage. Other possible causes include sepsis, Kawasaki syndrome, neuroleptic malignant syndrome, drug effects, serotonin syndrome, and thyroid storm.

Hyperthermia

Hyperthermia is an increase in body temperature over the body's thermoregulatory set-point, due to excessive heat production due to an outside source. ex-heatstroke, neuroleptic malignant syndrome, malignant hyperthermia, stimulants such as amphetamines and cocaine, idiosyncratic drug reactions, and serotonin syndrome.

A fever can be caused by many different conditions ranging from benign to potentially serious. Studies suggest that fever is useful as a defence mechanism as the body's immune response can be strengthened at higher temperatures, however, there are arguments for and against the usefulness of fever, and the issue is controversial. With the exception of very high temperatures, treatment to reduce fever is often not necessary; however, antipyretic medications can be effective at lowering the temperature, which may improve the affected person's comfort.

Fever in pregnancy is not a normal condition, it may be completely unrelated to pregnancy or may be manifestation of serious condition directly related to pregnancy and may adversely affect the fetus. It is easier to get fever in pregnancy as immune system is naturally suppressed.

Infections are the most common cause of fevers, however, as the degree of temperature rises other causes become more common. Infections commonly associated with hyperpyrexia include: Roseola, rubeola and enteroviral infections. Immediate aggressive cooling to less than 38.9°C (102.0°F) has been found to improve survival.

Temperature should be taken at every antenatal visit and women should be counselled to report whenever they have fever rather than simply taking some antipyretic and ignoring it. Fever in pregnancy could be due to simple strain like flu, UTI or due to some serious bacterial, viral infection affecting pregnancy outcome.

Causes of Pyrexia

1. *Infections*
   - *Parasitic and protozoal:* Malaria, toxoplasmosis, listerosis, intestinal worms, dengue.
   - *Viral:* Influenza, rubella, cytomegalovirus (CMV), measles, mumps, chickenpox (varicella), parvovirus, herpes simplex, HIV.
   - *Bacterial:* Group stertococci, urinary tract infection, respiratory tract infection, tuberculosis, gastroenteritis, gonorrhea, syphilis, Chlamydia, typhoid, hepatitis, typhoid.
   - Various skin inflammations, e.g. boils, or abscess.

2. *Immunological-lupus* erythematosus, sarcoidosis, inflammatory bowel disease.

3. *Tissue destruction:* Which can occur in hemolysis, surgery, infarction, crush syndrome, rhabdomyolysis, cerebral hemorrhage.

4. *Reaction to incompatible blood products*

5. *Cancers—leukemia, lymphoma*

6. *Metabolic—gout or porphyria*

7. *Thromboembolic processes:* Pulmonary embolism or deep venous thrombosis.

8. *Pyrexia of unknown origin:* Persistent fever that cannot be explained after repeated routine clinical examination.

To find out pathology behind fever we have to take detail history which itself give important clues for causes of fever. History should include—details of temperature, association of other symptoms with detailed past, personal and family history (Box 7.2).

Complete **clinical examination** should be done including general, abdominal and local examinations (Box 7.3).

Investigations
Routine
- Hb, total leukocyte count, differential leukocyte count, ESR, platelet count
- Complete urine examination
- Sputum examination and stool examination
- Blood sugar
- Ultrasound
- X-ray in 2nd trimester
- CT when indicated
- Peripheral blood smear
- Thick blood film for malaria
- Widal test for typhoid

1. Degree, duration and pattern of temperature (Table 7.1)
2. Associating symptoms
   - Chills and rigors—UTI, malaria, severe infection
   - Headache, sore throat—URTI
   - Running nose, malaise—influenza
   - Diarrhea, abdominal pain—gastroenteritis, typhoid
   - Leaking—chorioamnionitis
   - Vaginal discharge—gonorrhea, Chlamydia, group b streptococcus
   - Rashes—rubella, varicella
   - Burning micturition, abdominal pain—pyelonephritis
   - Convulsion and coma—cerebral malaria, hepatic, meningitis
3. Personal—sanitation, diet, occupation for tuberculosis
4. Sexual history—partners detail history, for HIV and STD
5. Past history of chronic illness/blood loss/hemorrhage/treatment—for tuberculosis/HIV
6. obstetrical history—history of recurrent abortion, stillbirth, delivery of congenital malformed baby
7. Family history

Box 7.3: Clinical examination

General examination
- Pallor, cyanosis, jaundice, pulse rate, blood pressure
- Throat examination
- Complete CVS, respiratory system, CNS examination
- Lymphadenopathy

Abdominal examination—splenomegally, hepatomegally
- Skin—rashes, pigmentation, any wound
- Local examination—vulva, vagina, cervix

Specific

IgG and IgM for suspected infections, specific test for q fever, brucellosis, listerosis, tuber-culosis, gonorrhea, Chlamydia, HIV, syphilis, whenever suspected.

Usually in pregnancy nowdays VDRL, HIV, HBsAg, HCV (hepatitis C) done in all cases.

COMMON CAUSES OF FEVER IN PREGNANCY

There are some common causes of fever in pregnancy which are temporary and treatable (Box 7.4).

Urinary Tract Infection (UTI)

Up to 10% of expectant mother will get a urinary tract infection (UTI) at some point during their pregnancies. Urinary tract system encompasses urethra, bladder, ureters, and kidneys. An infection occurs when bacteria gets into this system and multiplies. Most UTIs are bladder infections and are not serious if they are treated right away with antibiotics and lots of liquids. If left untreated, a bladder infection may travel to the kidneys and cause a variety of complications, including preterm labor, a low birth weight baby, and sepsis. Some UTIs are asymptomatic, but others come with symptoms such as a strong urge to urinate, a burning sensation with urination, cloudy urine, and/or blood in the urine, along with fever, chills, and pelvic pain.

Influenza

Fever, chills, achiness, coughing, nausea, and vomiting signals influenza (or the flu).

Table 7.1: Different pattern of rise of temperature with significance		
Pattern of temperature	*Character*	*Hints for diagnosis*
Continuous	Above normal throughout the day and not fluctuating >1° in 24 hrs	Pneumonia, typhoid, UTI, brucellosis
Intermittent	Elevation for only certain period later cyclically to normal	Malaria, kala-azar, pyraemia
Quotidian	Periodicity of 24 hrs	*Plasmodium falciparum*
Tertian	48 hrs periodicity	*P. vivax* or ovale
Quartan	72 hrs periodicity	*P. malarial*
Remittent	Remain above normal throughout day and fluctuate >1°C in 24 hrs	Infective endocarditis

Pregnant women have a higher risk of getting the flu and becoming severely ill from it, as their immune systems are suppressed. How to tell if it is the flu or just a cold? The flu comes on quickly and your symptoms are more severe then with a cold, recommended treatment rest and plenty of fluids, along with an antiviral medication to shorten the span of symptoms and preventing serious complications. Centers for Disease Control (CDC) recommend that all pregnant women get the flu shot.

Upper Respiratory Infection (Common Cold)

This is viral infection of the upper respiratory tract, which includes the sinuses, nasal passages, pharynx, and larynx. You may have symptoms that mirror the flu, as well as a runny nose, sore throat, cough, and breathing difficulty. An upper respiratory infection is not as serious as the flu and usually resolves spontaneously. The symptoms usually last from 3 to 14 days, and if persist for several days, it may be more serious infection (sinusitis, bronchitis, streptococcal throat or pneumonia).

Gastrointestinal Virus

The diarrhea and vomiting can cause serious consequences for pregnant women if left untreated, because dehydration can cause contractions and even preterm labor. Other potential side effects include hypotension, dizziness, weakness, fainting, and in severe cases, electrolyte imbalance. Most cases of these viruses will resolve on their own, but fluids such as water and electrolyte, as well as the BRAT diet (bananas, rice, applesauce and toast diet) are helpful. Signs of dehydration (a little or no urine, dry mouth, excessive thirst, dizziness), should be watched for assessing severity of diseases.

Box 7.4: Common causes of fever

- Influenza
- Urinary tract infection
- Upper respiratory tract infection
- In endemic areas—malaria, typhoid, tuberculosis, dengue
- Chorioamnionitis

Rare
- HIV, syphilis
- Toxoplasma, rubella, CMV
- Listerosis
- Gonorrhea
- Chlamydia

Fever causing abortion or congenital malformation
- Rubella
- CMV
- Syphilis
- Varicella
- Parvovirus
- High grade temperature, any origin

SERIOUS CAUSES OF FEVER AND/OR CHILLS

In rare cases, fever, chills, and pain are linked to medical conditions that affect only.

Pregnant women—not just common illnesses.

Chorioamnionitis

In addition to high fever and chills, this bacterial infection of the membranes surrounding the fetus (the chorion and amnion) and the amniotic fluid can cause sweating, rapid heartbeat, tender uterus, and unusual vaginal discharge. If chorioamnionitis is severe or left untreated, the mother may suffer from infections of the pelvic region and abdomen, endometritis, and blood clots, and her baby could have complications including sepsis, meningitis, and respiratory problems. Risk factors for chorioamnionitis include prior amniocentesis (usually in the previous two weeks), and premature or prolonged rupture of the membranes. Antibiotic and proper fetal surveillance for infection of fetus is required.

Septic Abortion

Septic abortion is when "the uterus and its contents become infected as a result of a surgically or medically treated miscarriage or abortion". It occurs in the first trimester, and symptoms include a high fever, chills, severe abdominal pain or cramping, vaginal bleeding and discharge, and backache. It should be treated with antibiotics with complete evacuation of uterus. If the condition is left untreated, potentially fatal septic shock may occur; signs include low blood pressure, low body temperature, a little urine output, and respiratory distress. Risk factors for septic abortion include poor surgical technique at the time of D&C, pre-existing cervical/uterine infection.

Listeria

Listeriosis is an infection that results from consuming contaminated food or water. Pregnant women, newborns, the elderly, and adults with impaired immune systems are most at risk. "Early symptoms of Listeria may include fever, muscle aches, nausea and diarrhea. Symptoms may occur a few days or even two months after eating contaminated food. If infection spreads to the nervous system, it can lead to headaches, stiff neck, confusion, loss of balance, or convulsions. Not all babies whose mothers are infected will have a problem, according to the American Pregnancy Association, but in some cases untreated listeriosis can result in miscarriage, premature delivery, serious infection in your newborn, or even stillbirth. A mother is advised antibiotics to keep her baby safe. To help prevent Listeria, avoid: Hot dogs, lunch meats unless they are reheated until steaming hot. Soft cheeses unless the label states that they are made from pasteurized milk. Refrigerated pot or meat spreads (canned are okay). Smoked seafood unless it is an ingredient in a cooked dish such as a casserole.

Fifth Disease (Parvovirus B19)

Fifth disease is a common childhood illness, so many adults are already immune to it. The most common symptom in is joint pain and soreness that can last for days or weeks. Athough it is rare—less than 5% of all pregnant women become infected with parvovirus B19, according to the CDC—the virus can cause a woman to miscarry or her baby to be born with severe anemia.

Dengue Fever

Women have fever, myalgia, abdominal pain with decreased platelet. It can affect pregnancy in form of abortion, pre-eclampsia, still-birth. Conservative treatment is advised.

TREATMENT OF PYREXIA IN PREGNANCY

General

Rest and Diet

Soup for the soul, sinuses, and throat, as well as any foods that make feel better like Scrambled eggs, applesauce, hot oatmeal, rice, or mashed potatoes are all comforting to you and good for your baby. Stay away from fat in all its as well as sugar (which can prolong diarrhea). And do not forget to revisit your old morning sickness pal, ginger, which works just as well when your nausea's triggered by a virus.

Fluid

In the short term, liquids are more important than solids—especially, if woman is losing them through a fever, a runny nose, vomiting, or diarrhea. Aim for at least one cup an hour, and though any liquid especially nutritious fluids—vegetables, juices, smoothies. Hot beverages will definitely soothe a sore throat.

Milk

Continue to take milk.

Vitamin C

Nature's most potent healer, so lay it on yourself in the form of C-rich fruits, vegetables, and juices. One can have less acidic choices (a mango or papaya, or honeydew, white grape juice that is C fortified.

Eat Smart

Stop colds before they even start—increase intake of fruits and veggies. Studies show that eating at least seven servings of fruits and veggies a day during pregnancy lowers your risk of developing upper respiratory infections like colds and sinus infections.

Colds are most commonly caused by rhinoviruses; cases of the flu are caused by influenza viruses. Decongestants should be avoided in pregnancy especially during the first trimester when the fetus's organs are forming should adopt more natural ways of relieving symptoms, including:

- Eating fresh garlic—known to have virus-fighting compounds (if you can actually get it down), or using anti-viral spices such as cardamom, cinnamon, and cloves in your cooking.
- Humidifiers to keep the air around you moist (consider a warm mist humidifier).
- Saltwater gargles to relieve sore throat pain (try one teaspoon of salt in eight ounces of warm water to get the fastest relief).

Steam Inhalation or Nasal Lavage

To relieve nasal congestion or sinus headaches (for lavage, dissolve a quarter teaspoon of salt and a tiny pinch of baking soda into eight ounces of lukewarm water, and use a nasal aspirator to irrigate, or clean out your nasal passages).

- *Flu shot* is a safe and important way to protect mother and baby health. According to a new study, babies born to mothers who were given the flu shot during the last trimester of pregnancy appear to be protected against the virus for the first six months of life.

Those babies whose moms got the flu shot while pregnant are also less likely to be born prematurely, are bigger and healthier, and are less likely to be hospitalized during the first year than babies whose moms were not vaccinated.

Medical Treatment

Antipyretic

Products containing aspirin or ibuprofen or naproxen are not recommended to take while pregnant; they can interfere with fetus development in the early months and create problems during labor later. Safe drugs during pregnancy are paracetamol, acetaminophen.

Safe Antibiotics during Pregnancy

- Ampicillin, amoxicillin, cephalosporin—URTI
- Nitrofurantoin, and netilmycin—UTI
- Chloramphenicol—typhoid, zidovudine—HIV
- Acyclovir, herpes, chloroquine, mefloquine—malaria
- Pyremethamine—sulphadoxine-toxoplasma
- Metronidazole—amoebiasis, trichomoniasis, bacterial vaginosis.

Antibiotics should be avoided in pregnancy are:

- Azithromycin
- Streptomycin

Fever in pregnancy

Do
- Do proper temperature charting to know exact pattern
- Take proper history to know disease behind temperature
- If temperature is not very high and duration is not long, start with conservative treatment
- Intensive workup should be done:
  - When conservative treatment fails
  - High grade temperature
  - Obstetric history
  - Bad give only safe antipyretics and antibiotics

Table 7.2: Details of infections causing fever in pregnancy

Infection	Associating feature	Effect on pregnancy	Diagnosis
Rubella	Rashes, lymphadenopathy, arthralgia	Abortion, stillbirth, congenital rubella syndrome	IgM, PCR
CMV	Arthralgia, lymphadeno-pathy	Abortion, IUGR, microcephaly intracranial calcification hepatosplenomegaly, thrombocytopenia	Culture of urine, nasopharyngeal secretions, IgM, PCR
Varicella	Rashes	Congenital varicella syndrome in early pregnancy	IgM, PCR
Parvo B19	Anemia, aplastic crisis	Fetal loss in early pregnancy, fetal hydrops	IgM, PCR of fetal and maternal blood
Toxoplasma	Asymptomatic, h/o recurrent abortion	Abortion, IUGR, stillbirth, microcephaly, cerebral calcification	IgM, PCR
Hepatitis	Flu-like illness, malaise, nausea, vomiting, rashes	Abortion, preterm, and intra-uterine death, postpartum hemorrhage, hepatic coma, renal failure, coagulopathy, infection	Serological detection of HBsAg, HBeAg, liver function test
Herpes	Skin lesion	Premature labor, IUGR, fetal affection—chorioretinitis, microcephaly	PCR
Group b streptococcus	Fever with sore throat, vaginal discharge	UTI, endometritis, preterm labor, neonatal infection causing sorethroat, pneumonia	Culture or PCR
Syphilis	Fever with rashes, rhinitis, genital ulcers	Abortion, preterm, intra-uterine death, nonimmune fetal hydrops	Serological test—VDRL, FTA-ABS, PCR
Malaria	Rigors, hypoglycemia, abdominal pain, headache, pallor (megaloblastic anemia), convulsion	Abortion, preterm, IUGR, IUD	Malarial parasites in thick blood smears
Listeria	Fever, nausea, diarrhea	Late miscarriage, preterm, stillbirth	Blood culture
Urinay tract infection	Fever with chills and rigor followed by hypothermia, burning and pain during micturition	Abortion, preterm labor, intrauterine death due to high temperature	Complete urine examination including culture
Upper respiratory tract infection, tuberculosis	Sore throat, cough, lymph nodes	Preterm, IUGR, neonatal transmission	Tuberculin test, early morning sputum, X-ray in late pregnancy, direct amplification tests and by gene probe
HIV	Fever, malaise, headache, sore throat, lymphadeno-pathy, protracted diarrhea, rash, candidiasis tuberculosis, lymphoma, sarcoma, h/o exposure, vaginal discharge, itching, abdominal pain	Prematurity, IUGR, perinatal morbidity and mortality, risk of neonatal transmission	Enzyme immunoassay (EIA), poly-merase chain reaction (PCR), Western blot (immunofluo-rescence)

- Doxycycline
- Clindamycin
- Tetracycline

Summary

- *Always keep in mind* that fever can affect pregnancy adversely, it is alarming sign so find out cause behind it earliest.
- In viral infections usually there is flu like illness or malaise but viruses are teratogenic so take care to suspect these infections by proper history.
- High grade temperature should be lowered immediately as it can leads to abortion.
- Associating symptoms are usually very helpful to reach to diagnosis.
- Clinician should remain updated regarding current infections and their latest available method for diagnosis and available treatment which is best and safe.
- Clinician should also remain updated regarding medicolegal part of termination.
- Most important part is to create awareness about high risk factors about particular infection and its prevention from prenatal period.

Table 7.2 shows different infections having varying intensity of fever with characteristic associating symptoms. It can be utilized to know exactly the diagnosis.

Bibliography

1. A, Sanz Moreno J, Valkova D, Domingo C, Anda P, de Ory F, Albarrán F, Raoult D. Q fever in pregnancy: case report after a 2-year follow-up. J Infect 1998 Jul;37(1):79–81.
2. Barone JE (August 2009). "Fever: Fact and fiction". *J Trauma* **67** (2): 406–9.doi:10.1097/TA.0b013e3181a5f335. PMID 1966789
3. *Harrison's principles of internal medicine.* (18th edn). New York: McGraw-Hill. 2011. p. 4012. ISBN 978-0-07-174889–6.
4. Ludlam H, Wreghitt TG, Thornton S, Thomson BJ, Bishop NJ, Coomber S, Cunniffe J. Q fever in pregnancy. J Infect 1997 Jan;34(1):75–78.
5. Racult D, Stein A. Q fever during pregnancy—a risk for women, fetuses, and obstetricians. N Engl J Med. 1994 Feb 3;330(5):371–371.
6. Stein A, Raoult D. Q fever during pregnancy: a public health problem in southern France. Clin Infect Dis. 1998 Sep;27(3):592–596.

8

Heart Disease in Pregnancy

• Usha Sharma

Cardiovascular disease in pregnancy is a matter of great concern for the obstetrician. The prevalence and incidence of all heart disease in pregnancy varies between 0.4% in developed countries to 1.5% in developing countries. The commonest cardiac lesion is of rheumatic origin followed by congenital ones. However, over the years, adequate treatment of rheumatic fever by appropriate antibiotics has decreased the incidence of this disease. Mitral stenosis is most common rheumatic valvular lesion while predominant congenital lesions are patent ductus arteriosus, atrial or ventricular septal defects, pulmonary stenosis and coarctation of aorta. Physiological changes during pregnancy make the diagnosis of heart disease more difficult. It is important to be vigilant on the diagnosis of heart disease during pregnancy and to treat it appropriately in time.

Hemodynamic Changes during Pregnancy

Pregnancy causes significant changes in cardiovascular physiology. Clark et al studied 10 healthy primiparous patients between 36 and 38 wks of gestation and between 11 and 13 wks postpartum using pulmonary artery catheterization. They found that main changes during pregnancy were:

1. Decreased peripheral vascular resistance (PVR)
2. Decreased pulmonary vascular resistance
3. Decreased colloid oncotic pressure
4. Increased cardiac output
5. Increased pulse rate

Hyperdynamic circulation: It is the most important finding during pregnancy which reflects as high cardiac output. The increase in cardiac output starts at 10 wks of the pregnancy, reaches a maximum at 24–28 wks and remains elevated until parturition. As pregnancy advances, there is an increase in heart rate of 10–15 beats/minute, a reflection of increased stroke volume. The cardiac output during pregnancy is sensitive to maternal positional changes and is significantly decreased in supine position due to compression of vena cava by pregnant uterus resulting in a decreased in venous return to the heart.

Increase in intravascular volume: It is another important feature in pregnancy. There is increase in both cell volume and plasma volume which start at about 8 wks of gestation and reaches maximum at 32–36 wks. The plasma volume increases first and then to a lesser degree red cell volume increase causing physiologic hemodilution during the mid-trimester of pregnancy which results in presence of grade 2/6 systolic ejection murmur on auscultation. This physiological murmur appears at 8–10 wks of gestation and disappears in early postpartum period. The increase in intravascular volume does not alter the central venous pressure but fulfills the need of developing better uteroplacental circulation and protects the mother against the potentially harmful effects of blood loss occurring at parturition.

Decrease in peripheral vascular resistance: It is most likely due to direct effect of placental hormones or prostaglandins on the blood vessels. The decreased PVR manifest clinically by decrease in both mean and diastolic blood pressure especially during 2nd trimester when mean average blood pressure is 10–15 mm Hg lower than in nonpregnant state.

Hemodynamic changes in 10 normal pregnant women were as follows:

Parameter	Changes (as compared with postpartum values)
Cardiac output	+43
Heart rate	+17
Left ventricular stroke work index	+17
Vascular resistance	
Systemic	– 21
Pulmonary	– 34
Mean arterial pressure	+04
Colloid osmotic pressure	– 14

EFFECT OF PREGNANCY ON CARDIAC DISEASE

Hemodynamic changes during pregnancy increase cardiac load and sometimes it may exceed the limited functional capacity of an ailing heart. If it occurs, sudden death, congestive heart failure (CHF) or pulmonary edema may occur. Due to deleterious effect of pregnancy on cardiac disease, maternal mortality may be as high as 10%, though it varies according to severity of cardiac problem.

There are certain periods when risk for cardiac compensation is maximum:

1. *Between 28 and 32 wks of gestation* when hemodynamic changes of pregnancy are at the peak.
2. *During labor and delivery:* During labor every contraction injects blood from uteroplacental circulation into maternal bloodstream increasing cardiac output by approximately 15–20% which may trigger congestive heart failure immediately after delivery. There is sudden transfusion of blood from the lower extremities and uteroplacental vascular tree to systemic circulation which is more than what many pregnant cardiac patients can tolerate and CHF occurs usually at this time.
3. *At postpartum period:* 4–5 days after delivery, decreased peripheral resistance with right to left shunting and pulmonary embolization are main complications.

EFFECT OF MATERNAL CARDIAC DISEASE ON PREGNANCY

Pregnancy outcome is compromised by cardiac disease. Fetal growth retardation, preterm delivery are common in pregnant cardiac patients due to inability to maintain adequate uteroplacental circulation. There is increased incidence of congenital heart diseases in fetus if mother has congenital cardiovascular anomalies. Fetal death occur in patients with cyanotic heart disease, Marfan's syndrome or in cardiac patients having significant functional impairment (Class III and IV NYHA classification).

DIAGNOSIS OF HEART DISEASE

Symptoms

Progressive dyspnea or orthopnea, nocturanl cough, hemoptysis, syncope, chest pain.

Signs

Cyanosis, clubbing, persistent neck veins engorgement, systolic murmur grade 3/6 or greater, diastolic murmur, cardiomegaly, persistent arrhythmia, persistent split second sound, pulmonary hypertension.

Diagnostic Measures

Chest radiography with lead shield: Cardiomegaly, increased pulmonary vascular markings, enlargements of pulmonary veins.

ECG: T wave inversion, dysarrhythmia.

ECHO (color flow Doppler): Evaluation of structural and functional cardiac factors. It detects atrial septal defects (ASD), ventricular septal defects (VSD), valve anatomy, valve area function, left ventricular ejection fraction, pulmonary artery systolic pressure.

Clinical Classification

Clinical classification was first introduced by New York Heart Association (NYHA) in 1928 and was revised for eighth time in 1979. This classifications are based on the cardiac response to physical activity of the person.

Class I: Uncompromised (no limitation of physical activities).

Class II: Slight limitation of physical activities. These women are comfortable on rest but slight exertion cause fatigue, palpitation.

Class III: Marked limitation of physical activities. These women are comfortable on rest but mild activity causes fatigue, dyspnea.

Class IV: Severely compromised (inability to perform any physical activity without discomfort).

Situ and associates in 2001 expanded NYHA classification and developed a scoring system for predicting cardiac complications.

Risk for maternal mortality caused by various types of heart disease	
Cardiac disorder	*Mortality*
Group 1: Minimal risk	0–1%
Atrial septal defect	
Ventricular septal defect	
Patent ductus arteriosus	
Pulmonic or tricuspid disease	
Fallot's tetralogy, corrected	
Bioprosthetic valve	
Mitral stenosis, NYHA class I and II	
Group 2: Moderate risk	5–15%
2A: Mitral stenosis, NYHA class III and IV	
Aortic stenosis	
Aortic coarctation without valvular involvement	
Fallot's tetralogy, uncorrected	
Previous myocardial infarction	
Marfan syndrome, normal aorta	
2B: Mitral stenosis with atrial fibrillation	
Artificial valve	
Group 3: Major risk	25–50%
Pulmonary hypertension	
Aortic coarctation with valvular involvement	
Marfan syndrome with aortic involvement	

NYHA: New York Heart Association.

Predictors are

1. Prior heart failure, ischemic heart attack, arrhythmia or stroke.
2. Baseline NYHA class III cardiac disease or greater with cyanosis.
3. Mitral value area <2 cm², aortic value area <1.5 cm² or peak left ventricular outflow tract gradient above 30 mm Hg by echo.
4. Ejection fraction less than 40%.

Preconception counseling: Women with cardiac disease may benefit from counseling before deciding to become pregnant. In some women cardiac abnormalities may be corrected by surgery and subsequent pregnancy may be less dangerous. In other cases when woman is taking warfarin, fetal consideration is more important. In general, risk of congenital heart disease in a offspring of such a woman is approximately 3–4%.

MANAGEMENT OF CARDIAC PATIENT WITH PREGNANCY

General Measures

Principles

1. Early diagnosis and evaluation of anatomical type and functional grade of the case.
2. To detect the predisposing factors for heart failure.
3. Care at tertiary hospital under supervision of obstetrician and cardiologist.

Role of Therapeutic Termination in a Cardiac Patient

Absolute Indications

1. Primary pulmonary hypertension
2. Eisenmenger's syndrome
3. Pulmonary veno-occlusive disease.

Relative Indications

1. Grade III and IV cardiac lesions in multiparous women.
2. Grade I or II cardiac lesion with previous history of cardiac failure in early months of pregnancy.

The termination should be done within 12 weeks by suction evacuation.

Antenatal care: Patient should be treated in a tertiary hospital in the supervision of a cardiologist. Counseling should be done and special care should be given to the patients having predisposing factors for cardiac failure as:

1. *Infection:* Urinary tract infections, dental infections.
2. Anemia
3. Obesity
4. Hypertension
5. Arrhythmias
6. Hyperthyroidism
7. Drugs: Betamimetics
8. Excess intake of high calorie diet, alcohol and caffeine.

Important components of care are:

a. *Bed rest:* It increases venous return to heart and improves renal perfusion and induces diuresis.

b. *Dietary salt restriction:* Prevent excessive retention of sodium and water.

c. *Diuretics:* Most commonly used diuretic is chlorothiazide which acts by inhibiting sodium resorption in distal tubule. Side effects are hypokalemia and neonatal thrombocytopenia. Most important concern with use of diuretic is that they may decrease the plasma volume to the point that fetal growth and placental perfusion are compromised. In these patients serial hematocrit levels may prove helpful. The dosage of diuretic may be adjusted to keep the hemotocrit value equal to or slightly above the value obtained before starting the therapy.

d. *Prophylactic digitalization:* Commonly used with severe heart disease who are not in overt congestive heart failure. It improves the contractility of the heart and relieve symptoms as fatigue and weakness. Other advantage is that it avoids ventricular tachycardia in those patients who have tendency to develop atrial arrhythmia.

Time of Admission at Hospital

Elective

- *Grade I cardiac disease:* 2 weeks prior to expected date of delivery.
- *Grade II cardiac disease:* At 28th week of pregnancy.
- *Grades III and IV:* As pregnancy is diagnosed.

Emergency Admission

1. Deterioration of functional grading
2. Appearance of dyspnea, cough or basal crepts.
3. Appearance of any pregnancy complication like anemia, pre-eclampsia.

Management of Cardiac Patient during Labor

Most of the pregnant cardiac patients go into spontaneous labor and deliver without difficulty. One should take care of pulmonary edema due to fluid overload and infection.

1. Pregnant cardiac patient should always be delivered in lateral supine position to avoid hemodynamic impairment.
2. Adequate pain relief should be given. Epidural narcotics may be used.
3. Continuous monitoring with pulse oximetry should be done, mild degree of desaturation may be corrected by oxygen through a mask.
4. All cardiac patients in labor should be given restricted intravenous fluid not more than 75 ml/hr to prevent pulmonary edema.
5. Antibiotic prophylaxis should be given to patients with congenital or acquired heart lesions with artificial valve prosthesis. Recommended regimes include intravenous ampicillin 2 gm and gentamicin 1.5 mg/kg (not to exceed 80 mg) at onset of labor followed by 8 hrly till 48 hrs after delivery. All high risk cases with structural heart disease, cyanotic congenital heart diseses and prosthetic valve need endocarditic prophylaxis.

6. Second stage of labor should be cut-short by ventouse under pudendal block anesthesia.
7. Oxytocin and ergot alkaloids should not be given intravenously. Oxytocin may cause sudden drop in peripheral vascular resistance and cause sudden hypotension. Ergot alkaloids cause significant vaso-constriction and elevation of blood pressure which can be deleterious as well.
8. To avoid thromboembolism prophylactic low dose heparin may be given during labor, delivery and immediate postpartum period. Early ambulation and pneumatic compression of lower extremities is also recommended to avoid embolism.

Place of cesarean section: In general there is no indication for cesarean section for heart patient except obstetrical indication. However, in coarctation of aorta, elective cesarean section is indicated to prevent rupture of aorta or mycotic cerebral aneurysm. Anesthesia should be given by expert anesthetist using either epidural or general anesthesia.

Puerperium: Patient should be observed closely for first 24 hrs. Oxygen should be administered if needed. Hourly pulse, BP and respiration should be recorded. Breastfeeding is not contraindicated.

Contraception: Barrier method of contraception is the best. Steroidal contraception is contraindicated. Sterilization should be done by minilaparotomy under local anesthesia.

SPECIFIC HEART PROBLEMS AND MANAGEMENT

A. Treatment of Acute Congestive Heart Failure during Pregnancy

In this situation one must try to find out cause of CHF:

1. If the cause is surgical correctable like mitral or aortic stenosis and undiagnosed

before pregnancy timely operative interventions may be life saving in such patients.

2. One must also rule out any precipitating factor like anemia, infections, arrhythmias, ingestion of salt retaining medications.

Once the potentially correctable precipitating factors have been ruled out, the management of pregnant patient consist of:

1. Bed rest to reduce cardiac load.
2. Use of diuretics to decrease preload.
3. Use of digitalis and other agents like dopamine or dobutamine to increase cardiac contractility.
4. Vasodilators to reduce afterload.

1. *Bedrest:* Bedrest is advocated to reduce metabolic rate, cardiac load though it may leads to harmful effects like pulmonary embolization or venous thrombosis. These side effects are more common in pregnant women with cardiac disease due to hypercoagulability state during pregnancy. Therefore passive leg exercise, prophylactic heparin (5000 IV subcutaneously every 12 hourly) and compression stockings should be used to avoid thromboembolic complication in these patients.

2. *Diuretics:* It Should be used with caution. One should start with mild diuretics as chlorothiazide 25–50 mg daily and potent diuretics as frusemide should only be given when necessary. Diuretic therapy should be monitored with daily weight check, serial measurement of hematocrit, electrolytes and creatinine.

3. *Digoxin:* can be used safely in pregnancy. It can be given orally as a loading dose 1–1.5 mg in 24 hrs. Maintenance dose is 0.25 mg/daily. Most serious side effect is Arrhythmias, diagnosed by ECG and require rapid treatment.

4. *Vasodilator therapy:* It is important part of treatment of patients with CHF. Use of vasodilator therapy reduce cardiac load by peripheral vascular resistance. Several drugs may be used in emergency like hydralazine, nitroglycerin and sodium nitroprusside. For maintenance, hydralazine or calcium channel blocker is drug of choice.

a. *Hydralazine:* It is arterial vasodilator and is drug that is relatively safe to use during pregnancy. It can be used in oral or intravenous form. If used in large doses, a marked decrease in blood pressure may cause alteration in placental perfusion and signs of fetal distress may appear subsequently.

b. *Nitrates:* Reduce both preload and after load but their predominant effect as on capacitance vessels. These drugs decrease the venous return to the heart and are useful in reducing pulmonary congestion. Side effects are in the form of decreased uteroplacental perfusion and fetal distress.

c. *Angiotensin converting enzyme inhibitor (ACE inhibitor):* It decreases peripheral vascular resistance, pulmonary capillary wedge pressure, heart size and increase stroke index and exercise tolerance time. ACE inhibitors are ideal drug as they reduce preload by impairing the retention of sodium and water. These drugs also reduce the vasoconstriction caused by angiotensin and block the increase in sympathetic tone mediated by renin angiotensin-aldosterone system. Fetal growth retardation and malformation have been noticed with this drug so it is contraindicated in pregnancy. In acute cardiac emergencies nitroglycerin, dopamine and dobutamine can be used in pregnant patients.

B. Management of Acute Pulmonary Edema during Pregnancy

Pulmonary edema is the condition in which there is mobilization of fluid from the pulmonary interstitium into the alveolar space. The majority of cases of pulmonary edema during pregnancy are caused in following conditions:

1. Administration of beta-adrenergic drugs for preterm labor.
2. Pre-eclampsia and eclampsia
3. Congestive heart failure

1. *Administration of beta-adrenergic drugs:* These drugs are used in preterm labor. Pulmonary edema is more common in patients taking drugs in intravenous infusion. Patients with multiple pregnancy, chorioamnionitis, intravascular volume expansion are more prone pulmonary edema.

   Treatment
   1. Discontinuation of drug
   2. Administration of frusemide
   3. Oxygenation

2. *In severe pre-eclampsia:* Pulmonary edema results from endothelial cell injury, altered capillary permeability and decreased plasma colloid oncotic pressure. Treatment is difficult as endothelial cell injury and capillary permeability problems cannot be corrected. In these cases supportive treatment and expectant management is required. Outcome is poor.

3. *In congestive heart failure:* Pulmonary edema results from inability of diseased heart to compensate for acute or chronic increase in intravascular volume. It is more common in patients with stenotic valvular lesion and fixed cardiac outputs.

   Treatment
   1. Decreasing preload fluid restriction with use of diuretics.
   2. Increasing contractility with digitalis or dobutamine.
   3. Decreasing afterload resistance with nitroglycerin.

C. Maternal Cardiac Arrhythmia during Pregnancy

It is due to premature beats, adaptation of heart to normal hemodynamic alterations. Most common type of arrhythmia during pregnancy is paroxysmal supraventricular tachycardia (PST) patients pulse rate is in between 200 and 250 bpm with palpitation and dyspnea.

ECG: Narrow QRS complex in majority due to atrioventricular node re-entry.

Treatment: Carotid sinus message for 10 seconds on left or right side accompanied by Valsalva's maneuver. If response is not satisfactory intravenous verapamil may be given 5–10 mg in a bolus for 1–3 minutes. Adenosine is drug of choice for treatment of paroxysmal supraventricular tachycardia (PST).

Cardioversion is rarely indicated. Digitalis and quinidine are commonly used for prophylaxis and maintenance therapy in patient with CHF. In paroxysmal supraventricular tachycardia (PST) treatment of choice is digoxin inspite of verapamil.

D. Cardiomyopathy in Pregnancy

Cardiomyopathy may arise *de novo* during pregnancy. It could be of the following types:

a. *Hypertrophic obstructive cardiomyopathy:* The pathological features are hypertrophy and disorganization of cardiac muscle especially of left ventricular outflow tract. Patient presents with cardiac failure. Diagnosis is based on echocardiography.

   Patients should not be allowed to become hypovolumic since it increases the risk of obstruction of left ventricular outflow tract. Particular care should be taken to give adequate fluid replacement especially in antepartum hemorrhage. During labor these patients should not be given epidural anesthesia to avoid relative hypovolemia.

b. *Peripartum cardiomyopathy:* It is rare form of congestive cardiac failure that is intimately related to pregnancy. There is no predisposing cause for heart failure and heart is grossly dilated. Signs and symptoms of this disease appear in the last month of pregnancy and up to 5 months after delivery. The majority of patients belong to age group 20–35 years and have complaints of cough, dyspnea specially paroxysmal nocturnal dyspnea and palpitation. Physical examination reveals tachycardia, cardiac arrhythmia, pulmonary rales and peripheral edema. Chest X-ray shows cardiac enlargement and pulmonary vascular redistribution. On Echocardiography there is enlargement of all chambers of heart especially of left ventricle. Ventricular wall motion, ejection fraction and cardiac output are decreased, while pulmonary wedge pressure is increased. Some patients may develop deep vein thrombosis and pulmonary embolization.

Bedrest, digitalis, diuretics and anticoagulant therapy are most important part of management. Prognosis of these patients is poor with low left ventricular ejection fraction. Patients who have dilated heart 6 months after the initiation of symptoms have very high mortality. Women who recover from postpartum cardiomyopathy are at high risk for recurrence in subsequent pregnancies.

E. Valvular Heart Disease (Rheumatic Heart Disease)

a. *Mitral stenosis:* It is most common rheumatic heart lesion and dangerous for pregnant women. The normal mitral valve surface area is 4 cm², when stenosis narrows this to less than 2.5 cm², symptoms usually develop. The most prominent complain is dyspnea due to pulmonary edema. Other common symptoms are fatigue, palpitations, cough and hemoptysis. It is usually observed that patients with mitral stenosis who are relatively asymptomatic at beginning of pregnancy, may develop pulmonary edema when the pregnancy advances and the hemodynamic changes become more apparent. Successful management of pregnant patients with mitral stenosis includes bed rest, diuretics and digitalization. During labor adequate pain relief, delivery in lateral supine position and adoption of measures to minimize the effect of autotransfusion that follows delivery is recommended. Vaginal delivery is preferable. Insertion of a pulmonary artery catherter may help in guiding the management decisions in women with severe stenosis. Intrapartum endocarditis prophylaxis may be required.

Valvotomy: It is better to avoid cardiac surgery during pregnancy. Surgery should be considered only in unresponsive cardiac failure with pregnancy beyond 12 wks. Best time of surgery is 14–18 wks. Valve replacement, commissurotomy and balloon valvotomy can be done.

b. *Aortic stenosis:* Most common cause is congenital, however, in some case, it is due to rheumatic heart disease. Pregnant patients with aortic stenosis have poor prognosis. Maternal mortality is approximately 17.4% and fetal loss is approximately 31.6%.

Patients with aortic stenosis develop left ventricular hypertrophy to generate the increased pressure necessary to pump blood through noncompliant valvular leaflets.

Hemodynamically these patients have fixed stroke volumes and increased left ventricular end-diastolic pressures. Eventually the left ventricular function fails to overcome the resistance to flow and the patients develops CHF. Angina and syncope frequently occur with the onset of CHF.

The key of management of these patients is bed rest. During labor, epidural anesthesia should be avoided because it will decrease peripheral vascular resistance and this will increase the pressure gradient across the narrow valve.

Patients with aortic stenosis should not be restricted to 75 ml/hours of IV fluids during labor. Intensive monitoring during labor is important. Intrapartum bacterial endocarditic prophylaxis is given if septicemia is suspected.

c. *Mitral valve prolapse:* Most common cardiac disease seen and affects 6–8% of all women of reproductive age. Mitral valve prolapse is incidentally found during echocardiography performed to investigate the common cardiac problems during pregnancy as palpitation and arrhythmia.

In mitral valve prolapse, the leaflets and chordae of mitral valve stretch and buldge into left atrium during systole. This is due to defect in collagen synthesis. The main symptoms of mitral valve prolapse are chest pain and cardiac arrhythmias reflected as palpitations or skipped beats on examination. One may find a midsystolic murmur appearing at the end of first trimester. Confirmed diagnosis is made by two-dimensional echocardiography which will show systolic displacement of mitral leaflets into left atrium. Doppler analysis also can demonstrate some degree of regurgitation.

Physiological changes during pregnancy will increase the left ventricular end diastolic volume and alleviate the signs and symptoms of mitral valve prolapse. There are more chances of thromboembolism and endocarditis. Most pregnant patients of mitral valve prolapse do not require treatment. Patients with severe arrhythmia require treatment with propranolol in dosage of 10–40 mg four times daily. Propranolol is safe for both mother and fetus. The patients having severe symptoms of mitral regurgitation should receive prophylactic antibiotics for prevention of endocarditis.

F. Septal Defects

Atrial septal defects: These are most common congenital cardiac lesions after bicuspid aortic valve. Most of these patients are asymptomatic until 3rd or 4th decade. Pregnancy is well-tolerated unless pulmonary hypertension develop. Usually risk of endocarditis with atrial septal defect is negligible. If congestive heart failure or arrhythmia develops, treatment is given.

Important cardiac valve disorders			
Type	Cause	Pathophysiology	Pregnancy
Mitral stenosis	Rheumatic	LA dilatation, pulmonary hypertension, and atrial fibrillation	Heart failure from fluid overload, tachycardia
Mitral insufficiency	Rheumatic Mitral valve prolapse LV dilatation	LV dilatation and eccentric hypertrophy	Ventricular function improves with afterload decrease
Aortic stenosis	Congenital Bicuspid valve	LV concentric hypertrophy, decreased cardiac output	Moderate stenosis tolerated; severe is life-threatening with decreased preload (e.g. hemorrhage, regional analgesia)
Aortic insufficiency	Rheumatic heart disease Connective tissue disease Congenital	LV hypertrophy and dilatation	Ventricular function improves with afterload decrease
Pulmonary stenosis	Congenital rheumatic	Severe stenosis associated with RA and RV enlargement	Mild stenosis usually well-tolerated; severe stenosis associated with right-sided heart failure and atrial arrhythmias

LA: Left atrial; LV: Left ventricular; RA: Right atrial; RV: Right ventricular

Ventricular septal defects: These defects spontaneously close in 90% of patients during childhood. Almost 75% of defects are para-membranous and physiological derangements are related to size of the defect. If defect is <1.25 cm², pulmonary hypertension and heart failure do not develop. Pregnancy is well tolerated with small to moderate left to right shunts. Bacterial endocarditis is more common with unrepaired defects and antimicrobial prophylaxis is often required.

Patent ductus arteriosus: Physiological consequences of this lesion are related to size. Significant lesions are repaired in child hood, those who do not under go repair, mortality is high due to pulmonary hypertension or heart failure. Sudden hypotension may lead to fetal collapse so it should be avoided.

G. Eisenmenger's Syndrome

Patients with Eisenmenger's syndrome have pulmonary hypertension with right to left shunt through an open ductus arteriosus and arterial or ventricular septal defects. The syndrome develops when pulmonary vascular resistance becomes greater than systemic vascular resistance and in which there is some right to left shunting.

Despite the best medical and obstetric care, these patients often die in postpartum period from irreversible cardiovascular collapse. Because of this poor prognosis, every pregnant patient with significant ventricular, atrial or ductus defects should have cardiac catheterization to determine the status of her pulmonary pressure. In addition to the general measures anticoagulation with heparin is advocated to avoid the formation of microthrombi in pulmonary circulation. Epidural narcotics can be used for pain relief during labor. To maintain peripheral vascular resistance and to avoid right to left shunting, it may be necessary to use intravenous fluids and peripheral vascular constrictors during delivery and puerperium.

H. Coarctation of Aorta and Marfan's Syndrome

In both these conditions the maternal risk is of dissection of aorta. Only those who already have evidence of dissection should have the coarctation repaired. In pregnancy any upper limb hypertension should be treated aggressively with beta-blocking antihypertensive drugs. If there is gross widening of ascending aorta, suggesting intrinsic disease, the baby should be deliverd by elective cesarean section to reduce risk of dissection associated with labor.

In Marfan's syndrome, there is also a risk of dissection of aorta. Dilatation of the aorta to more than 40 mm (determined echocardiographically) is the limit at which pregnancy is contraindicated. As in coarctation of the aorta, any associated hypertension should be treated aggressively with beta-blocker and delivery should be done by cesarean section if there is evidence of aortic disease.

I. Primary Pulmonary Hypertension

It is characterized by an increase in thickness of pulmonary arteriole. The consequence of lesion is marked increased in pulmonary vascular resistance that results in pulmonary hypertension. Etiology is unknown. Pregnancy is deleterious to patients with primary pulmonary hypertension. The maternal mortality is approximately 40% and fetal outcome is also poor. Termination of pregnancy is indicated. Bedrest is advocated from 20 wks of pregnancy. Anticoagulant (heparin) should be given. Oral nifedipine or IV prostacyclin helps in pulmonary vasodilatation. Epidural anesthesia may be used for pain relief.

J. Patients with Prosthetic Heart Valves

The pregnancy outcome in these patients will depend on the type of valves (mechanical, porcine, human allograft), the site and the number of valves that were replaced and the functional capacity of heart after surgery.

These patients suffer from thromboembolization, complications due to ingestion of anticoagulant regimes, valve dysfunction, endocarditis and heart failure.

Warfarin sodium has well-known teratogenic effects when administrated early in pregnancy. It is associated with spontaneous fetal intracranial bleeding and fetal death when it is taken in the second or third trimesters of pregnancy. It is used in the early first trimester may produce nasal hypoplasia, hypertelorism, prominence of frontal bone, short stature, abnormalities of central nervous system, mental retardation and stippling of the epiphyses of long bones. Due to these side effects of warfarin sodium, many clinicians are switching to heparin therapy though heparin is not as effective as warfarin sodium for clot prevention on the artificial valve. Side effects of heparin is osteoporosis and thrombocytopenia, if it is used in high dosage for more than 6 months. Heparin must be administrated subcutaneously every 8–12 hrs. Hence, some investigators recommend heparin during first 12 and last 4 weeks of pregnancy and warfarin in the interim months.

Conclusion

Heart disease is a significant cause of maternal mortality. It is best managed by obstetrician and physician in the hospital. Initial assessment can be clinical, supported by ECG and Echocardiography. Preconception counseling in known cardiac patients is important. Considering high maternal morality in certain heart diseases like Eisenmenger's syndrome and pulmonary hypertension, termination of pregnancy may also be advocated. Anticoagulation is a major problem. Heparin is the safest drug. Vaginal delivery is preferred but elective cesarean section can be done in selected cases. Because of the life-threatening complications the suspicion index regarding heart diseases with pregnancy should always remain high in the mind of an obstetrician as this may go a long way in saving many lives.

Thus, early diagnosis of heart diseases in pregnancy and prevention of its complications like heart failure and pulmonary edema can reduce maternal mortality and improve perinatal outcome.

Bibliography

1. American College of Obstetricians and Gynecologists: Prophylactic antibiotics in labor and delivery. Practice Bulletin No. 47, October 2003.
2. American College of Obstetricians and Gynecologists: Thromboembolism in pregnancy. Practice Bulletin No. 19, August 2000.
3. Arnoni RT, Arnoni AS, Bonini R. et al. Risk factors associated with cardiac surgery during pregnancy. Ann Thorac Surg 2003;76:1605.
4. Benitez RM: Hypertrophic cardiomyopathy and pregnancy: Maternal and fetal outcomes. J Matern Fetal Invest 1996;6:51.
5. Capeless EL, Clapp JF. Cardiovascular changes in early phase of pregnancy. Am J Obstet Gynecol 1989;161:1449.
6. Clark SL, Cotton DB, Lee W, et al. Central hemodynamic assessment of normal term pregnancy. Am J Obstet Gynecol 1989;161:1439.
7. Clark SL, Phelan JP, Greenspoon J, et al. Labor and delivery in the presence of mitral stenosis: Central homodynamic observations.
8. Clark SL, Porter TF, West FG. Coumarin derivatives and breastfeeding. Obstet Gynecol 2000;95:938.
9. Cunningham FG, Pritchard JA, Hankins GDV, et al. Peripartum heart failure: Idiopathic cardiomyopathy or compounding cardiovascular events. Obstet Gynecol 1986;67:157.
10. De Souza JL Jr, Frimm CD, Nastari L, et al. Left ventricular function after a new pregnancy in patients with peripartum cardiomyopathy. J Card Fail 200lb;7:30.
11. Easterling TR, Ralph DD, Schmucker BC. Pulmonary hypertension in pregnancy: Treatment with pulmonary vasodilators. Obstet Gynecol 1999;93:494.
12. Hoen B, Alla F, Selton-Suty C, et al. Changing profile of infective endocarditis: Results of a 1-year survey in France. JAMA 2002;288:75.
13. Iserin L. Management of pregnancy in women with congenital heart disease. Heart 2001;85:493.
14. Koscica KL, Anyaogu C, Bebbington M, et al. Maternal levels of troponin I in patients

undergoing vaginal and caesarean delivery Obstet Gynecol 2002;99:83S.

15. Lam GK, Stafford RE, Throp J, et al. Inhaled nitric oxide for primary pulmonary hypertension in pregnancy. Obstet Gynecol 2001;98:895.

16. Lao TT, Adelman AG, Sermer M, et al. Balloon valvuloplasty for congenital arotic stenosis in pregnancy. Br J Obstet Gynecol 1993a;100:1141.

17. Leyh Rg, Fischer S, Ruhparwar A, et al. Anticoagulant therapy in pregnant women with mechanical heart valves. Arch Gynecol Obstet 2003;268:1.

18. Mousa HA, McKinly CA, Thong J. Acute postpartum myocardial infarction after ergometrine administration in a woman with familial hypercholesterolaemia. Br J Obstet Gynaecol 2000;107:939.

19. Nishimura RA, Holmes DR, Jr. Hypertrophic obstructive cardiomyopathy. N Engl J Med 2004; 350:1320.

20. Riemold SC, Rutherford JD. Valvular heart disease in pregnancy. N Engl J Med 2003;349:52.

21. Robins K, Lyons G. Supraventrcular tachycardia in pregnancy. Br J Anaesth 2004;92:140.

22. Sadler L, McCowan L, White H, et al. Pregnancy outcomes and cardiac complications in women with mechanical, bioprosthetic and homograft valves. Br J Obstet Gynaecol 2000;107:245.

23. Sawhney H, Aggarwal N, Suri V, et al. Maternal and perinatal outcome in rheumatic heart disease. Int J Gynaecol Obstet 2003;80:9.

24. Schulte-Sasse U. Life-threatening myocardial ischaemia associated with the use of prosta-glandin E1 to induce abortion. Br J Obstet Gynaecol 2000;107:700.

25. Shere DM. Coarctation of the descending thoracic aorta diagnosed during pregnancy. Obstet Gynecol 2002;100:1094.

26. Siu SC, Colman JM. Congenital heart disease: Heart disease and pregnancy. Heart 85:710, 2001.

27. Siu SC, Sermer M, Colman JM, et al. Prospective multicenter study of pregnancy outcomes in women with heart disease. Circulation 2001; 104:515.

28. Siu SC, Sermer M, Harrison DA, et al. Risk and predictors for pregnancy-related complications in women with heart disease. Circulation 1997; 96:2789.

29. Weiss BM, Maggiorini Mm Jenni R, et al. Pregnant patient with primary pulmonary hypertension: Inhaled pulmonary vasodilators and epidural anesthesia for cesarean delivery. Anesthesiology 2000;92:1191.

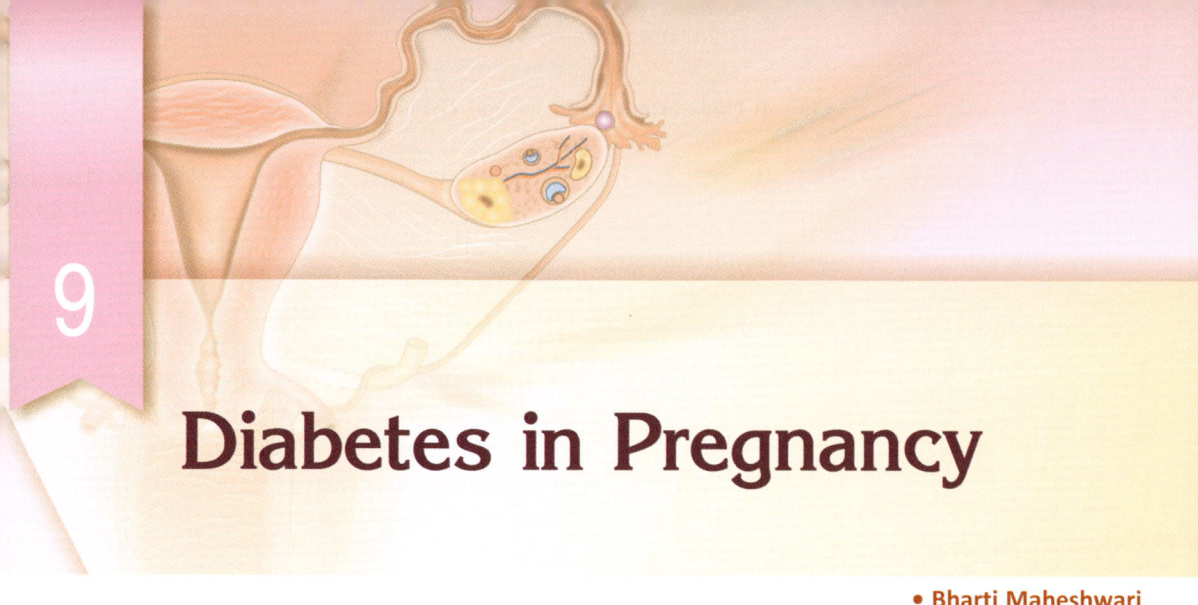

9

Diabetes in Pregnancy

• Bharti Maheshwari

Pregnancy induces progressive changes in maternal carbohydrate metabolism. As pregnancy advances, insulin resistance and diabetogenic stress due to placental hormones necessitate compensatory increase in insulin secretion. When this compensation is inadequate gestational diabetes develops. It is one of the most common complications of pregnancy, increasing day by day.

GESTATIONAL DIABETES MELLITUS (GDM)

Carbohydrate intolerance of varying degrees of severity developed during pregnancy is called gestational diabetes.

EFFECTS OF DIABETES ON PREGNANCY

In cases of GDM perinatal and neonatal mortality increased two- to four-fold with increased incidence of unexplained IUD at term which is more in **macrosomic babies**. There is increased incidence of **congenital abnormalities** like sacral agenesis, skeletal abnormalities and neural tube defect. The risk is related to the degree of glycemic control. During pregnancy HbA1c should not be >6%. Evidence shows that risk for congenital malformation is 5% with HbA1c >8% which increase up to 25% with HbA1c >10%. Macrosomia is associated with increased risk of operative delivery, **birth trauma, and**

shoulder dystocia. Diabetic pregnant women has hyperglycemia which causes fetal polyuria and polyhydramnios leads to PROM and preterm delivery. There are more chances of **prematurity** due to delayed production of pulmonary surfactant in babies of diabetic mother. There is increase risk of **future diabetes** in their children.

Why Screening is Important

Timely screening of all pregnant women for glucose intolerance results in better maternal and perinatal outcome and also prevents its transmission from one generation to other generation.

Whom to Screen?

We can divide women in 2 groups:
1. Low risk
2. High risk

Low Risk

- Age <25 years
- Weight normal before pregnancy
- Member of ethnic group with low prevalence of GDM
- No known diabetes in first-degree relatives
- No history of abnormal glucose tolerance and poor obstetric outcome.

High Risk for GDM

- Polycystic ovary syndrome
- A previous diagnosis of gestational diabetes or prediabetes, impaired glucose tolerance, or impaired fasting glycemia
- A family history of first-degree relative with type 2 diabetes
- Maternal age—a woman's risk factor increases as she gets older (especially for women over 35 years of age).
- Ethnic background (African-Americans, Afro-Caribbeans, Native Americans, Hispanics, Pacific Islanders, and people originating from South Asia)
- Being overweight, obese or severely obese increases the risk by a factor 2.1, 3.6 and 8.6, respectively.
- A previous pregnancy which resulted in a child with a macrosomia (high birth weight: >90th centile or >4000 g (8 lbs 12.8 oz))
- Previous poor obstetric history
- *Other genetic risk factors:* There are at least 10 genes where certain polymorphism are associated with an increased risk of gestational diabetes, most notably TCF7L2.

Types of Screening

1. Universal
2. Selective
   Which one is better—still controversial?

Selective screening cost effective and convenient but 37–50% of women with GDM may remain undiagnosed. Even if we exempt women with low risk for diabetes, 90% of pregnant women will require screening. Hence, the practice of **universal screening is advocated**, specially for countries like India with high prevalence of diabetes, universal screening is mandatory.

When to Screen?

Insulin is detected in fetal pancreas as early as 9 wks after conception. Increase in pancreatic beta cell mass and insulin secretion occurs by 16th wks of gestation due to maternal hyperglycemia. The priming of fetal beta cells may cause persistence of fetal hyperinsulinemia throughout the pregnancy and may result in accelerated fetal growth even if mother enjoys good metabolic control in later month of pregnancy. Considering above facts it is recommended to screen/test in first trimester, as early detection and management results in better fetal outcome because if screening is done at 24–28 wks of pregnancy only, then there are chances of diabetes being missed.

Even if screening test is normal in first trimester of pregnancy, they should all be screened again at 24–28th wks and 32–34th wks of pregnancy.

Difference in Screening and Diagnostic Test

Screening test identifies women at greater or lower risk but do not identify the women with or without the disease, in contrast-diagnostic test (OGTT) provides a definite answer for presence or absence of diabetes.

How Screening should be Done?

The controversy concerning optimal strategy still continues for the detection and diagnosis of GDM. American Diabetes Association (ADA) recommends two step procedures for screening and diagnosis of diabetes and that too in selective (high risk) population. Universal screening for GDM detects more cases and improves maternal and neonatal prognosis compared with selective screening. In the Indian context, screening is essential in all pregnant women as the Indian women have 11-fold increased risk of developing glucose intolerance during pregnancy compared to Caucasian women. The recent data on the prevalence of GDM in our country was 16.55% by WHO criteria of 2 hrs PG = 140 mg/dl. As such universal screening during pregnancy has become important in our country. Hence, we need a simple procedure which is economical and feasible.

Commonly used screening and diagnostic procedures for gestational diabetes are recommended by:

- American Diabetes Association (ADA)
- WHO
- Single step method—recently introduced in India.

1. ADA Recommendations

Two-step procedure:

Step 1: 50 gm glucose challenge test (GCT) is used for screening irrespective of the time of last meal.

Step 2: If 1 hour GCT value is >140 mg/dl than 100 gm oral glucose challenge test (OGTT) is recommended and plasma glucose is estimated 0, 1, 2, 3, hrs.

Gestational diabetes is diagnosed if any two values are equal or more than:

- FPG ≥95 mg/dl, 1 hr PG ≥180 mg/dl
- 2 hrs PG ≥155 mg/dl, 3 hr PG ≥140 mg/dl

Drawbacks of ADA recommendation

- 4 blood samples are required to complete the procedure
- At least two visits are required

2. WHO Recommended Criteria

Fasting blood sugar is estimated in pregnant women, if more than 100 mg/dl, 75 gm of oral glucose is given as in nonpregnant woman and after 2 hrs glucose level are taken if plasma glucose level equal or more than 140 mg/dl, significant.

Significance of cut-off point of 2 hrs plasma glucose level of 140 mg/dl.

Studies show that cumulative risk of type 2 diabetes depend on 2 hrs plasma glucose levels.

Plasma glucose level	Cumulative risk
120–139 mg/dl	19%
140–199 mg/dl	30%

Single step test according to Indian guidelines—recommended in India.

- Pregnant women is given 75 gm oral glucose without regard to time of last meal
- Venous sample is collected at 2 hrs for estimating plasma glucose.
- Gestational diabetes is diagnosed if plasma glucose is >140 mg/dl.

Advantages of single step test

- It is simple, economical and feasible
- Pregnant women need not be fasting
- Only 1 visit is required, causes least disturbances in a pregnant woman's routine activities serves as both screening and diagnostic procedure.

Rationale for skipping fasting level in single step test: In normal glucose tolerant pregnant women glucose levels are minimally effected by the time of last meal, as compared to woman with GDM, on glucose challenge test, normal glucose tolerant woman will be able to maintain euglycemia due to brisk and adequate insulin response, while in cases of GDM glycemic excursion is exaggerated further due to impaired insulin secretion and response.

Gestational weeks at which screening is recommended: Practically all the pregnant women should undergo screening for glucose intolerance. The usual recommendation for screening is between 24 and 28 weeks of gestation. The recent concept is to screen for glucose intolerance in **the first trimester** itself as the fetal beta cell recognizes and responds to maternal glycemic level as early as 16th week of gestation. If found negative at this time, the screening test is to be performed again around 24–28th weeks and finally around 32nd–34th weeks.

Management of GDM

A team approach is ideal for managing women with GDM. The team would usually comprise an obstetrician, diabetes physician,

Plasma glucose mg/dl	In pregnancy	Outside pregnancy
Important facts: Glycemic criteria with 75 gm 2 hrs OGTT (WHO criteria)		
2 hrs >200	Diabetes	Diabetes
2 hrs >140–199	GDM	Impaired glucose tolerance
2 hrs >120–139	GGI	—
2 hrs <120	Normal	Normal

a diabetes educator, dietitian, midwife and pediatrician. In practice, however, the team approach is not always possible due to limited resources. In such circumstances, management by an obstetrician and physician, with the assistance of an appropriately skilled dietitian, diabetes educator, is acceptable.

Principles of Management

a. Patient Education

The importance of educating women with GDM (and their partners) about the condition and its management cannot be overemphasized. The compliance with the treatment plan depends on the patient's understanding of:

- The implications of GDM for her baby and herself
- The dietary and exercise recommendations
- Self-monitoring of blood glucose
- Self administration of insulin and adjustment of insulin doses
- Identification and treatment of hypoglycemia (patient and family members)
- Incorporate safe physical activity
- Development of techniques to reduce stress and cope with the denial
- Care should be taken to minimize the anxiety of the women.

b. Medical Nutrition Therapy (MNT)

The expected weight gain during pregnancy is 300 to 400 gm/week and total weight gain is 10 to 12 kg by term. All women with GDM should receive nutritional counseling to provide sufficient calories to sustain adequate nutrition for mother and fetus and to avoid excess weight gain and postprandial hyper-glycemia. Pregnancy is not ideal time for obesity correction. Women are advised to distribute their calorie consumption especially the breakfast. In pregnant woman due to "dawn phenomenon" insulin response is less in the morning that is why breakfast should be distributed in two meals to avoid undue peaking of plasma glucose interval of two hours is recommended. Fat should be curtailed if patient is obese. Fiber containing diet is increased. Usually 3 meals with breakfast—25%, lunch—30%, dinner—30% of total calorie is recommended. Rest 15% calorie can be taken in form of snacks.

Insulin Therapy

Insulin is essential if medical nutrition therapy fails to achieve euglycemia. Various criteria have been proposed for the initiation of insulin therapy. Fourth International Workshop on GDM recommended lowering capillary blood glucose concentration to 140 mg/dl at 1 hour and 120 mg/dl at 2 hours, whereas ADA recommended the option of measuring 1 hour post-meal values with cut-off of 120 mg/dl. These recommendations are based on one single determination, which reflects a "snap shot" of glucose evaluation rather than a "video" of continuous glucose profile. The continuous glucose monitoring system has established that in normal pregnancy, peak plasma glucose occurs at 60 minutes and the value was 108.7 ± 16.9 mg/dl. In a woman with GDM, the peak occurs between 70 and 110 minutes (at approximately 90 minutes) and with a good glycemic control the value was 103 ± 26 mg/dl. However, being interstitial fluid glucose it has its own limitation. herself inulin is indicated if postprandial (2 hrs) blood sugar >140 mg% even on diet control to achieve 90 mg% FBG and PP 120 mg%. For stabilization of insulin dose, create awareness for self glucose monitoring and dose adjustment by the patient.

If the FPG concentration on the OGTT is >120 mg/dl, then the patient is started on insulin immediately along with meal plan. Other GDM women are seen within 3 days and are also taught self-monitoring of blood glucose (SMBG). SMBG is to be performed in fasting and 1½ hours after each meal. GDM women usually have high post-breakfast plasma glucose level compared to post-lunch and post-dinner. A few GDM women do have post-dinner plasma glucose also high. Insulin is started within 1 to 2 weeks, if the majority (i.e., at least four of seven per week) of fasting values exceed 90 mg/dl. Similarly, if the majority of postprandial values after a particular meal exceed 120 mg/dl, insulin is started. Pen injectors are very useful and the patient's acceptance is excellent. The initial dose of NPH insulin could be as low as 4 units and the dose of insulin can be adjusted on follow-up. A few GDM patients may require combination of short-acting insulin and intermediate acting insulin in the morning and evening.

If a patient has elevated prelunch blood sugar, regular insulin is usually necessary in the morning to handle the post-breakfast hyperglycemia, as there is a lag period before the intermediate-acting insulin begins to work. The above regimen of regular and intermediate-acting insulin in the morning controls hyperglycemia in most cases. If the post-dinner blood sugar is high, a small dose of regular insulin is necessary before dinner in addition to the regular and intermediate-acting insulin given in the morning. Combination of regular and intermediate-acting insulin before dinner may be necessary if fasting blood sugar is high. This combination of short- and intermediate-acting insulin in the morning and as well as in the evening

is known as mixed and split dose of insulin regimen. In this regimen two-thirds of the total daily dose of insulin is given in the morning and one-third in the evening. For each combination one-thirds dose should be regular insulin and two-thirds intermediate acting insulin. With this regimen if the patient continues to have fasting hyperglycemia, the intermediate-acting insulin has to be given at bedtime instead of before dinner. Insulin dose is individualized.

As pregnancy advances a 'double mixed regime "may be given. Aim is to maintain blood sugar level as near to normal as possible without causing hypoglycemia.

Target Blood Glucose Levels

Maintenance of mean plasma glucose (MPG) level ~105 mg% is ideal for good fetal outcome. This is possible if FPG and post-prandial peaks are around 90 mg/dl and 120 mg/dl respectively (MPG should not be <86 mg/dl as this may cause small for gestational age infants).

Species of Insulin

It is ideal to use human insulins are least immunogenic. Though insulin does not cross the placenta, the insulin antibodies due to animal source insulin can cross the placenta, and stress the fetal beta cell, increase insulin production and induce macrosomia. Rapid acting insulin analogues (Novorapid/Humalog) have been found to be safe and effective in achieving the targeted post-prandial glucose value during pregnancy. Lyspro the first analogue to get category B approval by US FDA and aspart has also been used in pregnancy.

Oral Antidiabetic Drugs

Recently reports have shown good fetal outcome in GDM women who were on glyburide (micronised form of Glibenclamide). A randomized unblinded clinical trial compared the use of insulin and glyburide in women with GDM who were not able to meet glycemic goals on meal plan. Treatment with either agent resulted in similar perinatal outcomes. All these patients were beyond the first trimester of pregnancy at the initiation of therapy. More studies are required before routinely recommending glibenclamide during pregnancy especially during the first trimester itself. Metformin has been found to be useful in women with polycystic ovarian disease (PCOD) who failed to conceive. Continuing this drug after conception is still a controversy. But there are a few studies favoring continuation of metformin through-out pregnancy.

Currently, oral agents are not routinely recommended during pregnancy though emerging data on glibenclamide and metformin is interesting.

MONITORING GLYCEMIC CONTROL

The success of the treatment for a woman with GDM depends on the glycemic control maintained with meal plan or pharmaco-logical intervention. To know the effectiveness of treatment, monitoring of glycemic control is essential.

Once diagnosis is made, medical nutritional therapy (MNT) is advised initially for two weeks. If MNT fails to achieve control, i.e. FPG = 90 mg/dl and/or 1 ½ hr PPG = 120 mg/dl, insulin may be initiated. Once target blood glucose is achieved, woman with GDM till the 28th week of gestation require lab monitoring of both fasting and 1 ½ hr post-breakfast once a month and at other time of the day as the clinician decides.

After the 28th week of gestation, the laboratory monitoring should be more frequent at least once in 2 weeks, if need be more frequently. After 32 weeks of gestation, lab monitoring should be done once a week till delivery. In high risk pregnancies, frequency of monitoring may be intensified with SMBG. Continuous glucose monitoring devices are available but these equipment need special training and are expensive. These devices may be useful in high risk pregnancies to know the glycemic fluctuations and to plan proper insulin dosage. Throughout the stages and phases of a diabetic woman, her health status is directly dependent on her nutritional status and her blood glucose control. As a woman ages, to prevent the increased risk of osteoporosis and cardiovascular disease of the diabetic woman, exercise and hormonal replacement therapy can minimize the ravages of diabetes per se on the aging process. Normoglycemia throughout the lifecycle of a diabetic woman results in a lifecycle of health.

HbA1c Levels

If the glucose intolerance is detected in the early pregnancy, HbA1c level will be helpful to differentiate between a pre-gestational diabetic and GDM. If the HbA1c level is more than 6%, she is likely to be a pre-GDM. HbA1c is useful in monitoring the glucose control during pregnancy, but not for the day to day management. A1c level may serve as a prognostic value.

Estimation of fructosamine during pregnancy is less frequently used.

- Glycosylated hemoglobin (HbA1c) should be determined at the end of first trimester and trimonthly thereafter.
- HBA1c <6% is desirable

Measuring Other Parameters

The blood pressure has to be monitored during every visit. Examination of the fundus and estimation of microalbuminuria, every trimester.

OBSTETRIC CONSIDERATIONS

Fetal Evaluation

An **ultrasound** scan has to be performed around 18–20 weeks of gestation focusing on structures namely the spine, skull, kidney and heart. **Fetal echocardiography** has to be done around 20–24 weeks which allows to view all the four chambers of the heart. From 26th week onwards, fetal growth and liquor volume has to be monitored every 2–3 weeks. **Fetal abdominal circumference** provides baseline for further serial measurements which gives growth acceleration or restriction. Fetal movements are monitored from 20 weeks onwards. Screening for chromosomal anomalies is necessary in pre-GDM. Screening should be done for Down's syndrome, alpha fetoprotein for neural defects and human chorionic gonadotrophin to identify any chromosomal abnormalities (16–20 weeks of gestation). The obese fetus of GDM mother is also hyper-insulinemic, interaction between leptin and insulin may be a link between maternal diabetes and increased adiposity in the fetus. Sonographic evaluation in pregnancy:

- 7 wks—first USG for cardiac activity
- 11–14 wks—diabetic congenital anomalies
- 18–20 wks—structural congential anomalies
- 32–36 wks—weekly for macrosomia and growth restriction.

Assessment of fetal well-being is made from 28 wks onward by

- Biophysical profile
- NST
- Doppler velocimetery

TIMING OF DELIVERY

Sudden intrauterine fetal demise in the third trimester of diabetic pregnancy is not uncommon. To avoid this risk, preterm delivery is recommended. But with this, respiratory distress syndrome (RDS) is likely to occur. Administering steroids for lung maturity or β adrenoreceptor agonist to inhibit premature uterine contractions are likely to induce adverse metabolic effects due to their glycolytic, glycogenolytic and lipolytic effects. In this situation, extra insulin may be required to maintain euglycemia. Fetal demise can also occur due to pre-eclampsia, which can produce fetal hypoxia via decreased uteroplacental perfusion. Some centres allow women with uncomplicated diabetes to go into spontaneous labor irrespective of the gestational age, but most still advocate delivery at 38 weeks as perinatal mortality and morbidity appear to increase after this time. Induction at 38 weeks gestation may be slow or unsuccessful due to unfavorable conditions of the cervix but this has to be balanced against the poorly defined and predictable risk of late intrauterine death, if pregnancy is allowed to continue more than 38 weeks. Fetal health may deteriorate suddenly, hence obstetric management should not be rigid and each case needs individual care and attention. Having a neonatologist support at the time of delivery is advisable. In uncomplicated cases advocated at 34–36 wks.

Hospitalization

Early hospitalization is useful for:

- Stabilization of diabetes
- Minimizes the incidence of pre-eclampsia, polyhydramnios, preterm labor
- To select appropriate time and method of delivery.

Place of Spontaneous Labor at Term

- Young pregnant woman with good obstetric history
- Diabetes well-controlled and without any fetal and maternal complication.

In any case pregnancy should not be allowed to overrun the expected date or should be terminated before term till there is any complication like macrosomia, poly-hydramnios, poor metabolic control or other obstetric indication as IUGR or PE indication for induction of labor:

- Diabetic women controlled on insulin after 38 wks of pregnancy
- Women with vascular complications like pre-eclampsia, IUGR after 37 wks.

Method of Induction

- Prior to day of induction the usual bed time dose of insulin is given

- No morning dose of insulin is given on day of induction. Once labor begins, insulin is not necessary. In a gestational diabetic the requirement of insulin is likely to fall precipitously and no insulin may be required immediately after expulsion of placenta.
- An intravenous drip of 1 litre of 5% dextrose is setup with 10 U of soluble insulin.
- Infusion rate of 100–125 ml/hr will maintain good glucose control to approx 100 mg. Blood glucose level is estimated hourly to decide insulin dose
- Normal saline infusion can be given
- Induction is done by usual method as low rupture of membrane with oxytocin or by misoprostol
- Epidural analgesia is ideal for pain relief
- If labor fails to start within 6–8 hrs or if labor progress unsatisfactorily, cesarean section should be done.

Indication of Cesarean

- Elderly primigravida
- Multigravida with bad obstetric history
- Diabetes with complications or difficult to control
- Obstetric complications like pre-eclampsia, polyhydramnios, malpresentation and fetal macrosomia (>4 kg)

Role of Spontaneous Labor at Term

- Young pregnant woman with good obstetric history
- Diabetes well-controlled either by diet or insulin and without any obstetrical complication
- *In any case pregnancy should not be allowed to overrun the expected date.*

Fetal Monitoring during Labor

- Constant watch to note the fetal condition is mandatory preferably with CTG
- Labor should not be allowed for more than 12 hrs and should be augmented by low

rupture of membrane and oxytocin or delivered by cesarean section
- Take care of shoulder dystocia
- Cord should be clamped immediately. within 20 seconds of delivery, to avoid erythrocytosis.

Conclusion

As fetal morbidity can start even at lower maternal glycemic level (<140 mg/dl) and macrosomia is possible when 2 hrs plasma glucose increased from 120 mg/dl. Screening is essential especially for all Indian pregnant women due to high prevalence. DIPSI recommends that as a pregnant woman walks into the antenatal clinic in the fasting state, she has to be given a 75 g oral glucose load and at 2 hrs a venous blood sample is collected for estimating plasma glucose. This one step procedure of challenging women with 75 gm glucose and diagnosing GDM is simple, economical and feasible. Screening is recommended between 24 and 28 weeks of gestation and the diagnostic criteria of ADA are applicable. A team approach is ideal for managing women with GDM. The team would usually comprise an obstetrician, diabetes physician, a diabetes educator, dietitian, midwife and pediatrician. Intensive monitoring, diet and insulin is the corner stone of GDM management. Oral agents or analogues though used are still controversial. Until there is evidence to absolutely prove that ignoring maternal hyperglycemia when the fetal growth patterns appear normal on the ultrasonogram, it is prudent to achieve and maintain normoglycemia in every pregnancy complicated by gestational diabetes. The maternal health and fetal outcome depends upon the care by the committed team of diabetologists, obstetricians and neonatologists. A short-term intensive care gives a long-term pay off in the primary prevention of obesity, IGT and diabetes in the offspring, as the preventive medicine starts before birth.

Bibliography

1. Alberti K, Zimmett P. WHO Consultation. Definition, diagnosis and classification of diabetes mellitus and its complications, diagnosis and classification of diabetes mellitus. Diabet Med 1998;15:539-53.

2. American Diabetes Association. Gestational diabetes mellitus. Diabetes Care 2003;26 (suppl):S103–5.

3. Ben-Haroush A, et al. The post prandial glucose profile in the diabetic pregnancy. Am J Obstet Gynecol 2004;191:576–81.

4. Cornblath M, Ichord R. Hypoglycemia in the neonate. Semin Perinatol 2000;24:136–49.

5. Cosson E, et al. Screening and insulin sensitivity in gestational diabetes. Abstract volume of the 40th Annual Meeting of the EASD, September 2004: A 350.

6. Coustan, Donald R. MD, "Making the diagnosis of Gestational Diabetes Mellitus (Diabetes and Pregnancy)". Clin Obstet Gynecol 2000;43:99–105.

7. de Sereday MS, et al. Diagnostic criteria for gestational diabetes in relation to pregnancy outcome. J Diabetes Complications 2003;17:115–9.

8. Dornhost A, Paterson CM, Nicholls JS, Wadsworth J, Chiu DC, Elkeles RS, Johnston DG, Beard RW. High prevalence of GDM in women from ethnic minority groups. Diabetic Med 1992;9:820–2.

9. Dornhost A, Rossi M. Risk and prevention of type 2 diabetes in women with gestational diabetes. Diabetes Care 1998;21: Suppl 2,B43–B49.

10. Jakubowicz DJ, Iuorno MJ, Jakubowicz S, Roberts KA, Nestler JE. Effects of metformin on early pregnancy loss in the polycystic ovary syndrome. J Clin Endocrinol Metab 2002;87:524–9.

11. Jovanovic. Medical management of pregnancy complicated by diabetes: 3rd edn, Alexandria, VA: ADA 2000.

12. Langer L, Conway DL, Berkus MD, Xenakis EMJ, Gonzales O. A comparison of glyburide and insulin in women with gestational diabetes mellitus. N Engl J Med 2000;343:1134–8.

13. Langer O, Levy J, Brustman L, Anyaegubunam A, Merkatz R, Divon MY. Glycemic control in gestational diabetes mellitus: How tight is tight enough: small for gestational age versus large for gestational age? Am J Obstet Gynecol 1989;161: 646–53.

14. Metzger BE, Coustan DR. Summary and recommendations of the fourth international workshop-conference on gestational diabetes mellitus. Diabetes Care 1998;21(suppl):B161–7.

15. Nahum GG, Wilson SB, Stanislaw H. Early-pregnancy glucose screening for gestational diabetes mellitus. J Reprod Med 2002;47:656–62.

16. Patmore JE, Mason EA, Brash PD, Boxter M, Caldwell G, Gallen J, Price PA, Vice PA, Walker J, Lindow SW. Maternal outcome in type 2 diabetic pregnancy treated with insulin lispro. Abstract 2275 PO, the 61st Scientific sessions, American Diabetes Association, 2001; Philadelphia PA. June 22–26.

17. Paul W Franks, et al. Gestational glucose tolerance and risk of type 2 diabetes in Young Pima Indian Offspring. Diabetes 2006;55:460–65.

18. Ravi Retnakaran, et al. Impaired Glucose Tolerance of Pregnancy is a Heterogeneous Metabolic Disorder as Defined by the Glycemic Response to the Oral Glucose Tolerance Test. Diabetes Care 2006;29:57–62.

19. Sermer M, et al. The Toronto Tri Hospital Gestational Diabetes Project—a preliminary review. Diabetes Care 1998;21 suppl 2:B33–42.

20. Seshiah V, Balaji V, Madhuri S Balaji, Sanjeevi CB, Green A. Gestational Diabetes Mellitus in India. J Assoc Physic of India 2004;52:707–11.

21. Seshiah V, et al. Diabetes in Pregnancy Awareness and Prevention (DIPAP) Project. Data presented at WDF Diabetes Summit; Hanoi, 21st-23rd February 2006.

22. Seshiah V, et al. One step procedure for screening and diagnosis of gestational diabetes mellitus. J Obstet Gynecol India 2005;55:525–9.

23. Sunil Gupta. Gestational Diabetes Mellitus (GDM): We Need to Revise the Standard Criteria for Diagnosis—Indian Experience. Australian Diabetes in Pregnancy Group (ADIP) meet: Sydney; August 2004.

24. Vijayam Balaji, Shyam Mukundan, Madhuri S Balaji, Veerasamy Seshiah. "Correlation between Maternal Glycemic Levels and Birth Weight in Asian Indians" At The 36th Annual Meeting Of the Diabetes and Pregnancy Study Group, Luso, Portugal, September 2004.

25. Yogev Y, Chen R, Langer O, Hod M. Diurnal glycemic profile characterization in nondiabetic nonobese subjects during the first trimester. The 37th Annual Meeting of the Diabetes and Pregnancy Study Group, Myconos–Hellas: September 2005.

10

Fetal Growth Disorder

• Usha Sharma

Overview

Intrauterine growth restriction (IUGR) refers to a condition in which a fetus is unable to achieve its genetically determined potential size. This functional definition seeks to identify a population of fetuses at risk for modifiable but otherwise poor outcomes. This definition intentionally excludes of fetuses that are small for gestational age (SGA) but are not pathologically small (Fig. 10.1). SGA is defined as growth at the 10th or less percentile for weight of all fetuses at that gestational age. Not all fetuses that are SGA are pathologically growth restricted, and in fact, may be constitutionally small. Similarly, not all fetuses that have not met their genetic growth potential are in less than the 10th percentile for estimated fetal weight (EFW).

Of all fetuses at or below the 10th percentile for growth, only approximately 40% are at high risk of potentially preventable perinatal death (see image below). Another 40% of these fetuses are constitutionally small. Because this diagnosis may be made with certainty only in neonates, a significant number of fetuses that are healthy but SGA will be subjected to high-risk protocols, and potentially, iatrogenic prematurity.

The remaining 20% of fetuses that are SGA are intrinsically small secondary to a chromosomal or environmental etiology. Examples include: Fetuses with trisomy 18, cytomegalovirus infection, or fetal alcohol syndrome. These fetuses are less likely to benefit from prenatal intervention, and their prognosis is most closely related to the underlying etiology.

The clinician's challenge is to identify IUGR fetuses whose health is endangered *in utero* because of a hostile intrauterine environment and to monitor and intervene appropriately. This challenge also includes identifying small

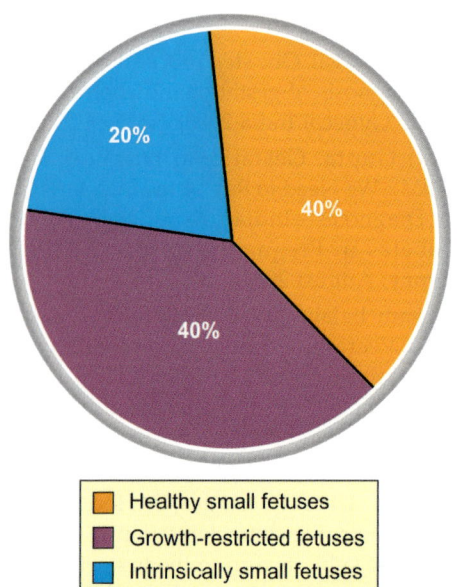

Fig. 10.1: Fetal growth restriction. Distribution of small fetuses

but healthy fetuses and avoiding iatrogenic harm to them or their mothers.

Maternal causes of IUGR (adapted from Severi et al, 2000) include the following:

- Chronic hypertension
- Pregnancy-associated hypertension
- Cyanotic heart disease
- Class F or higher diabetes
- Hemoglobinopathies
- Autoimmune disease
- Protein-calorie malnutrition
- Smoking
- Substance abuse
- Uterine malformations
- Thrombophilias
- Prolonged high-altitude exposure

Placental or umbilical cord causes of IUGR include the following:

- Twin-to-twin transfusion syndrome
- Placental abnormalities
- Chronic abruption
- Placenta previa
- Abnormal cord insertion
- Cord anomalies
- Multiple gestations

IUGR occurs when gas exchange and nutrient delivery to the fetus are not sufficient to allow it to thrive *in utero*. This process can occur primarily because of maternal disease causing decreased oxygen-carrying capacity (e.g., cyanotic heart disease, smoking, hemoglobinopathy), a dysfunctional oxygen delivery system secondary to maternal vascular disease (e.g., diabetes with vascular disease, hypertension, autoimmune disease affecting the vessels leading to the placenta), or placental damage resulting from maternal disease (e.g. smoking, thrombophilia, various autoimmune diseases).

Evaluation of causative factors for intrinsic disorders leading to poor growth may include a fetal karyotype, maternal serology for infectious processes, and an environmental exposure history.

Perinatal Implications

IUGR causes a spectrum of perinatal complications, including fetal morbidity and mortality, iatrogenic prematurity, fetal compromise in labor, need for induction of labor, and cesarean delivery. In a cohort study in Sweden, a 10-fold increase in late fetal deaths was found among very small fetuses. Similarly, Gardosi et al noted in 1998 that nearly 40% of stillborn fetuses that were not malformed were SGA. Fetuses with IUGR who survive the compromised intrauterine environment are at increased risk for neonatal morbidity. Morbidity for neonates with IUGR includes increased rates of necrotizing enterocolitis, thrombocytopenia, temperature instability, and renal failure. These are thought to occur as a result of the alteration of normal fetal physiology in utero.

With limited nutritional reserve, the fetus redistributes blood flow to sustain function and to help in the development of vital organs. This is called the brain-sparing effect and results in increased relative blood flow to the brain, heart, adrenals, and placenta, with diminished relative flow to the bone marrow, muscles, lungs, GI tract, and kidneys. The brain-sparing effect may result in different fetal growth patterns.

In 1977, Campbell and Thoms introduced the idea of symmetric versus asymmetric growth. Symmetrically small fetuses were thought to have some sort of early global insult (e.g. aneuploidy, viral infection, fetal alcohol syndrome). Asymmetrically small fetuses were thought to be more likely small secondary to an imposed restriction in nutrient and gas exchange. Investigators since then have disagreed on the importance of this differentiation. Dashe et al examined this issue among 1364 infants who were SGA (20% were asymmetrically grown, 80% symmetrically grown) and 3873 infants who were in the 25–75th percentile (i.e. appropriate for gestational age). Table 10.1 includes a selected list of statistically significant perinatal outcomes and events among these groups.

Table 10.1: Perinatal events and outcomes

Event	Asymmetrically SGA	Symmetrically SGA	Appropriate for gestational age
Anomalies	14%	4%	3%
Survivors: No serious morbidity	86%	95%	95%
Labor induction (<36 wks)	12%	8%	5%
Intrapartum high blood pressure (<32 wks)	7%	2%	1%
Cesarean delivery for nonreassuring fetal heart rate	15%	8%	3%
Intubated in delivery room	6%	4%	3%
Neonatal ICU admission	18%	9%	7%
Respiratory distress syndrome	9%	4%	3%
Intraventricular hemorrhage (grade III or IV)	2%	<1%	<1%
Neonatal death	2%	1%	1%
Gestational age at delivery	36.6 wk ± 3.5 wks	37.8 wks ± 2.9 wks	37.1 wks ± 3.3 wks
Preterm birth ≤32 wks	14%	6%	11%

The symmetrically grown infants who were SGA had outcomes very similar to the infants who were appropriate for gestational age and very different prognoses than the asymmetrically SGA fetuses, thus reinforcing the concept of using growth parameters for diagnostic and outcome counseling.

Several studies have addressed prognostic factors influencing outcome and have consistently reported that the dominant influence on survival is gestational age at birth. Madazli reported experience with IUGR fetuses with absent end-diastolic flow. No fetus less than 28 weeks' and less than 800 g survived. Madazli also noted that all fetuses with absent end-diastolic flow greater than 31 weeks' survived. The variable period for survival occurred between these gestational ages, with antenatal and neonatal survival rates at 28–31 weeks' of approximately 54%.

The stress that results in IUGR has been postulated to also result in advanced maturation of the fetus, resulting in decreased perinatal morbidity compared with age-matched normally grown neonates. Bernstein et al examined this issue by identifying almost 20,000 white or African American neonates from 196 centers who were born at 25–30 weeks' gestation without major anomalies. They categorized infants as IUGR at less than the 10th percentile using race- and sex-specific growth charts. These results do not support the concept of a stress-related protective effect of IUGR.

Relative risks associated with IUGR using morbidity and mortality parameters, from the study by Bernstein et al, are as follows:
- Relative risk of death, 2.77; 95% confidence interval (CI), 2.31–3.33
- Relative risk of respiratory distress syndrome, 1.19; 95% CI, 1.03–1.29
- Relative risk of intraventricular hemorrhage, 1.13; 95% CI, 0.99–1.29
- Relative risk of severe intravascular hemorrhage, 1.27; 95% CI, 0.98–1.59
- Relative risk of necrotizing enterocolitis, 1.27; 95% CI, 1.05–1.53.

Increasingly, data support the idea that long-term consequences of IUGR last well into adulthood. Several authors have noted that these individuals have a greater predisposition to develop a metabolic syndrome later in life, manifesting as obesity, hypertension, hypercholesterolemia, cardiovascular disease, and type 2 diabetes. Several hypotheses have been proposed to explain this relationship. Hales and Barker proposed the so-called thrifty phenotype in 1992. This idea suggests that intrauterine malnutrition results in insulin resistance, loss of pancreatic beta cell mass, and an adult predisposition to type 2 diabetes.

Other authors found that prepubertal individuals who had IUGR at birth show a greater insulin response than prepubertal individuals who had healthy growth as infants. This suggests that the increased risk of type 2 diabetes in adults who had restriction as infants stems, instead, from increased peripheral insulin resistance allowing the brain-sparing physiology to occur but with a permanent reduction in skeletal-muscle glucose transport. This ultimately results in beta cell burnout. Although the causative pathophysiology is uncertain, the risk of a metabolic syndrome in adulthood is clearly increased among individuals who had IUGR at birth.

Organ system specific morbidity, as a result of growth restriction, is now being evaluated using different animal species and models. Human studies have clearly show organ specific sequelae of IUGR. Kaijser et al, using a large cohort, were able to demonstrate an association between low birth weight and adult risk of ischemic heart disease. Hallan et al demonstrated that adult kidney function is adversely affected by restricted intrauterine growth.

In addition to an increased risk for physical sequelae, mental health problems have been found more commonly in children with growth restriction. In a study performed in Western Australia, Zubrick et al showed that children born below the second percentile for weight were at significant risk for mental health morbidity (odds ratio, 2.9; 95% CI, 1.18–7.12), academic impairment (odds ratio, 6; 95% Cl, 2.25–16.06), and poorer general health (odds ratio, 5.1; 95% Cl, 1.69–15.52).

Specifically, Tideman et al have shown that impaired fetal circulation, as demonstrated by Doppler studies, in association with IUGR, results in worsened cognitive function in adulthood.

Diagnosis and Surveillance

Criteria for Diagnosis of IUGR

For most purposes, an EFW at or below the 10th percentile is used to identify fetuses at risk. Importantly, however, understand that this is not a definitive cut-off for utero-placental insufficiency. A certain number of fetuses at or below the 10th percentile may be constitutionally small. In these cases, short maternal or paternal height, the neonate's ability to maintain growth along a standardized curve, and a lack of other signs of uteroplacental insufficiency (e.g. oligohydramnios, abnormal Doppler findings) can be reassuring to the clinician and parents. Customized growth curves for ethnicity, parental size, and gender are in development so as to improve sensitivity and specificity of diagnosing IUGR.

Importantly, review the dating criteria before offering intervention to treat growth restriction in a fetus. If dates are uncertain or unknown, obtaining a second growth assessment over a 2- to 4-week interval may be of value unless strong supportive data or risk factors warrant an immediate change in management plans.

Screening the Fetus for Growth Restriction

Although no single biometric or Doppler measurement is completely accurate for helping make or exclude the diagnosis of growth restriction, screening for IUGR is important to identify at-risk fetuses. Dependent upon the maternal condition associated with IUGR (see maternal causes of IUGR) patients may undergo serial sonography during their pregnancies. An initial scan may be obtained in the middle of the second trimester (at 18–20 wks) to confirm dates, evaluate for anomalies, and identify multiple gestations. A repeat scan may be scheduled at 28–32 weeks' gestation to assess fetal growth, evidence of asymmetry, and stigmata of brain-sparing physiology (e.g. oligohydramnios, abnormal Doppler findings).

Screening for IUGR in the general population relies on symphysis—fundal height measurements. This is a routine portion of prenatal care from 20 weeks' until term. Although recent studies have questioned the accuracy of fundal height measurements, particularly in obese patients, a discrepancy of greater than 3 cm between observed and expected measurements may prompt a growth evaluation using ultrasound. The clinician should be aware that the sensitivity of fundal height measurement is limited, and he or she should maintain a heightened awareness for potential growth-restricted fetuses. In an unselected hospital population, only 26% of fetuses that were SGA were suggested to be SGA based on clinical examination findings.

One study using fundal height curves that customized for maternal weight, height, and ethnicity was able to increase the detection rate from 29.2% in the control group to 47.9% in the study population. As Yoshida et al indicated, these inaccuracies occur:

1. Because of the limited accuracy of predicting birth weight within 10% using ultrasonography in the third trimester
2. Because not all fetuses that are SGA have IUGR
3. Because individual and unpredictable changes in growth potential occur, and
4. Because growth distribution is a continuum.

Biometry and Amniotic Fluid Volumes

Most ultrasonographic machines report aggregate gestational age measurements and individual parameters. Assessing individual values is important to identify a fetus that is growing asymmetrically. In the presence of normal head and femur measurements, abdominal circumference (AC) measurements

of less than 2 standard deviations below the mean appear to be a reasonable cut-off to consider a fetus asymmetric. Baschat and Weiner showed that a low AC percentile had the highest sensitivity (98.1%) for diagnosing IUGR (birth weight <10th percentile). The sensitivity of EFW (birth weight below the 10th percentile) is 85.7%; however, an AC below the 2.5 percentile had the lowest positive predictive value (36.3%), while a low EFW had a 50% positive predictive value.

Supporting evidence of a hostile intrauterine environment can be obtained by specifically looking at amniotic fluid volumes (AFVs). Chauhan et al found that in a group of normal pregnancies greater than 24 weeks', the rate of IUGR was 19% with an amniotic fluid index (AFI) of less than 5 and 9% with an AFI higher than 5 (odds ratio, 2.13; 95% CI, 1.10–4.16). Banks and Miller also noted a significantly increased risk of IUGR in a group of fetuses with borderline amniotic fluid (AFI of 5–10) relative to a group of normal fetuses (AFI >10) (13% vs 3.6%; rate ratio, 3.9; 95% CI, 1.2–16.2). These results confirm much earlier work by Chamberlain et al.

These authors showed an increased rate of IUGR among fetuses with decreasing maximum vertical pocket (MVP) values. An MVP measurement of larger than 2 cm was associated with an IUGR rate of 5%, an MVP value smaller than 2 cm was associated with an IUGR rate of 20%, and an MVP measurement of smaller than 1 cm was associated with an IUGR rate of 39%. Chamberlain et al concluded that decreased AFI may be an early marker of declining placental function.

Uterine Artery Doppler Measurement

Both arterial Doppler and venous Doppler have been used in recent literature to support expectant management or delivery of IUGR fetuses and to identify fetuses at risk. Doppler velocimetry has been shown to contribute to the identification of fetuses at risk of IUGR. To follow is an overview of the various

Doppler techniques and their clinical applications.

Flow patterns of maternal uterine arteries have been shown to reflect the impact of placentation on maternal circulation. Albaiges et al suggest that a one-stage uterine artery screening at 23 weeks' gestation is effective in identifying pregnancies that will have poor perinatal outcomes prior to 34 weeks' gestation related to uteroplacental insufficiency. In their study of 1751 women who were seen at 23 weeks' gestation for any reason, an abnormal uterine artery study result included bilateral uterine artery notches or a mean pulsatility index (PI) of greater than 1.45 in both arteries.

These criteria were observed in approximately 7% of the population. Within this 7% were 90% of the women who later developed pre-eclampsia and required delivery before 34 weeks' gestation, 70% of women with a fetus below the 10th percentile who required delivery before 34 weeks' gestation, 50% of placental abruptions, and 80% of fetal deaths. Importantly, the negative predictive value for these adverse events prior to 34 weeks' gestation was higher than 99%.

Chien and colleagues conducted an overview of published studies on the efficacy of uterine artery Doppler findings as a predictor of pre-eclampsia, IUGR, and perinatal death. In reports of studies performed on low-risk women, an abnormal uterine artery Doppler result yielded a likelihood ratio (LR) of developing IUGR of 3.6 (95% CI, 3.2–4), while a normal test result reduced the risk to below background, with an LR of 0.8 (95% CI, 0.08–0.09). For women at high risk, an abnormal test result indicated an LR of 2.7 (95% CI, 2.1–3.4), while a normal result reduced the risks by 30% (LR of 0.7; 95% CI, 0.6–0.9).

Although these measurements appear promising, the sensitivity and specificity of uterine artery Doppler measurements is relatively low, because no proven interventions are available to prevent IUGR, uterine artery blood flow measurements are not included in routine surveillance protocols.

Umbilical Artery Doppler Measurement

In normal pregnancies, umbilical artery (UA) resistance shows a continuous decline; however, this may not occur in fetuses with uteroplacental insufficiency. The most commonly used measure of gestational age-specific UA resistance is the systolic-to-diastolic ratio of flow, which changes from a baseline value to an elevated value with worsening disease. As the insufficiency progresses, end-diastolic velocity is lost, and finally, reversed. The clinical significance of this progression has been well-documented by Mandruzzato et al, who reported a significant difference in mean birth weight and perinatal mortality for absent end-diastolic velocity (20%) versus reversed end-diastolic velocity (68%).

The status of UA blood flow corroborates the diagnosis of IUGR and provides early evidence of circulatory abnormalities in the fetus, enabling clinicians to identify the high risk status of these fetuses and to initiate surveillance (see Management and Delivery Planning).

UA Doppler measurements may help the clinician decide whether a small fetus is truly growth restricted.

Baschat and Weiner looked at UA resistance to determine, if it can help improve the accuracy of diagnosing IUGR and help identify a small fetus at risk of chronic hypoxemia. These investigators identified 308 babies greater than 23 weeks' at the time of delivery who had an AC of less than the 2.5 percentile, an EFW of less than the 10th percentile, or both criteria. UA measurements were obtained on all of these fetuses. The positive predictive values of AC alone and EFW alone for the diagnosis of IUGR were 36.6% and 50%, respectively. An elevated UA systolic-to-diastolic ratio yielded a positive predictive value of 53.3% for postnatally confirmed IUGR.

Among all 138 identified fetuses with an elevated UA systolic-to-diastolic ratio, a 10-fold increase occurred in the rate of admission to and the duration of stay in neonatal ICUs and in the frequency and severity of respiratory distress syndrome. Equally importantly, no fetus with normal Doppler measurements was delivered with documented metabolic acidemia.

Middle Cerebral Artery Doppler

Fong and colleagues identified 297 singleton pregnancies in which EFW was below the 10th percentile in anatomically normal fetuses. These investigators studied middle cerebral artery (MCA), renal artery, and UA Doppler findings. They addressed outcomes, including cesarean delivery for fetal distress, cord pH less than or equal to 7.10, and Apgar score less than or equal to 7 at 5 minutes. They concluded that a normal MCA Doppler finding may be useful to help identify small fetuses that are not likely to have a major adverse outcome with a reported negative predictive value of 86%.

Hershkovitz et al also looked at MCA Doppler finds in small fetuses. They found that those fetuses with abnormal MCA study results had earlier deliveries, lower birth weights, fewer vaginal deliveries, and increased admissions to neonatal ICUs. Importantly, only 7 of 16 fetuses with Doppler evidence of brain-sparing physiology had elevated UA Doppler findings. This emphasized the possible presence of a gradient in the degree of fetal redistribution and that when performing Doppler studies, evaluating only the UAs may not be sufficient.

Specific MCA Doppler changes were evaluated by Mari et al. They specifically evaluated MCA peak systolic velocity (PSV) and pulsatility index (PI) in growth-restricted fetuses that were longitudinally evaluated. They found that while an abnormal PI preceded an abnormal PSV, the PI demonstrated an inconsistent pattern. MCA-PSV, however, consistently showed an increase in blood velocity and immediately prior to demise, a decrease. They concluded that MCA-PSV is a better predictor of IUGR-associated perinatal mortality than any other single measurement.

Venous Doppler Waveforms

Venous Doppler has been measured at the ductus venosus (DV), umbilical vein (UV), inferior vena cava (IVC), and 7 other sites. This provides information about fetal cardiovascular and respiratory responses to its intrauterine environment. These measurements have been reported to become consistently abnormal when a fetus is severely compromised, thus providing evidence in support of an expedited delivery. Bilardo et al completed a prospective study of the cardiotocography, UA, and DV values of 70 IUGR fetuses and their outcomes. They reported that only the DV measurements consistently predicted adverse perinatal outcomes from 0–7 days prior to delivery. While the optimal vessel for use for venous Doppler evaluations has not been identified, the knowledge gained from these measurements may provide additional information for the timing of delivery, especially in extremely premature (<32 wks) gestations.

Three-dimensional Ultrasonography

With the introduction and use of obstetrical 3-dimensional ultrasonography, many new applications for this technology are constantly explored. The use of these techniques in the evaluation of the growth-restricted fetus has been evaluated as well. As fetal femur dysplasia is associated with IUGR, Chang et al used 3-dimensional ultrasonography to measure fetal femur volume as a predictor of IUGR. They found a 10th percentile femur volume threshold, which differentiates growth-restricted fetuses from normal fetuses.

Using this technique, they obtained a sensitivity of 71.4%, specificity of 94.1%, positive predictive value of 62.5%, negative predictive value of 96.0%, and accuracy of 91.3% in prediction of growth restriction. As a single biometric measurement, fetal femur volume is better in prediction of growth restriction than fetal AC and biparietal diameter. Chang et al also evaluated 3-dimensional ultrasonographic measurement of fetal humerus volume in evaluation of IUGR. Again, a 10th percentile humerus volume threshold was found to differentiate growth-restricted fetuses from normal fetuses.

Therapeutic Options

Although multiple therapeutic strategies have been tested to promote intrauterine growth and decrease perinatal morbidity and mortality, limited, if any, success has been achieved in this area. Gülmezoglu et al reported results of meta-analyses of studies, the goals of which were to treat impaired growth. In this review, 3 interventions were shown to be helpful. First, behavioral strategies to quit smoking result in a lower rate of low birth weight in babies at term among mothers who smoke. Second, balanced nutritional supplements in undernourished women and magnesium and folate supplementation (in some studies) decrease the rate of SGA newborns. Third, if malaria is the etiologic agent, maternal treatment of malaria can increase fetal growth.

Pollack et al additionally examined in-hospital bedrest as a way to promote fetal growth and found no improvement. Newnham et al studied women receiving 100 mg of aspirin versus placebo after a diagnosis of IUGR based on abnormal UA Doppler findings, and they did not find a clinically significant difference.

Other options have been considered with a goal of decreasing perinatal morbidity and mortality. In 2003, Say et al reviewed maternal estrogen administration, maternal hyper-oxygenation, and maternal nutrient supplementation as therapies for suspected impaired fetal growth. They concluded that evidence to evaluate the risks and benefits of these therapies was lacking. However, they did suggest that further trials of maternal hyperoxygenation seem warranted.

Additional therapies that have been proposed and may warrant further study are maternal hemodilution and intermittent abdominal negative pressure. These are also poorly studied, carry potential maternal and fetal harm, and should be considered experimental.

The only intervention that has been shown to decrease neonatal morbidity and mortality is the administration of steroids to premature fetuses when delivery is anticipated. Bernstein et al described the effect of maternal prenatal glucocorticoid administration in growth-restricted fetuses and found the benefits to be similar to those found in gestational age-matched, normally grown fetuses.

Odds ratio reduction with steroids, from Bernstein et al, is as follows:

- Relative risk of death, 0.54; 95% CI, 0.48–0.62
- Relative risk of respiratory distress syndrome, 0.51; 95% CI, 0.44–0.58
- Relative risk of intraventricular hemorrhage, 0.67; 95% CI, 0.61–0.73
- Relative risk of severe intravascular hemorrhage, 0.5; 95% CI, 0.43–0.57
- Relative risk of necrotizing enterocolitis, no difference noted.

Recently, several studies have questioned the metabolic and cardiovascular response of IUGR fetuses to maternal glucocorticoid administration. Simchen et al performed a prospective longitudinal study of chromosomally normal IUGR fetuses at 24–34 weeks' with absent or reversed end-diastolic flow. They found a divergent response between the 2 groups of fetuses as measured by UA Doppler. Almost 45% of these fetuses had transient improvement in their Doppler waveforms, and these fetuses had significantly better outcomes than their counterparts who had no improvement of their waveforms, even transiently. These authors suggest that daily Doppler-based monitoring after the administration of steroids can help delineate a group of fetuses at extremely high risk of acidosis and mortality. They also suggest that further work is needed to elucidate the efficacy of steroids versus immediate delivery in this very high-risk subset of IUGR fetuses.

Management and Delivery Planning

Once IUGR has been detected, the management of the pregnancy should depend on a surveillance plan that maximizes gestational age while minimizing the risks of neonatal morbidity and mortality. This should include steroid administration when at all feasible, based on the monitoring and delivery strategies discussed below (see image below and Harman and Baschat's integrated fetal testing for IUGR). Fetal lung maturity studies by amniocentesis, in fetuses greater than 34 weeks', may additionally influence delivery timing.

The goal in the management of IUGR, because no effective treatments are known, is to deliver the most mature fetus in the best physiological condition possible while minimizing the risk to the mother. Such a goal requires the use of antenatal testing with the hope of identifying the fetus with IUGR before it becomes acidotic. Developing a testing scheme, following it, and having a high index of suspicion in this population when results of testing are abnormal is important. The positive predictive value of an abnormal antenatal test result in fetuses with IUGR is relatively high because the prevalence of acidemia and chronic hypoxemia is relatively high.

Although numerous protocols have been suggested for antenatal monitoring of IUGR fetuses, the mainstay includes a weekly nonstress test (NST). Additional modalities may include amniotic fluid volume determination, biophysical profiles, and/or Doppler assessments. Other more complex protocols have been proposed. The protocol for antenatal testing suggested by Kramer and Weiner (Fig. 10.2) is one example. It relies heavily on the use of UA Doppler testing because severely abnormal Doppler findings (absent or reversed end-diastolic flow) can precede an abnormal fetal heart rate by several weeks. Harman and Baschat suggested a different proposed antenatal testing strategy. This protocol integrates multiple venous and arterial Doppler measurements and the

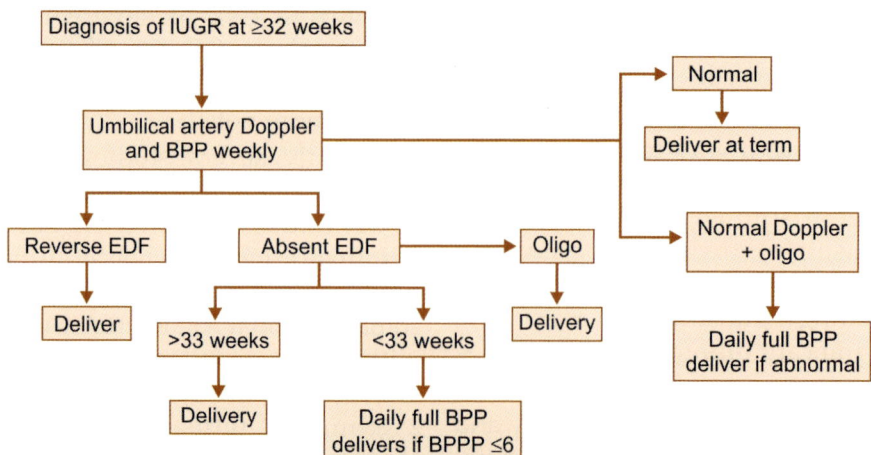

Fig. 10.2: Management of IUGR ≥32 weeks

biophysical profile score (BPS); this strategy may be used at institutions where these measurements are routinely obtained by qualified technicians.

Fetal growth restriction. Sample protocol for antenatal testing for intrauterine growth restriction at 32 weeks' gestation or after. IUGR is intrauterine growth restriction, BPP is biophysical profile, and EDF is end-diastolic flow.

Harman and Baschat's integrated fetal testing for IUGR, in increasing order of severity from 1 (least severe) to 5 (most severe), is as follows:

Situation 1

- Test results—AC less than fifth percentile, low AC growth rate, high ratio of head circumference to AC; BPS greater than or equal to 8 and AFV normal; abnormal UV and/or cerebroplacental ratio; normal MCA.
- Interpretation—IUGR diagnosed, asphyxia extremely rare, increased risk for intrapartum distress.
- Recommended management—intervention for obstetric or maternal factors only, weekly BPS, multivessel Doppler every 2 weeks.

Situation 2

- Test results—IUGR criteria met, BPS greater than or equal to 8, AFV normal, UA with absent or reversed end-diastolic velocities, decreased MCA.
- Interpretation—IUGR with brain sparing, hypoxemia possible and asphyxia rare, at risk for intrapartum distress.
- Recommended management—Intervention for obstetric or maternal factors only; BPS 3 times a week; weekly UA, MCA, and venous Doppler.

Situation 3

- Test results—IUGR with low MCA PI; oligohydramnios; BPS greater than or equal to 6; normal IVC, DV, and UV flow.

- Interpretation—IUGR with significant brain sparing, onset of fetal compromise, hypoxemia common, acidemia/asphyxia possible.
- Recommended management—if at more than 34 weeks' gestation, deliver (route determined by obstetric factors). If at less than 34 weeks' gestation, administer steroids to achieve lung maturity and repeat all testing in 24 hours.

Situation 4

- Test results—IUGR with brain sparing, oligohydramnios, BPS greater than or equal to 6, increased IVC and DV indices, UV flow normal.
- Interpretation—IUGR with brain sparing, proven fetal compromise, hypoxemia common, acidemia/asphyxia likely.
- Recommended management—If at more than 34 weeks' gestation, deliver [route determined by obstetric factors and oxytocin challenge test (OCT) results]. If at less than 34 weeks' gestation, individualize treatment with admission, continuous cardiotocography, steroids, maternal oxygen, and/or amnioinfusion and then repeat all testing up to 3 times a day depending on status.

Situation 5

- Test results—IUGR with accelerating compromise, BPS less than or equal to 6, abnormal IVC and DV indices, pulsatile UV flow.
- Interpretation—IUGR with decompensation, cardiovascular instability, hypoxemia certain, acidemia/asphyxia common, high perinatal mortality, death imminent.
- Recommended management—if fetus is considered viable by size, deliver as soon as possible at tertiary center. Route determined by obstetric factors and OCT results. Fetus requires highest level of natal ICU care.

The diagnosis of severe IUGR before 32 weeks' gestation is associated with a poor prognosis, and therapy must be highly individualized. Once a decision has been made to effect delivery, the mode of delivery is governed by evidence of acidemia, gestational age, and Bishop score. Cesarean delivery without a trial of labor may be appropriate (i) in the presence of evidence of fetal distress by nonstress testing or reversed diastolic flow or (ii) for traditional obstetrical indications for cesarean delivery (i.e. mal-presentation, prior cesarean delivery).

Li, et al investigated the success rate of induction of labor in IUGR fetuses with and without UA blood flow changes and the neonatal outcomes of induced fetuses with a negative result after an OCT. They found that fetuses with abnormal (but not absent or reversed) UA blood flow who had a normal OCT result had similar success in induction of labor, without indications of detrimental fetal hypoxia or distress. This suggests that in fetuses with altered UA blood flow, an OCT may be appropriate to select fetuses that will tolerate labor induction.

When a trial of labor is undertaken, continuous heart rate monitoring should optimize the success of the induction.

Future Directions and Prevention

Prevention of IUGR is highly desirable, and several studies have addressed this potential. Investigators have looked at altering the thromboxane-to-prostacyclin ratio by administering aspirin with or without dipyridamole to mothers of fetuses with IUGR. The studies examining these agents for prevention of IUGR are difficult to compare. Different doses of aspirin, different times of administration in pregnancy, and different indications for use make comparisons difficult; however, the following is a summary of the studies:

- Wallenburg, et al studied a population of women at high risk for IUGR in a non-randomized trial using historic controls.

They noted a decline in the rate of IUGR from 61.5% in the historic controls to 13.3% in those treated with aspirin and dipyridamole.

- Sibai, et al studied low-risk nulliparous women in a double-blinded, placebo-controlled, randomized trial. Patients were treated from weeks 13–26 with either placebo or 60 mg/d of aspirin. This study showed a small decrease in the rate of pre-eclampsia but not IUGR (4.6% vs 5.8% in controls), at the risk of increased chance of abruption.

- In the Essai pre-eclampsia dipyridamole aspirin (EPREDA) randomized controlled trial, high-risk patients received placebo, aspirin only, or aspirin plus dipyridamole. No difference in the rate of IUGR was found between those receiving aspirin alone and those receiving aspirin plus dipyridamole. The control rate of IUGR was 26%; in the 2 groups receiving aspirin with or without dipyridamole, the rate was 13%.

- In an Italian study, women considered to be at moderate risk of IUGR or pregnancy-induced hypertension at 16–32 weeks' gestation were randomly assigned to receive either 50 mg aspirin or no treatment. No difference in any outcome studied was found between the 2 groups.

- Harrington et al identified patients with abnormal uterine artery Doppler findings at 20 weeks' gestation. Participants were started on aspirin, and therapy was discontinued at 24 weeks' if repeat Doppler results normalized. No difference in the rate of fetuses that were SGA below the 10th or third percentile was found between the treated and control groups.

- Trudinger et al performed a double-blinded, randomized clinical trial using 150 mg of aspirin in pregnant women with abnormal UA Doppler findings. The result was an increase in birth weight of 516 g and an increase in placental weight.

- The Collaborative Low-dose Aspirin Study in Pregnancy trial, which investigated both prevention and treatment of IUGR, showed no change in the rate of IUGR in treated and control patients with the administration of 60 mg of aspirin.
- Leitich et al performed a meta-analysis of 13 trials in which women were enrolled for prophylactic aspirin therapy. In women treated, the odds ratio for IUGR was 0.82 (95% Cl, 0.66–1.08). Among those trials in which women were hypertensive or had other risk factors, the risk of IUGR was clearly decreased. Leitich et al found that beginning 100–150 mg/d of aspirin at less than 17 weeks' gestation decreased the rate of IUGR by approximately 65% and the rate of perinatal mortality by approximately 60%.
- The disproportionate intrauterine growth intervention trial at term (DIGITAT) suggests that women who have had a previous singleton pregnancy beyond 36 weeks' gestation can safely choose expectant management with intensive maternal and fetal monitoring if induction is not wanted. Choosing induction to prevent neonatal morbidity or stillbirth is reasonable.

Despite the theoretical benefit of aspirin in many studies, the role of aspirin, if any, in the prevention of IUGR is still unclear. A large randomized controlled trial using a standardized high risk population with a standardized treatment regimen could serve to better answer this question.

Conclusion

IUGR remains a challenging problem for clinicians. Most cases of IUGR occur in pregnancies in which no risk factors are present; therefore, the clinician must be alert to the possibility of a growth disturbance in all pregnancies. No single measurement helps secure the diagnosis; thus, a complex strategy for diagnosis and assessment is necessary. The ability to diagnose the disorder and understand its pathophysiology still outpaces the ability to prevent or treat its complications. The current therapeutic goals are to optimize the timing of delivery to minimize hypoxemia and maximize gestational age and maternal outcome. Further study may elucidate preventive or treatment strategies to assist the growth-restricted fetus.

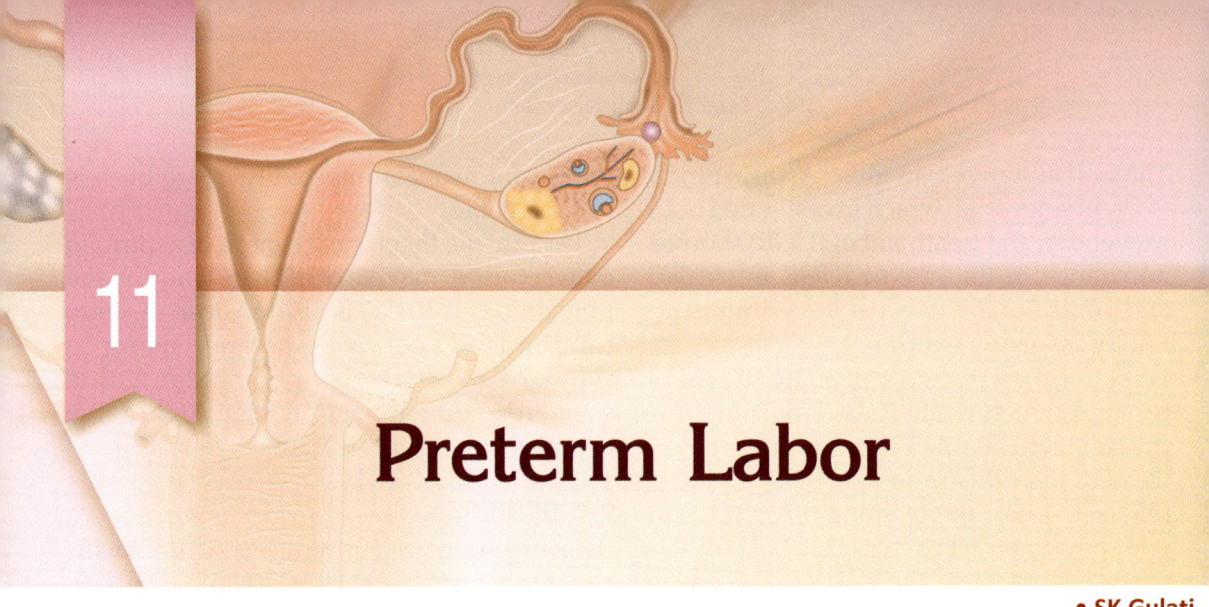

11

Preterm Labor

• SK Gulati

Definition

Preterm labor is *defined as* initiation of regular, palpable uterine contractions with increasing frequency and intensity, associated with progressive cervical changes in effacement and dilatation during the gestation between 20–37 weeks.

HERRON'S[1] CRITERIA OF PRETERM LABOR

Uterine contraction should last longer than 30 seconds and occur at least four times per 20 min or eight in one hour and cervical changes of dilatation of at least 2 cm and effacement of cervix at least 80%.

Threatened Preterm Labor

Onset of uterine contractions between 20 and 37 weeks of gestation without any cervical changes. In 80% of women with threatened preterm labor, preterm delivery will not occur.

Incidence: The incidence of preterm delivery varies between 5% and 11% (Andrews et al. 2000)[2] in developed countries and 25% in developing countries and 2/3 of preterm labors occur between 34 and 37 weeks.

In the past 20 to 30 years, there has been an increase in preterm delivery rates in most of developed countries (Craig, et al. 2002)[3] largely as a result of:

1. More and more high risk mothers are daring to get pregnant
2. Increased incidences of multiple pregnancy due to IVF.
3. An increasing trend towards elective preterm delivery (iatrogenic) as neonatal intensive care has improved.

In 2008 (the latest year for which data are currently available), the overall preterm birth rate in the United States was 12.3%. (Mathews et al.)[4] This represents a 35% increase in overall preterm births over the past 25 year.

Type of Preterm Labor Clinically

1. Spontaneous preterm labor—40–45%
2. Indicated/induced preterm labor—30–35%
3. Preterm rupture of membranes—30–35% (Goldenberg and colleagues, 2008).[4]

Etiology

The causation of preterm delivery is multifactorial and comprises a complex interaction of previous obstetric history, sociodemographic risk factors and obstetric complications in the pregnancy.

Iatrogenic

A significant and increasing number of preterm deliveries are iatrogenic, especially in the developed world where they may account for as many as 30% of all preterm births (Olsen et al. 1995).[5] Clinicians will elect to undertake preterm delivery if it is felt that continuation of the pregnancy is a greater risk to the life or health of the mother or fetus. Maternal conditions commonly causing such a decision to be considered would include severe pre-eclampsia or eclampsia; major obstetric hemorrhage; chorioamnionitis; and severe or deteriorating maternal cardiac, respiratory or renal disease. Preterm delivery may also be necessary for any fetal condition that is deteriorating, and for which early delivery would confer benefit, either by removing the fetus from an adverse intrauterine environment (e.g. infection) or by allowing treatment of the condition only possible *ex utero*. Such complications that may necessitate preterm delivery include rhesus isoimmunization, severe IUGR, and any other evidence of fetal compromise, e.g. abnormal fetal heart rate.

Idiopathic

A large variety of etiological factors have been implicated but in majority of cases no definite cause is found. Approximately one half of all preterm births are idiopathic with no recognized precipitating factor.

Genetics

Genetic factors influence preterm birth. A family history of preterm birth is a key risk factor, such that women whose mothers and sisters have had a preterm delivery are more likely to enter labor prematurely. A small but significant association also links the paternal genome to preterm labor; this is probably because of the influence of paternally contributed fetal genes, as demonstrated by segregation analyses and twin studies.

Maternal Factors

1. *Medical disorders:* Pre-eclampsia, anemia and malnutrition.
2. *Antepartum hemorrhage:* Placenta praevia— abruptio placentae.
3. *Uterine anomalies:* Septate uterus, incompetent cervix, fibroid uterus.
4. Psychological or hormonal.
5. *Infections:* Genital bacterial vaginosis (BV), group B Streptococcus, Chlamydia, Mycoplasma's intrauterine ascending (from genital tract), transplacental (blood-borne), transfallopian (intraperitoneal), iatrogenic (invasive procedures), extra-uterine pyelonephritis, malaria, typhoid fever, pneumonia and asymptomatic bacteriuria.

Fetal Factors

Congenital anomalies, polyhydramnios, multiple pregnancy, Rh-isoimmunization and premature rupture of membranes.

Reproductive Factors

Previous preterm delivery, previous pPROM, previous miscarriage/abortion, short inter-pregnancy interval.

Sociodemographic Factors

Primiparity, poor antenatal weight gain/low maternal weight, low or high maternal age, lack of social support, low socioeconomic status, substance abuse, environmental pollution.

Biology of Preterm Labor

Romero et al (1997)[6] propose that the fundamental difference between term and preterm labor is that the term labor results from physiological activation of the components of a common terminal pathway, while preterm labor results from disease processes activating one or more of the components of common terminal pathway (Fig. 11.1).

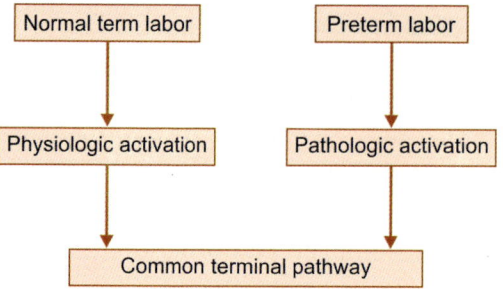

Fig. 11.1: Type of activation for common terminal pathway for term and preterm labor

Common terminal pathways of term and preterm labor are:

1. Increased myometrial contractility
2. Cervical ripening (dilatation and effacement)
3. Decidual/membrane activation

Physiologic activation of term labor: We all understand the role of estrogen, progesterone, oxytocin. Prostaglandins, relaxin and corticotropin-releasing hormone.

Pathologic activation of preterm labor: Preterm labor is a pathological condition with multiple etiologies and has recently been termed the preterm parturition syndrome. This has various:

- Risk factors which have been discussed in etiology
- Probable causes

Probable Causes of Preterm Parturition Syndrome

1. ***Uterine distension*** (multifetal gestation or hydramnios): Early uterine distension initiate expression of contraction associated protein (CAP) in myometrium which increases the gap junction, that in turn causes premature loss of myometrial quiescence. Uterine distension also causes early cervical changes.
2. ***Maternal-fetal stress:*** Studies show correlation between maternal psychological stress and placental-adrenal endocrine axis leading to stress-induced preterm birth. It has been observed that women who are destined for preterm labor has rise in CRH level 2 to 6 weeks before parturition.
3. a. ***Intrauterine infections:*** There is a strong correlation between infection within the uterus and the onset of spontaneous preterm labor. Infection within the uterus has the potential to activate all of the biochemical pathways ultimately leading to cervical ripening and uterine contractions. Intrauterine infections (both clinically evident and subclinical) are associated with increased amniotic fluid concentrations of proinflammatory cytokines. In addition to culture-proven intrauterine infection, there may be an "intrauterine inflammatory response syndrome" that could account for cases preterm labor in which no infectious organism can be identified.

   b. ***Extrauterine infection:*** Generalized maternal infections such as pyelonephritis (Lang et al 1996)[7], and malaria (Luxemburger et al 2001)[8] remain relatively common antecedents of preterm delivery, and timely anti-microbial treatment usually reduces the risk.

4. ***Cytokines:*** Perhaps the area of most recent interest and potential diagnostic usefulness has been the role of cytokines in preterm labor. It has been demonstrated that a variety of cytokines are detectable in amniotic fluid and an increased production of many of these cytokines is observed in association with intrauterine infection. These would include: IL-1, IL-2, IL-6, IL-8, tumor necrosis factor-α (TNF-α), and granulocyte-macrophage colony stimulating factor (GM-CSF) (Keelan et al).[9] There are now numerous studies to demonstrate that, in amniotic fluid, IL-6 is a reliable index of intrauterine infection and its levels are increased and can predict preterm labor in these cases. TNF-α would seem to be second most important in terms of studies performed and its use as an indication of infections (Baud O et al),[10] (Romero R et al).[11]

Prediction of Preterm Labor

Can we predict preterm labor?

A number of scoring systems has been proposed combining various risk factors but their clinical utility is poor. The two most promising markers currently available are ultrasound assessment of cervical length and fetal fibronectin levels.

1. *Fetal fibronectin (fFN):* It is an extracellular glycoprotein secreted by the chorionic tissue at maternal-fetal interface. It is present in amniotic fluid, placental tissue and decidua basalis. It acts as a biological glue which binds blastocyst to endometrium interface. It can be normally present in cervicovaginal secretions up to 20–22 wks. Around 22 wks chorion fuses completely with underlying decidua. This prevents fibronectin to leak into the vaginal secretions any further, until at term, a few weeks before labor when cervix dilates or membranes rupture. Therefore presence of fFN between 24 and 34 wks can provide important marker of preterm labor. However, in women experiencing preterm uterine activity, a negative test reduces the likelihood of delivery within 7–10 days of presentation from 3% to less than 1%; a positive test increases the likelihood of delivery within 7–10 days from 3 to 14% (Honest et al 2002).[12] A negative test therefore implies a low risk for delivery in the near future and might form the basis for withholding interventions with subsequent reductions in hospital admissions, inter-hospital transfers and costs (Joffe et al 1999).[13] A cut-off of 50 ng/ml is considered positive. Swabs can be taken from ectocervix or post-vaginal fornix. ELISA with FDC-6 monoclonal antibody is used to detect fetal fibronectin.

2. *Cervical length:* When compared with digital examination, transabdominal scanning, transperineal and TVS, trans-vaginal ultrasound has a higher sensitivity for the detection of cervical shortening (Iams et al 1996),[14] (Berghella et al 1997).[15]

   a. *Length of cervix (TVS):* ACOG recommend TVS at 22 weeks and if cervical length is less than 25 mm between 20 and 28 weeks POG there is increased risk of preterm labor and reduction in cervical length >06 mm between two ultrasound have higher risk of preterm delivery (Figs 11.2 and 11.3). Funneling (internal os diameter >05 mm) is also independent risk factor.

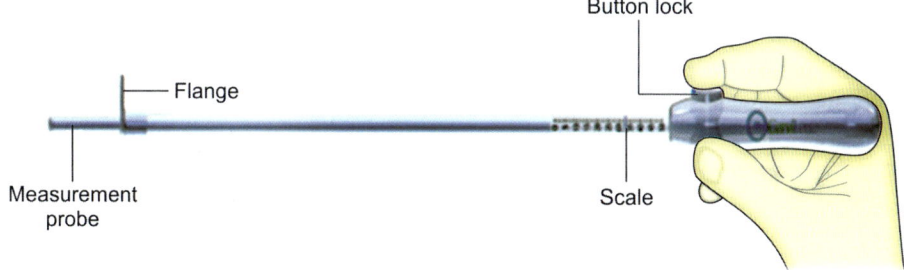

Fig. 11.2: Measuring cervical length by CerviLenz

Approaches for the prevention of preterm birth		
Component	*Test*	*Treatment*
Myometrium	Uterine monitoring	Tocolysis
Cervix	Ultrasound	Cervical circlage
Decidua/ membranes	Fetal fibronectin	Antibiotics

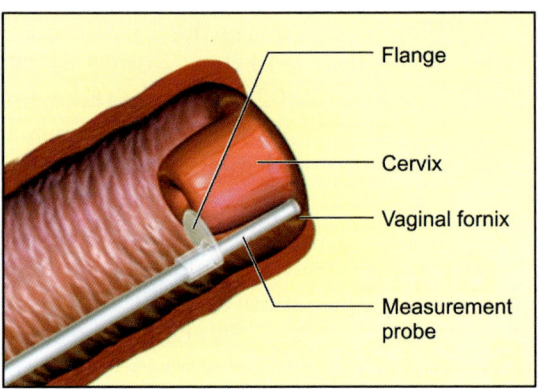

Fig. 11.3: Measuring cervical length with CerviLenz

b. *CerviLenz:* A simple new device, called *CerviLenz*, can provide a reliable cervical length measurement during prenatal visit without ultrasound (Moller M et al).[16]

Research has shown good correlation between CerviLenz and transvaginal ultrasound.

Importance of predictive tests: When fibronectin is negative and cervical length by transvaginal ultrasound is 2.5 cm and above than tocolytic therapy should be withheld.

Prevention of Preterm Birth

Recent reports, suggest that prevention in selected populations may be achievable.

- Interventions have been aimed at general improvement in nutrition, rest, discourage cigarette smoking, and psycological support.
- Adequate antenatal care including supplementation of iron, folic acid, calcium and protein.
- *Antibiotis:* Only proven beneficial strategy is eradication of asymptomatic bacteriuria and bacterial vaginosis in preventing preterm labor.
- *Progesterone:* On February 3, 2011, the US Food and Drug Administration (FDA)[17] approved the use of progesterone supplementation (hydroxyprogesterone caproate) during pregnancy to reduce the risk of recurrent preterm birth in women with a history of at least one prior spontaneous preterm delivery.

ACOG committee opinion on use of progesterone to reduce preterm birth

a. *Progesterone for women with prior h/o preterm births:* Weekly intramuscular injections of 17-hydroxyprogesterone caproate were given from 16 to 36 weeks. (Approved by FDA). Rates of preterm delivery significantly reduced by giving progestrone (Meis and colleagues, 2003).[18]

b. *Progesterone for women with sonographically short cervices 15–25 mm:* Cervical shortening is a known risk factor for preterm birth in both low and high risk populations (Fonseca EB et al).[19] 200 mg micronized progesterone vaginal suppositories from 24 to 34 weeks significantly reduced spontaneous delivery before 34 weeks (Hassan SS et al).[20]

Cervical Encerclage

Three circumstances when cerclage placement may be used to prevent preterm birth.

a. *History indicated:* History of recurrent mid-trimester losses and who are diagnosed with an incompetent cervix.

b. *Sonographically indicated:* Women have a short cervix <15 mm on sonographic examination.

c. *Physical examination indicated* (rescue cerclage): "Rescue" cerclage, done in emergency when cervical incompetence is recognized in the women with preterm labor.

Diagnosis of Preterm Labor

1. Uterine contractions should have:
   a. Frequency every 10 minutes or less,
   b. Duration at least 30 seconds, and
   c. Continue for at least one hour.
2. Uterine contractions of whatever the frequency and duration but with:
   a. Rupture membranes,

b. Effacement 80% or more, and

c. Cervical dilatation 2 cm or more.

In addition to painful or painless uterine contractions, symptoms such as pelvic pressure, menstrual-like cramps, watery vaginal discharge, and lower back pain have been empirically associated with impending preterm birth. Such complaints are thought by some to be common in normal pregnancy and are therefore often dismissed by patients, clinicians.

Management of Preterm Labor

Management objectives are:

a. Early diagnosis of preterm labor

b. Identify the cause of preterm labor—treat the underlying cause when possible

c. Attempt to arrest labor when appropriate

d. Intervene to minimize neonatal morbidity and mortality.

Management

1. *Bedrest:* To reduce the mechanical stimuli from the pressure of the presenting part on the lower uterine segment.

2. Hydration with a rapid IV infusion of 0.9% NaCl (normal saline) in a rate of 120 ml/hour. This will decrease the release of oxytocins as well as antidiuretic hormone from the posterior pituitary.

3. *Sedation:* With diazepam

4. *Tocolysis*

   Aim of tocolysis

   a. Primary aims of tocolytic therapy

      i. To delay delivery to allow the administration of a complete course of antepartum glucocorticosteroids in order to primarily reduce the incidence and severity of idiopathic respiratory distress syndrome.

      ii. To arrange *in utero transfer* to a center with neonatal intensive care unit facilities.

   b. Secondary aim of tocolytic therapy is to delay delivery to reduce the perinatal mortality and morbidity associated with severe prematurity.

- Before you start tocolysis, if time permits, an ultrasound scan should be done to check for fetal viability, fetal morphology, fetal number, fetal presentation, placental site, an estimate of fetal weight and amniotic fluid volume index because all of which might affect the management.

Tocolytic Drugs

a. The following drugs shows some evidences for efficacy but with high maternal side effects hence used with cautions. Beta-agonists: Ritodrine, terbutaline and isoxsuprine.

   PG synthetase inhibitors: Indomethacin, nitroglycerin and $MgSO_4$.

b. The following drugs are more effective and safe as tocolytics: Calcium-channel blockers (nifedipine) and oxytocin antagonist (atosiban).

   i. *Nifedipine:* Many investigators have concluded that calcium-channel blockers, especially nifedipine, is safer and more effective tocolytic than other available tocolytics agents.[21-23] Calcium channel blockers are able to prolong the pregnancy for 3.83 days on an average. Nifedipine to be considered as first-line tocolytic agent as incidences of neonatal respiratory distress syndrome, necrotizing enterocolitis, intraventricular hemorrhage and neonatal jaundice were reduced. Nifedipine has recently been included as an anti-oxytocic in the WHO model of list of essential medicines.[24] Nifedipine—doses 20–30 mg stat followed by 10–20 mg 06 hourly.

   ii. *Atosiban:* Oxytocin antagonist inhibits the activity of oxytocin on uterus. Licenced in Europe, where this drug is widely used as a first-line treatment as tocolytic. Delay in delivery occurs up to 07 days. Dose—6.75 mg IV bolus over 1 minute, 18 mg/hr in infusion for 03 hrs, 06 mg/hr for

45 hrs, duration of treatment should not exceed 48 hrs. Total dose given during a full course should preferably not exceed 330 mg of atosiban.[25,26]

- Maintenance tocolysis is not recommended for routine practice.
- Contraindication of tocolysis

Absolute contraindications *includes clinically* apparent intrauterine infection, congenital malformation, fulminating pre-eclampsia urgent fetomaternal indication for delivery.

Relative contraindications are those in which a debate exists about the risks and benefits of intervention such as antepartum hemorrhage, ruptured membranes, intrauterine growth restriction, insulin-dependent diabetes, multiple pregnancy.

Role of Corticosteroids

Corticosteroids for fetal lung maturation: American College of Obstetricians and Gynecologists[27] recommend single course of corticosteroids therapy from 24 to 34 weeks period of gestation.

Single versus weekly corticosteroids: Weekly repeated courses of corticosteroids can cause increase incidences of cerebral palsy, maternal and neonatal infection, adrenal suppression, impaired glucose tolerance hence single course of corticosteroids therapy recommended.

Which corticosteroid: Betamethasone versus dexamethasone.

Previous observational data indicated that betamethasone has decreased the incidence of periventricular leukomalacia compared with dexamethasone, so betamethasone was preferred till recently. Elimian and co-workers (2007)[28] did randomized double-blinded trial study (betamethasone versus dexamethasone), which included 299 women between 24 and 33 weeks period of gestation and found these two drugs were comparable in reducing the rates of major neonatal morbidities in preterm infants.

Doses: Inj betamethasone two doses 12 mg IM 24 hours apart and inj dexamethasone four doses 6 mg IM 12 hrs apart.[29]

Evidence does not support the use of inj vit K and phenobarbital prior to preterm birth.

Conclusion

The clinical importance of preterm labor dictates us that we should understand the *biology of preterm labor* and its diagnostic usefulness. Future should give us more options and hopefully better choices to predict and manage the preterm labor. We would expect to see CRH as possible test to predict the labor. Another promising test to predict preterm labor is interleukin-6 and TNF-α. Future of preterm labor treatment will probably revolve around anticytokine therapy.

References

1. Herron MA , Katz M, Creasy RK. Evaluation or preterm birth prevention program. Preliminary report. Obstet Gynaecol, 1982;59:452–6.
2. Andrews WW, Goldenberg RL, Mercer B, et al. The Preterm Prediction Study: association of second-trimester genitourinary Chlamydia infection with subsequent spontaneous preterm birth. Am. J. Obstet. Gynecol. 2000a;183:662–8.
3. Craig ED, Thompson JM and Mitchell EA (2002). Socioeconomic status and preterm birth: New Zealand trends, 1980 to 1999. Arch. Dis. Child. Fetal Neonatal Ed. 86.
4. Mathews TJ, Miniño AM, Osterman MJ, et al. Annual summary of vital statistics: 2008. Pediatrics 2011;127:146–57. [PubMed]
5. Olsen P, Laara E, Rantakillio P, et al. Epidemiology of preterm delivery in two birth cohorts with an interval of 20 years. Am. J. Epidemiol 1995;142: 1184–93, 21.
6. Romero R, Avela C, Brehies CA, et al. The role of systemic and intrauterine infection in preterm parturition. Ann NY Acad Sci 1991;622:355–75.
7. Lang JM, Lieberman E, Cohen A. A comparison of risk factors for preterm labor and term small-for-gestational-age birth. Epidemiology 1996;7: 369–76.
8. Luxemburger C, McGready R, Kham A, et al. Effects of malaria during pregnancy on infant mortality in an area of low malaria transmission. Am. J. Epidemiol. 2001;154, 459–65.

9. Keelan JA, Coleman M, Mitchell UD. The molecular mechanisms of term and preterm labor: Recent progress and clinical implications. Clin Obstet Gynecol, 1997;40:460–78, 43.

10. Baud O, Emilie D, Pelletier E, et al. Amniotic fluid concentrations of interleukin-1 beta, interleukin-6 and TNF-alpha in chorioamnionitis before 32 weeks of gestation: Histological associations and neonatal outcome. Br J Obstet Gynaecol. 1999;106:72–77.

11. Romero R, Mazor M, Sepulveda W, et al. Tumor necrosis factor in preterm and term labor. Am J Obstet Gynecol 1992;166:1576–87.

12. Honest H, Bachmann LM, Gupta JK, Kleijnen J and Khan KS. Accuracy of cervicovaginal fetal fibronectin test in predicting risk of spontaneous preterm birth systematic review. BMJ 2002;325, 301–4.

13. Joffe GM, Jacques D, Bemis-Heyes R, et al. Impact of the fetal fibronectin assay on admissions for preterm labor. Am. J. Obstet. Gynecol. 1999;180: 581–6.

14. Iams JD, Goldenberg RL, Meis PJ, et al. The length of the cervix and the risk of spontaneous preterm delivery. N. Engl. J. Med. 1996;334:567–72.

15. Berghella V, Tolosa JE, Kuhlman K, et al. Cervical ultrasonography compared with manual examination as a predictor of preterm delivery. Am. J. Obstet. Gynecol 1997;177:723–30.

16. Moller M, Henderson jj, Nathan EA, Pennell CE. CerviLenz is an effective tool for screening cervical-length in comparison to transvaginal ultrasound.J Maternal Fetal Neonatal Med 2012 Nov 21; early online:1–5.

17. Statement on Makena [press release] Silver Spring, MD: US Department of Health and Human Services, Food and Drug Administration; 2011 Mar 30 [Accessed on May 9, 2011].

18. Meis PJ, Klebanoff M, Thom E, et al. Prevention of recurrent preterm delivery by 17-alpha hydroxyprogesterone caproate. National Institute of Child Health and Human Development Maternal-Fetal Medicine Units Network. N Engl J Med 2003;348:2379.

19. Fonseca EB, Celik E, Parra M, et al. Fetal Medicine Foundation Second Trimester Screening Group. Progesterone and the risk of preterm birth among women with a short cervix. N Engl J Med 2007;357:462–9.

20. Hassan SS, Romero R, Vidyadhari D, et al. For the pregnant trial, authors. Vaginal progesterone reduces the rate of preterm birth in women with a sonographic short cervix: a multicenter, randomized, double-blind, placebo-controlled trial. Ultrasound Obstet Gynecol 2011;38:18–31.

21. King JF, Flenady V, Papatsonis D, Dekker G, Carbonne B. Calcium-channel blockers for inhibiting preterm labor; a systematic review of the evidence and a protocol for administration of nifedipine. Aust N Z J Obstet Gynaecol 2003;43:192–8.

22. Gaunekar NN, Crowther CA. Maintenance therapy with calcium-channel blockers for preventing preterm birth after threatened preterm labor. Cochrane Database Syst Rev 2004;3:CD004071.

23. Khan K, Zamora J, Lamont RF, et al. Safety concerns for the use of calcium-channel blockers in pregnancy for the treatment of spontaneous preterm labor and hypertension: a systematic review and meta-regression analysis. J Matern Fetal Neonatal Med 2010 Feb 25 [Epub ahead of print].

24. WHO Model List of Essential Medicines, 14th edition. MedIDName=228@nifedipine (revised in March 2005) (accessed on 04 October 2005) .

25. Coomarasamy A, Knox EM, Gee H, Khan KS. Oxytocin antagonists for tocolysis in preterm labor—a systematic review. Med Sci Monit 2002 Nov;8(11):RA268–73.

26. Papatsonis D, Flenady V, Cole S, Liley H (2005). Papatsonis, Dimitri, ed. "Oxytocin receptor antagonists for inhibiting preterm labor". *Cochrane database of systematic reviews (Online)* (3): CD004452.

27. ACOG Committee on Obstetric Practice. ACOG Committee Opinion No. 475: antenatal corticosteroid therapy for fetal maturation. Obstet Gynecol 2011;117:422.

28. Elimian A, Figueroa R, Spitzer AR, et al. Antenatal corticosteroids: Are incomplete courses beneficial? Obstet Gynecol. 2003;102:352.

29. Brownfoot FC, Gagliardi DI, Bain E, et al. Different corticosteroids and regimens for accelerating fetal lung maturation for women at risk of preterm birth. Cochrane Database Syst Rev 2013; 8:CD006764.

12

Multiple Pregnancy

• Neerja

Definition: Twin pregnancy result from fertilization of two different ova—dizygotic or fraternal twins. Less often twins arise from division of single fertilized ovum monozygotic or identical twins. Either or both processes may be involved in the formation of higher numbers, e.g. quadruplets may arise from as few as one to as many as four ova.

Types (Figs 12.1 and 12.2)

1. *Dizygotic twins or fraternal twins:* It results from fertilization of two ova probably ruptured from two distinct graafian follicles fertilized by two sperms and are not in a strict sense true twins. Nearly two-thirds (67%) of all twins are dizygotic.
2. *Monozygotic or uniovular twins:* It results from fertilization of ovum by a single sperm and occurs in 33% of all twin pregnancies. It is of many types depending on time when splitting occurs in the embryo as described below:
   a. *Dichorionic-diamniotic twins:* Develop if division occurs within 3 days (7 hrs) at 8-cell stage: Embryo will have two separate or single-fused placentae, two chorions and two amnions.
   b. *Monochorionic-diamniotic twins:* Develop if division occurs between 4 and 7 days when inner cell mass is forming. It is the commonest type seen in two-thirds of monozygous twins.
   c. *Monochorionic-monoamniotic twins:* If splitting occur 8–12 days after fertilization, accounts for only 1–5% of monozygotic twins.
   d. *Conjoined twins:* Rare type, seen if splitting occurs after the appearance of the primitive streak, i.e. after 13 days of fertilization.

Superfetation and superfecundation: In Superfetation there is fertilization of two ova released in two different menstrual cycles and is yet to be proved in human beings. Superfecundation refers to the fertilization of two ova in the same cycle but by two different acts of coitus.

Incidence: The frequency of monozygotic twin births is relatively constant throughout the world at approximately one in 250 births and is independent of race, heredity, age and parity. Hellin's law(1895) propounds the following rates of multiple pregnancy, viz: twins 1:80, triplets $1:80^2$, quadruplets $1:80^3$, quintruplets $1:80^4$, conjoined twins 1:60,000 births.

Etiology: Though exact etiology is not clear, various factors associated with twin pregnancy are: Racial (more common in

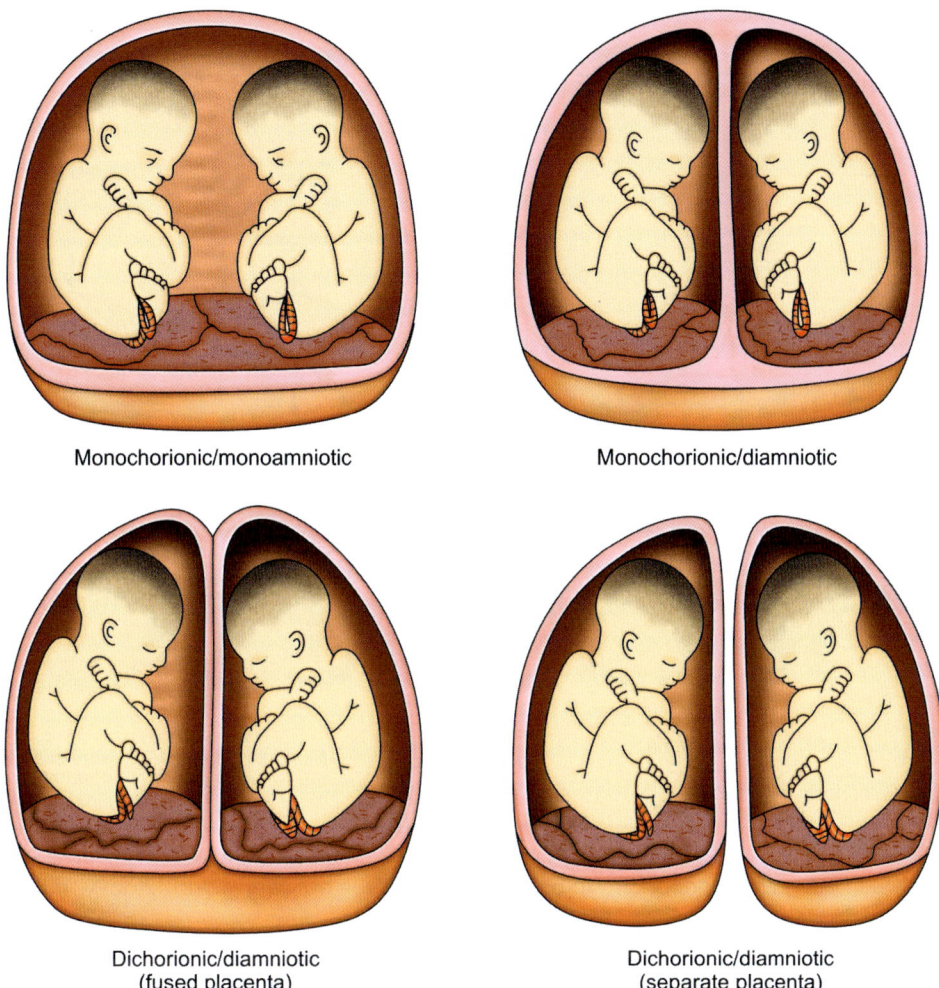

Monochorionic/monoamniotic

Monochorionic/diamniotic

Dichorionic/diamniotic
(fused placenta)

Dichorionic/diamniotic
(separate placenta)

Fig. 12.1: Types of twins

Africans than Japanese), seen in mother and sister, high parity (in para 5 and above), rising maternal age: With a peak of 37 years, 25–35% more in taller, heavier women with good nutritional status.

Iatrogenic; 6–8% risk of multiple pregnancy with ovulation induction with clomiphene and 16–40% risk with gonadotropin in ART.

Prognosis: Maternal mortality increases 3–7 times in multiple pregnancy than singleton pregnancy. Postpartum hemorrhage, anemia, pre-eclampsia and increased incidence of operative interferences increases maternal morbidity.

Perinatal mortality: Perinatal mortality increases 3–11 times due to prematurity, growth restriction and infection. 2nd twin is at higher risk. The monozygotic twins have 2.5 times higher mortality due to higher chances of congenital anomalies, discordant growth, twin-to-twin transfusion syndrome and malpresentation.

DIAGNOSIS OF MULTIPLE PREGNANCY

History

1. Family or past history of multiple pregnancy
2. History of ovulation induction drugs, ART like IVF.

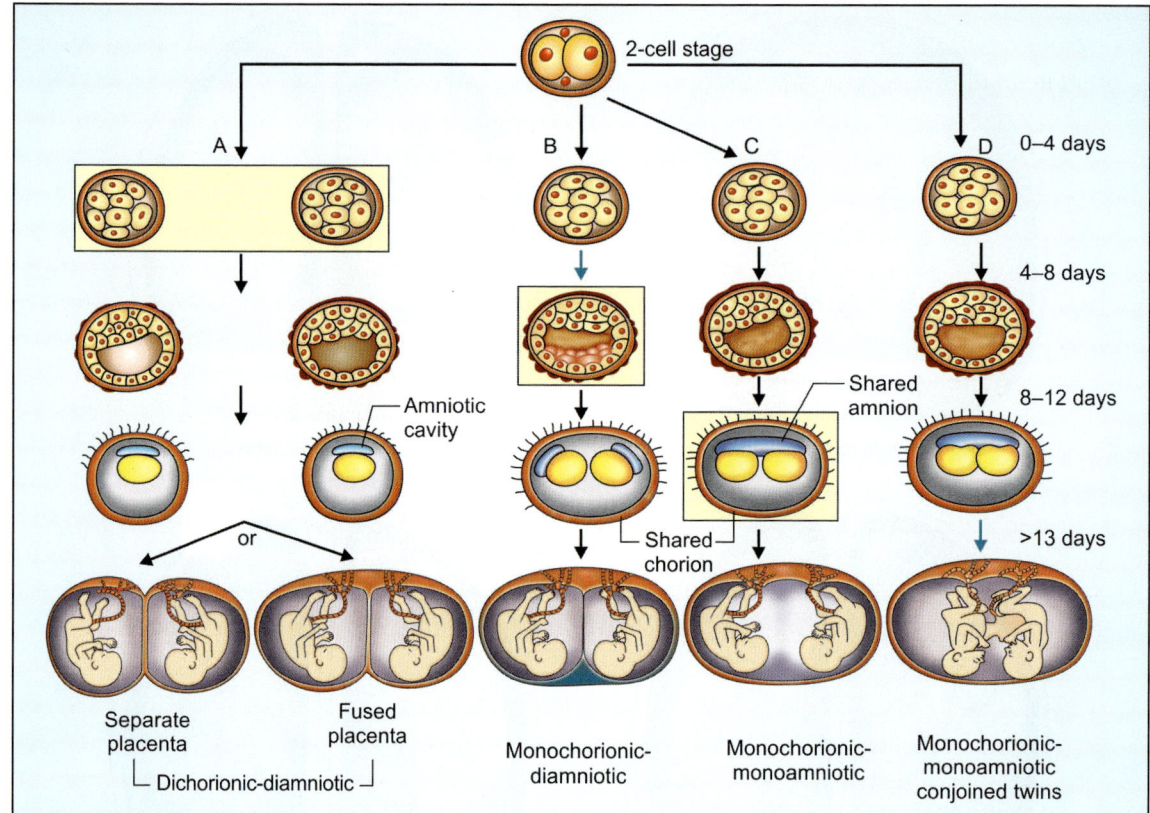

Fig. 12.2: Mechanism of monozygotic twinning. A. Division at 0–4 days postfertilization—diamniotic-dichorionic; B. Division between 4–8 days—monochorionic-diamniotic; C. Division between 8 and 12 days—monochorionic-monoamniotic; D. Division after 13 days—conjoined twinning.

Clinical Features

1. Due to excess of hCG there is increased nausea, vomiting and hyperemesis during early pregnancy.
2. Due to excessive distension cardio-respiratory symptoms like palpitation and dyspnea are more common in later pregnancy.
3. Swelling and varicosity of legs and vulval veins, hemorrhoids are more common due to excessive enlargement of uterus.

Abdominal Examination

1. Symphysiofundal height is more than the period of gestation.
2. Abdominal girth is increased (>100 cm at term).

3. Multiple fetal parts are palpable. Palpation of two fetal heads or three fetal poles is diagnostic of multiple pregnancy.

Auscultation

Presence of two fetal heart sounds at two different areas at least 10 cm apart by two independent observers, is diagnostic of twin pregnancy, provided the difference in heart rate is at least 10 bpm.

Vaginal examination: Depending upon the presentation of two fetuses, one fetal head is usually felt on vaginal examination while the other fetal head may be higher up.

Investigations

Ultrasonography: It is the diagnostic modality of 1st choice for multiple pregnancy.

1. Multiple pregnancy can be diagnosed in 1st trimester with ultrasound seeing two or more gestation sacs. It can also demonstrate vanishing twin with fetal pole in one sac and no pole in the other sac. Later two heads are seen.
2. Chorionicity of placenta by "Twin peak or lambda sign" (Fig. 12.3)
3. Fetal growth monitoring
4. Presentation and lie of fetuses
5. AFI of two sacs
6. Localization of placenta
7. Fetal wellbeing

Differential Diagnosis

1. Mistaken dates
2. Hydramnios
3. Fetal macrosomia
4. Fibroid with pregnancy
5. Ovarian tumor with pregnancy

6. Ascitis with pregnancy
7. Full bladder
8. Hydatidiform mole

Effects on Mother

During antenatal period

1. Miscarriage
2. Aggravated early pregnancy symptoms, hyperemesis (3 times)
3. Anemia—iron deficiency and folate deficiency
4. Hypertension and pre-eclampsia (up to 25%)
5. Antepartum hemorrhage
   a. Placenta previa (due to large placenta)
   b. Abruption placentae (due to pre-eclampsia)
6. Hydramnios
7. Gestational diabetes (2–3 times)
8. Cholestatic jaundice
9. Malpresentation
10. Preterm labor
11. Mechanical distress

During labor

1. Early rupture of membranes
2. Ineffective labor
3. Cord prolapse
4. Increased risk of operative delivery
5. Abruptio placentae (due to sudden shrinkage of uterus after delivery of first twin)
6. Postpartum hemorrhage (due to large uterus and more operative interference, retained placenta)

During puerperium

1. Subinvolution of uterus
2. Infection
3. Failing lactation

EFFECTS OF MULTIPLE PREGNANCY ON FETUSES

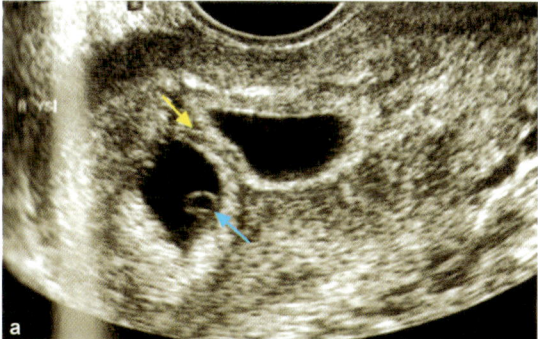
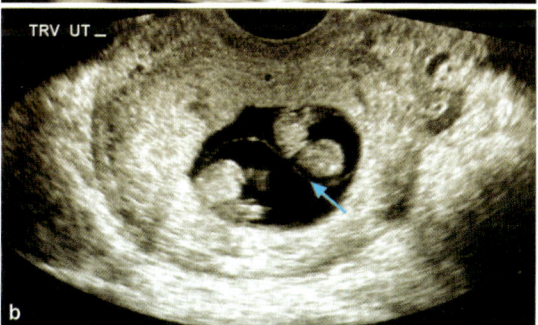

Fig. 12.3: Sonogram of 1st trimester twins. a. Dichorionic-diamniotic twins at 6 wks gestation showing thick dividing chorion; b. Monochorionic diamniotic twin pregnancy at 8 wks gestation showing thin dividing membrane—amnion

The various complications in multiple pregnancy are shown in Table 12.1 and important complications are discussed.

Table 12.1: Fetal risks in multiple pregnancy
1. Abortion
2. Fetal growth restriction
3. Vanishing twin and single fetal death
4. Preterm labor and delivery
5. Stillbirth
6. Congenital malformations
7. Discordant growth
8. Conjoined twins
9. Monoamniotic twins
10. Twin-to-twin transfusion syndrome
11. Twin reversed arterial perfusion (TRAP)
12. Malpresentations
13. Stuck twin
14. Asphyxia
15. Neonatal death
16. Operative vaginal delivery (especially for second baby)
17. Twin entrapment

1. Vanishing Twin

When in a twin pregnancy, one of the fetuses aborts or gets reabsorbed within 10 weeks of pregnancy, it is called vanishing twin. When fetal death occurs during the second trimester, the remains of the baby get compressed and become paper like and flattened by pressure from the survivor (fetus compressus or papyraceous).

2. Prematurity

Preterm labor is the most important complication of multiple pregnancies and the main reason for higher perinatal mortality. It may be spontaneous or iatrogenic. Patients with twin-to-twin transfusion and those showing a discordant fetal growth may require a preterm delivery as soon as lung maturity is achieved. The mean gestational age at delivery is 37 weeks for twins, 33.5 weeks for triplets, 30 weeks for quadruplets and 29 weeks for quintuplets.

3. Growth Restriction

Growth restriction is more marked in monozygotic twins and occurs at and after 30 weeks of pregnancy. Almost 90% twins are low birth weight due to growth restriction (25%) or due to prematurity.

4. Discordant Twins

Discordant twins are due to unequal division of the zygote resulting in unequal placental mass, umbilical cord abnormalities, genetic diseases, twin-to-twin transfusion or placental insufficiency. The difference of birth weight 25% or more amongst the twins is termed as discordant growth. The smaller twin has a higher risk of perinatal complications, long term physical and intellectual growth restriction and risk of death.

Pathology

In monochorionic twins discordancy is usually due to placental vascular anastomosis that cause hemodynamic imbalances between twins. Occasionally discordancy can be due to structural anomalies.

Dizygotic twins may be discordant due to different genetic potential, suboptimal implantation site, *in utero* crowding and placental abnormalities.

The criteria for diagnosis on ultrasound examination are as follows:

a. A difference in the head circumference of >5%.

b. A difference in the abdominal circumference of >20 mm.

c. Increased head to abdomen and femur to abdomen ratios.

d. A difference of >25% in estimated fetal weight.

e. Abnormal umbilical artery Doppler waveforms.

5. Single Fetal Death (Acute Intertwin Transfusion)

Single fetal death may occur either early in pregnancy or later as the pregnancy progresses. However, it is uncommon. Morbidity of the surviving fetus depends to a great extent on the chorionicity of the pregnancy. When one monochorionic twin dies *in utero*, there is a 25% risk of necrotic neurological lesions including cerebral palsy and renal lesions in the survivor. There is high (25%) risk of intrauterine death of the healthy co-twin. These complications are usually due to consequence of severe hypotension occurring during the death of the other twin.

6. Twin-to-twin Transfusion Syndrome (TTTS)

Twin-to-twin transfusion syndrome is a condition that complicates up to 15% of monochorionic twin pregnancies. It is characterized by a relative lack of superficial bilateral vascular anastomoses, which protect against hemodynamic imbalances caused by unidirectional deep arteriovenous vessels.

Antenatal criteria recommended for defining the twin-twin transfusion syndrome include the following:

1. Same sex fetuses
2. Monochorionicity with placental vascular anastomoses
3. Weight difference between twins greater than 20%
4. Hydramnios in the larger twin, oligo-hydramnios in the smaller twin
5. Stuck smaller twin
6. Hemoglobin difference >5 g/dl.

All of these criteria, except hemoglobin levels, can be determined ultrasonographically.

Quintero Staging System for Twin-twin Transfusion Syndrome

- Stage I—discordant amniotic fluid volume but urine still visible sonographically within donor twin's bladder.
- Stage II—stage I + but urine not visible within donor's bladder.
- Stage III—stage II + abnormal Doppler studies of umbilical artery, ductus venosus or umbilical vein.

- Stage IV—ascites or frank hydrops in either twin.
- Stage V—it is most severe form with demise of either twin.

If untreated, the perinatal mortality is extremely high (>80%). Although twin-twin transfusion is usually a gradual process, it can happen suddenly with the death of one twin, usually the recipient, due to heart failure. Hence, recipient twin is at higher risk of death than donor.

7. Twin Reversed Arterial Perfusion (TRAP) Sequence and Acardiac Twinning

Twin reversed arterial perfusion sequence and acardiac twinning is a complication which occurs in approximately 1% of monochorionic pregnancies. It is characterized by an acardiac twin, which receives its blood supply via a large arterio-arterial anastomosis from a normal 'pump' co-twin. This results in absent or rudimentary development of the upper body structures like head or neck. The perinatal mortality of the pump twin is high with death usually occurring from cardiac failure, hydrops or polyhydramnios induced preterm delivery.

8. Monoamniotic Twin Pregnancies

Monoamniotic twin pregnancies are rare, occurring once in every 12,500 births. The main factors associated with perinatal mortality are umbilical cord entanglement, cord accidents, congenital malformations, preterm delivery and twin to twin transfusion.

Sonographic diagnosis is based on the absence of a dividing amniotic membrane and twins of the same sex with the presence of a single placenta. Color Doppler examination is valuable in detecting umbilical cord entanglement. Presence of variable decelerations is also suggestive of cord entanglement. The optimal route of delivery is by cesarean section after giving a course of two doses of betamethasone after 34 weeks of gestation to avoid umbilical cord problems.

9. Congenital Malformations

The incidence of congenital malformations is significantly increased in twins and higher-order multiple gestations compared with singleton pregnancy. Major malformations develop in 2% and minor malformations in 4% of twins.

10. Conjoined Twins

Conjoined twins, also called Siamese twins, affect 1 in every 200 monozygotic twins. Conjoined twins are uniovular and have the same sex and karyotype. The different types of conjoined twins (Fig. 12.4) are:

a. *Thoracopagus:* Fusion at the chest (40%). It is the most common type.
b. *Omphalopagus (xiphopagus):* Fusion at the anterior abdominal wall (33%).
c. *Pyopagus:* Fusion at the buttocks (18%).
d. *Ischiopagus:* Fusion at the ischium (6%).
e. *Craniopagus:* Fusion of heads (2%). It is least common.

The outcome of conjoined twins is poor and is dependent largely on the feasibility of surgical separation. Antenatal USG shows, both twins facing each other or on repeated examination heads are at same level and plane. The thoracic cages are in unusual

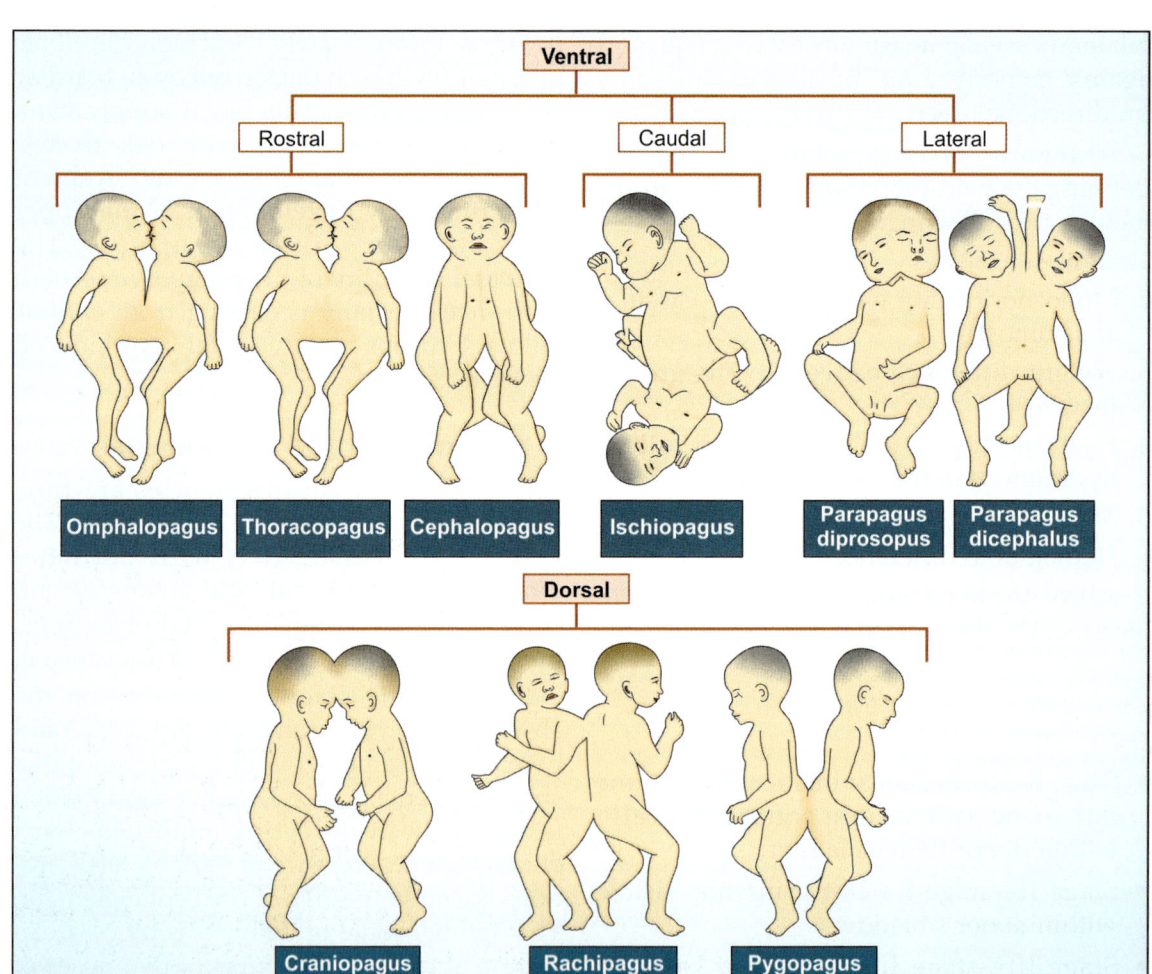

Fig. 12.4: Types of conjoined twins

proximity. There is no change in relative fetal positions with time or manipulation.

11. Umbilical Cord Problems

Umbilical cord problems are more frequent in twin pregnancies and include single umbilical artery and velamentous insertion of the cord. Cord entanglements, cord prolapse and torsion due to focal absence of Wharton's jelly are more common in monoamniotic twins.

12. Malpresentations

There is a high incidence of fetal malpresentations at the time of delivery in twin gestations. The frequency of different fetal presentations reported is as follows:

a. Vertex-vertex   40% (most common)
b. Vertex-breech   28%
c. Vertex-transverse   7.5%
d. Breech-vertex   9%
e. Breech-breech   6.5%
f. Breech-transverse   2.5%
g. Other combinations   6%
h. Both transverse   (0.5%/least common)

Malpresentations are more common in the second fetus. During labor, early rupture of membranes and cord prolapse are likely to occur due to a higher prevalence of malpresentations.

Prevention of Multiple Pregnancy

Placing three instead of two embryos increases the risk of triplets by 15-fold, from 0.4 to 6% with no increase in the take home baby rate. Legislation to allow only one or two embryo transfer can help to reduce incidence of multiple pregnancies. Similarly, avoiding high risk factors like minimizing use of ovulation induction can lower rates.

Management

During antenatal period: Successful outcome of a twin pregnancy depends on an early diagnosis. High index of clinical suspicion and liberal use of ultrasound examination are the keys to the diagnosis.

Antenatal Advice and Care

1. *Nutrition:* An additional 300 kilocalories per day dietary supplementation should be advised. Requirement of protein, minerals, vitamins and essential fatty acids is also increased.

2. Extra rest and early stopping of work is recommended to prevent preterm labor.

3. *Iron and other supplements:* (a) She should be given therapeutic dose (200 mg) of elemental iron per day, (b) extra vitamins, calcium should be prescribed. She should be given 5 mg folic acid per day.

4. Antenatal visits should be more frequent (every 2 weekly) to pick up pregnancy complications at the earliest.

5. Fetal monitoring is done by 4 weekly ultrasounds for fetal growth and amniotic fluid volume. Non-stress test, Doppler study and biophysical score (Manning's score) are performed regularly.

Admission to Hospital

1. Routine hospitalization for bedrest has not been shown to be helpful.

2. Evidence based medicine does not support prophylactic cervical cerclage or routine sympathomimetics to prevent preterm labor in multiple pregnancy.

3. Guidelines for the use of corticosteroids are same for multiple pregnancy as for singleton pregnancy (American College of Obstetricians and Gynecologists, 2004).

4. Limited physical activity, early work leave, more frequent antenatal visits and ultrasonographic examination for cervical length and maternal education on the risks of preterm delivery have been advocated to reduce preterm births with a little evidence.

5. Emergency admission is needed in case of complications.

Labor Management

Patients with multiple pregnancy should preferably be taken care of in tertiary health care centres with anesthesia services and intensive neonatal care unit facilities. During labor the following precautions are to be taken.

1. The patient should be kept nil by mouth to avoid anesthesia complications in the event of operative interference.
2. Adequate caloric supplementation with intravenous fluids using Ringer lactate or dextrose saline solution.
3. Blood should be cross-matched and kept ready.
4. Continuous intrapartum fetal monitoring using two CTG machines is preferable to detect any signs of fetal distress.
5. An experienced obstetrician skilled in intrauterine identification of fetal parts and in intrauterine manipulations of the fetus should be available at all times.
6. Pain relief, if required, can be given. Epidural anesthesia is ideal as second fetus may need intrauterine manipulations for delivery. An experienced anesthetist should be kept informed and should be available.
7. Two neonatologists should preferably be present at the time of delivery.

DELIVERY OF THE FIRST TWIN

The delivery of the first baby is conducted as in normal labor. Intramuscular or intravenous oxytocin for active management of third stage is withheld. The cord should be clamped at two places and cut in between and kept long for administration of drugs or blood transfusion, if needed. The baby is handed over to the attending neonatologist and labeled as the first twin.

DELIVERY OF THE SECOND TWIN

After first baby is born, abdomen is carefully palpated to know the lie and presentation of the second twin. An ultrasound may be used to confirm the presentation and for fetal heart sounds. A vaginal examination is performed gently for confirmation of presentation, membrane status and to rule out cord presentation and cord prolapse.

1. For longitudinal lie and vertex presentation with head in pelvis, amniotomy is performed. If there is uterine inertia, a controlled intravenous oxytocin infusion can be used to augment labor. In 80% cases, the second twin is born within 30 minutes of the first. As long as the fetal heart rate remains normal, there is no reason to expedite delivery. If vaginal bleeding occurs suggesting abruptio placentae or there are late decelerations indicating fetal distress or there is cord prolapse, delivery should be conducted immediately by forceps or cesarean section.
2. For longitudinal lie with breech presentation, with good fetal heart condition, amniotomy is done and assisted breech delivery is performed. For fetal distress or placental abruption, breech extraction is done.
3. When the lie is transverse or oblique, an external cephalic version should be performed to convert it into longitudinal lie and vertex presentation followed by amniotomy when head is in pelvis and vaginal delivery is accomplished. If membranes are ruptured or if external cephalic version cannot be done or fails or there is fetal distress or abruption, an internal podalic version should be performed preferably under general anesthesia in operation theatre, followed by breech extraction. Infact, an internal podalic version done by an expert for the transverse lie of the second twin is the only acceptable indication for internal podalic version in a live fetus in modern obstetrics. Indications of cesarean delivery are given in Table 12.2.

Management of the Third Stage of Labor

These women are at high risk of postpartum hemorrhage due to large placenta and bigger

Table 12.2: Indications of cesarean delivery in twin pregnancy

Indications of elective cesarean delivery

1. First baby in noncephalic, especially shoulder presentation
2. Conjoined twins
3. Congenital abnormality precluding safe vaginal delivery
4. Fetal growth restriction in dichorionic twin
5. Chronic twin-twin transfusion syndrome in monochorionic twins
6. Monoamniotic twins (high risk of cord prolapse or entanglement and fetal deaths)
7. Placenta previa
8. Contracted pelvis
9. Previous cesarean section
10. Severe pre-eclampsia

Indications of emergency cesarean delivery

1. Fetal distress
2. Cord prolapse in first baby
3. Non-progress of labor
4. Collision of both twins

Indications of cesarean for second twin

1. Second twins transverse, both external cephalic and internal podalic version failed after delivery of first twin
2. For a large second twin weighing more than 3.5 kg
3. Prompt closure of cervix after delivery.

placental site, overdistension of uterus, anesthesia and uterine manipulations. Active management of third stage is practiced by administration of 10 units of oxytocin intramuscularly or intravenously after delivery of the second baby (rule out triplet pregnancy before giving it). The placenta is delivered by controlled cord traction method. It is better to continue oxytocin drip for 1–2 hours and carefully observe the patient.

Postpartum

Special attention is needed in puerperium because there can be subinvolution, greater chances of infection and failure of lactation. Cooperation of all family members is essential to rear multiple births.

Care of the Newborns

Care of the newborns is according to their birth weight and gestation. They are mostly treated as preterm neonates and may require admission or more frequent care in nursery.

LOCKING OF TWINS

Locking of twins is a rare situation (occurring 1 in 8,000 twin gestations) in which one baby impedes the descent and common in primigravida and in smaller babies. For twins to lock, the first fetus must present as breech and the second as cephalic. With descent of the breech through the birth canal, the chin of the first fetus locks between the neck and chin of the second cephalic fetus. Cesarean delivery is recommended when the potential for locking is identified.

Management of Triplets and other High-order Multiple Pregnancies

There is excessive distension of abdomen and increased frequency of all the maternal and perinatal complications than twin pregnancy. Mean gestation in triplets is 34 weeks.

Cesarean delivery (section) is recommended with triplets and quadruplets, mainly because of difficulties in ensuring adequate monitoring in labor. These fetuses are also more premature, growth retarded and have malpresentations. The fetal mortality and morbidity is closely related to the fetal weight, birth order and fetal position.

In the recent years, selective fetal reduction of high order multifetal pregnancies has developed as an alternative.

Key Points

1. Multiple pregnancy is the simultaneous development of two or more fetuses in the uterus. The incidence of multiple pregnancies is about 1 in 80 and rising due to assisted reproductive technology.
2. Determination of chorionicity is important to allocate pregnancy risk.

Prenatal diagnosis using amniocentesis or CVS is suitable in multiple pregnancy.

3. Cervical length measurement may be useful in predicting preterm birth in multiple pregnancy (level ll evidence).

4. Maternal complications include higher incidence of anemia, pre-eclampsia and postpartum hemorrhage. The intra-partum complications in twin pregnancy include: Abnormal presentations, uterine inertia, cord prolapse, abruptio placentae, interlocking of twins and postpartum hemorrhage.

5. Fetal complications in twin pregnancy include: Increased incidence of miscarriage, congenital malformations, malpresenta-tions, twin-to-twin transfusion syndrome and low birth weight. Monochorionic monoamniotic placentation may be associated with twin- to twin-transfusion syndrome, twin reversed arterial perfusion (TRAP) and conjoined twins and need management in a higher center.

6. Antenatal management includes more frequent antenatal visits, higher dose of iron (200 mg elemental) and folic acid (5 mg) per day, regular ultrasound examination 3–4 weekly for fetal growth and well-being, fetal surveillance by NST and biophysical scoring.

7. Multiple pregnancy is a high-risk pregnancy and should be managed in a tertiary referral or specialized unit.

8. Vaginal delivery is aimed for if the first twin is presenting by vertex. However, cesarean delivery is recommended if first twin is presenting by breech or transverse lie or other malpresentation or for obstetric indications.

9. After vaginal delivery of the first twin, the presentation of second twin is confirmed. For vertex and breech, vaginal delivery is performed after amniotomy and oxytocin administration. If second twin is presenting by transverse or oblique lie then external version is performed failing which internal podalic version and breech extraction are performed. Infact it is the only indication of internal podalic version for a live fetus in modern obstetrics.

10. The mothers are at high risk of PPH which should be prevented by active management of third stage (using 10 units of oxytocin IM) after delivery of all fetuses. PPH should be energetically treated if it occurs.

Bibliography

1. American College of Obstetricians and Gyneco-logists: Multiple Gestation: Complicated Twin, Triplet and High Order Multiple Pregnancy: Practice Bulletin No. 56, October 2004.

2. American College of Obstetricians and Gyneco-logists: Special Problems of Multiple Gestation. Education Bulletin No. 253, November 1998.

3. Nice Clinical Guidelines 129, Sept 2011.

4. Quintero RA, Morales WJ, Allen MH, et al. Staging of twin-twin transfusion syndrome. Journal of Perinatology 1999;19:550.

5. Royal College of Obstetricians and Gynaeco-logists: Management of monochorionic twin pregnancies. Green top Guideline No. 51, London: RCOG; 2008.

6. RCOG Guidelines No.14 Clinical Practice Guideline Management of Multiple Pregnancy, June 2014.

7. Williams Obstetrics, Cunningham, Levend, Bloom, Hauth, Rouse 7 Spong, 24th Edition.

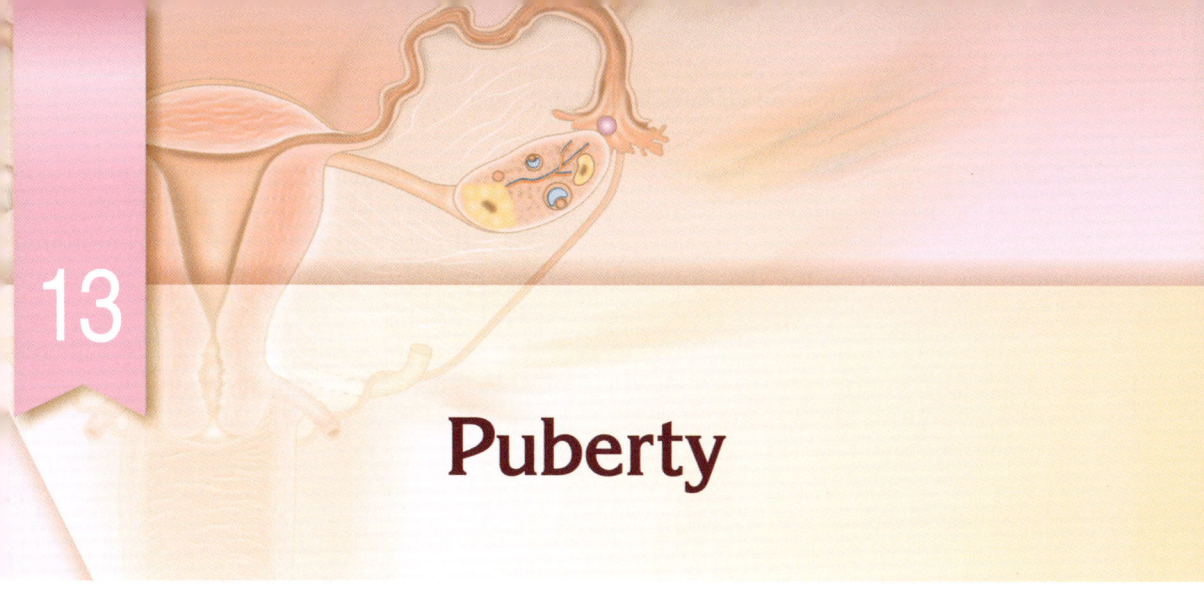

13

Puberty

• Mamta Tyagi

Puberty (latin-pubertus means adulthood) is the state of becoming functionally capable of procreation. This is usually accepted as occurring at the age of 12 years in girls and 14 years in boys, but full reproductive capacity is not usually attained until later. Puberty is the process of cognitive, psychosocial, and biological maturation. At puberty as a result of the increased secretion of releasing factors by hypothalamus and increased responsive of the pituitary gland to these factors all activities are increased phase of active physical growth thereafter, the figure becomes fuller and feminine shrill voice of the child changes to deeper and melodious tone of adult peak height velocity takes place early in puberty before menarche (GH, insulin like growth factor I and gonadal steroids play major role) long bone lengthen, and the epiphyses closes. Changes in the body contour with accumulation of fat at the thighs hips, and buttocks. Psychological changes are profound. The sex urge becomes manifest. Temporary enlargement of the thyroid takes place. Acne of the face is mainly the result of increased androgen secretion.

ENDOCRINOLOGY IN PUBERTY

The levels of gonadal steroids and gonado-trophins are low until the 6–8 years of age. This is due to the negative feedback effect of oestrogen to the hypothalamic pituitary system which remains very sensitive 6–15 times to the negative feed back effect.

As puberty approaches this negative feedback effect of estrogen is gradually lost.

Although hormone concentrations are low throughout infancy and the prepubertal child, FSH and LH display evidence of pulsatile secretion.

Generally, the beginning of adrenarche—the clinical sign of adrenal androgen activity precedes by 2 years the linear growth spurt, the rise in estrogen and gonadotropins of early puberty, and menarche at midpuberty. Because of this temporal relationship, activation of adrenal androgen secretion has been suggested as a possible initiating event in the ontogeny of the pubertal transition.

However, studies of adrenal activity are more consistent with a gradual increase in activity beginning in childhood, indicating that clinical adrenarche represent the achievement over time of steroid levels that are sufficient to produce somatic changes.

Considerable evidence supports a dissociation of the control mechanisms that initiate adrenarche and those governing GnRH-pituitary-ovarian maturation (gonad-arche).

The Menarche (Greek: Month + origin)

It is the onset of menstruation and is merely one manifestation of puberty. During the two years before the menarche the development of the genital tract proceeds apace.

Menstrual flow itself is often preceded by mucoid vaginal discharge and hypogastric pain. Rarely ovulation and conception can proceeds menstruation.

Age of menarche varies to some extent with family, race, social class, family size, birth order, environment, diet and general health.

PUBERTY

Period varies between 13 and 16 years.

Duration of puberty lasts approximately about 2 to 3 years and pubertal changes occur slowly over this period.

WHO has defined adolescence as progression from appearance of secondary sexual characters to sexual and reproductive maturity and development of adult mental process.

Phenotypic Puberty

Plasma levels of sex steroids rise gradually over many years and when threshold has been attained secondary sexual characteristics develop.

There is normally a fixed sequence of acquisition of the various characteristics of sexual maturation.

After initial phase of spurt in growth, there follows development of breasts, pubic and axillary hair.

In women, body weight and reproductive function are closely linked with onset of puberty.

Clinical adrenarche represent the achievement over the time of steroid levels that are sufficient to produce somatic changes.

Physical, endocrinological, genital organs, psychological and emotional changes that occur during puberty are modulated by the interaction of various hormones secreted through hypothalamus-pituitary-ovarian axis as well as thyroid and adrenal glands.

Heredity, enviornment, nutrition, emotional stress and childhood illness can influence onset of puberty.

Tanner and Marshall described five stages of pubertal changes (Fig 13.1):

1. Physical growth
2. Development of secondary sex organs and breast development
3. Pubic and axillary hair growth
4. Development of ovaries and the genital organs
5. Growth spurt and menstruation

Management of Normal Puberty

In many societies throughout history, puberty has been a time of celebration. It announce the transition from childhood to adulthood and the development of fertility. Puberty can be the difficult transition for many adolescents.

Management of adolescent is difficult. The girl should not be teased, but her move towards independence is respected and controlled within limits.

Affection and trust should take the place of orders.

She should be encouraged to be occupied in healthy recreation.

Girls should be well-primed in what to expect. Sex education should come naturally an piecemeal throughout childhood. Their curiosity should be satisfied, questions asked by them should be answered simply but truthfully.

Adolescent needs to be explained with sufficient information to be protected against the HIV infection and genital tract infection.

Common disorders of puberty and adolescence:

- Obesity
- Precocious puberty
- Delayed puberty
- Menstrual abnormalities

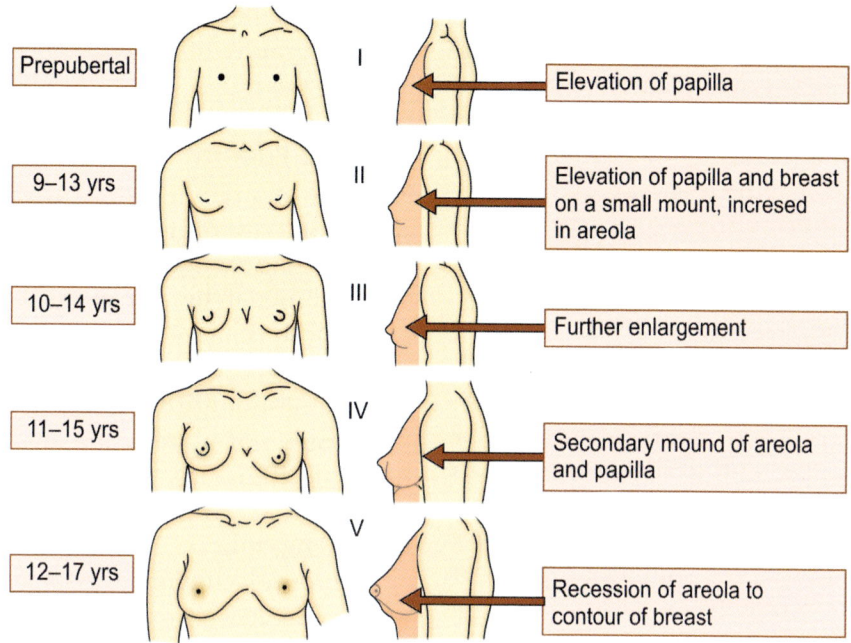

Prepubertal		I	Elevation of papilla
9–13 yrs		II	Elevation of papilla and breast on a small mount, incresed in areola
10–14 yrs		III	Further enlargement
11–15 yrs		IV	Secondary mound of areola and papilla
12–17 yrs		V	Recession of areola to contour of breast

Fig. 13.1: Tanner staging of breast development—Marshal and Tanner (1969)

Obesity

Adolescence is sometimes accompanied by a rapid increase in weight and the development of fat. Obesity in children and adolescents, irrespective of the underlying metabolic processes of the individual, is nearly always associated with overeating.

Adolescent obesity of a minor degree tend to disappear by the age of 20 years if the appetite is curbed.

Obesity of a gross degree however, requires strict dietetic control.

Precocious Puberty (Fig. 13.2)

It is defined as onset of menstruation accompanied by other evidence of puberty before the age of 8 years.

Epiphyseal closure is likely to occur early, so the individual maybe short in stature.

Mental development may be retarded or advanced.

These girls commonly show abnormal EEG.

Leptin-adipocyte derived hormone product of obesity (ob gene) also plays an important role. Therefore in an obese girl growth spurt and menarche start earlier.

Premature release of GnRH from hypothalamus and of gonadotrophins from the anterior pituitary.

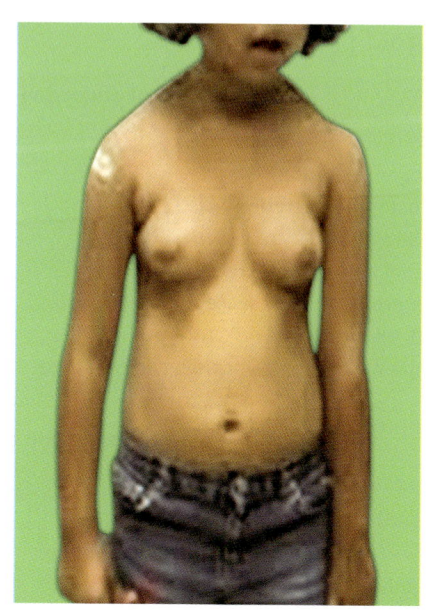

Fig. 13.2: Precocious puberty

In this the signs of puberty usually appear in correct order, and bone age and height are several years in advance of chronological age.

Gonadotrophins are found in concentrations that are normal for adults.

These cases may be treated with administration of either cyproterone acetate or a GnRH analogue.

Causes of Precocious Puberty

- Constitutional—80% it is due to premature activation of hypothalamopituitary-ovarian axis. There is precocious appearance of pubic and axillary hair before 8 years.
- A large glycoprotein has been identified that also displayed adrenal androgen stimulating activity.
- Pitutary tumors
- Feminizing tumors of ovary
- Adrenal tumors
- Hypothyroidism

Investigations

- Radiography of pituitary fossa, CT scan, MRI
- USG
- Thyroid profile

- FSH, LH, oestrogen levels
- Radiography of bones
- Treat the cause

Delayed Puberty

Defined as girls who fail to develop any secondary sex characteristics by age of 13, have not had menarche by age 16, or have not attained menarche 5 or more years since the pubertal development.

Hyperprolactinemia

In prepubertal women the levels can range from 2 to 12 ng/ml.

In normal women levels are usually less than 20 ng/ml.

Hyperprolactinemia can cause:
- Disruption of normal folliculae development
- Premature destruction of corpus luteum.

ELISA Test or Radioimmunoassay Advised

- Medical management—bromocriptine 1.25 mg—at bedtime. Dose to be increased if required.
- Cabergoline—half life of 65 hours.

1. *Puberty menorrhagia:* Menarche usually occurs at age of 12–14 years.

Relationship of endocrine events and secondary sexual characteristics	
Endocrine events	*Sexual maturation*
Estrogen secretion	Breast development
Testosterone secretion	Penile and scrotal development
FSH secretion	Testicular enlargement
Adrenal androgen secretion	Pubic and axillary hair
Sex steroids and GH secretion	Growth acceleration
Estrogen withdrawl	Menarche, initial ovulatory cycles
Complex mechanism including an LH surge	Ovulatory menstrual cycles

Classification of premature sexual maturation	
Gonadotrophin dependent	*Gonadotrophin independent*
Constitutional (idiopathic) CCP	Testotoxicosis in boys
Suprasellar tumors/cysts	McCune-Albright syndrome in girls
Secondary to cranial irradiation	Feminizing tumors in girls
Primary hypothyroidism	Premature thelarche/variant

Menstrual problems are common in adoloscence due to slow maturation of HPO axis.

Menorrhagia: Denotes regularly timed episodes of bleeding that are excessive in amount (>80 ml) and or duration of flow (>5 days).

Dysmenorrhea: Painful cramping pain accompanying menstruation.

Amenorrhea: Absence of menstruation.

2. *Central precocious puberty due to intra-cranial lesions*

Premature release of gonadotrophins from pituitary but caused by existence of n intracranial lesion or disease such as meningitis, encephalitis, cerebral tumor, hydrocephalus, sequelae following a head trauma or radiation therapy.

Phenomenon is more common in boys.

3. *Isolated premature thelarche*

Breast development under the age of 2 years without any other signs of puberty.

No pubic hair development. Growth and bone age are normal.

Breast development commonly cycles up and down at 6 weekly interval.

It does not require any treatment.

4. *Variants of premature thelarche*

Breast changes are similar as to those in premature thelarche but they also have accelarated bone age and growth velocity.

Bibliography

1. Clinical Gynecologic Endocrinology and Infertility (7th edition)—Leon Speroff and Marc A Fritz.
2. Counts DR. Pescovitz OH, Barnes KM, Hench MD, Chrousos GP, Sherins RJ, Comite F, Loriaux DL. Cutler GB (Jr), Dissociation of adrenarche and gonadarche in precocious puberty and in isolated hypogonadotropic hypogonadism. J Clin Endocrinol Metabolism 1987;86:1174.
3. DC Dutta's Textbook of Gynaecology (6th edition).
4. Dunkel L, Alfthan H, Stenman U-H, Selstam G, Rosberg S, Albertsson-Wikland K. Developmental changes in 24-hour profiles of leuteinizing hormone and follicle stimulating hormone from prepuberty to midstages of puberty in boys. J Clin Endocrinol Metabolism 1992;74:890.
5. Frisch RE, Revelle R. Menstural cycle: fatness as a determinants of minimum weight-for-height for their maintenance or onset. Science 1974.
6. Jakachi RI, Klech RP Sander SE, Lloyd JS, Hopwood NJ, Marshall JC. Pulsatile secretion of leuteinizing hormone in children, J Clin Endocrinol Metab 1982;53:453.
7. Jeffcoate's Principles of Gynaecology (8th edition).
8. Kaplan SL, Grumbach MM, Aubert ML, The ontogenesis of the pituitary hormones and hypothalamic factors in human fetus : Maturation of central nervous system regulation of anterior pituitary function, Recent Program Hormone Research 1976;32:161.
9. Maclure M, Travis LB, Willett W, MacMahon B. A prospective cohort study of nutrient intake and age at menarche. Am J Clin Nutr 1991;54:649.
10. Marti-Henneberg C, Vizmanos B. The duration of puberty in girls is related to the timing of its onset. J Peditar 1997;131:618.
11. Palmert MR, Hayden DL, Mansfield MJ, Crigler JF (Jr), Crowley WF (Jr) Chandler DW, Boepple PA. The Longitudnal study of adrenal maturation during gonadal suppression evidence that adrenarche is a gradual process. J Clin Endocrinol Metabolism 2001;86:4536.
12. Parker LN, Lifrak AT, Odell WD, A 60,000 molecular weight glycoprotein stimulates adrenal androgen secretion. Endocrinology 1983;113:2092.
13. Shaw's Textbook of Gynaecology (15th edition).
14. Sizonenko PC, Paunier L, Carmignac D, Hormonal changes during puberty: IV. Longitudnal study of adrenal androgen secretion. Hormone Research 1976;7:288.
15. Sklar CA. Kaplan SL, Grumbach MM. Evidence for dissociation between adrenarche and gonadarche: studies in patients with idiopathic precocious puberty, gonadal dysgenesis, isolated gonadotroph deficiency, and constitutionally delayed growth and adolescence. J Clin Endocrinol Metabolism 1980;51:548.
16. Suter KJ, Phol CR, Wilson ME. Circulating concentrations of nocturnal leptin, growth hormone and insulin like growth factor 1 increase before the onset of puberty in agonadal male monkeys: potential signals for the initiation of puberty, J Clin Endocrinol Metabolism 2000;85:808.
17. Tanner JM. Growth at Adolescence, 2nd edn. Blackwell Scientific Publications. Oxford, 1962.
18. Winter JSD, Faiman C. The development of cyclic pituitary gonadal function in adolescent females, J Clin Endocrinol Metabolism 1973;37:714.

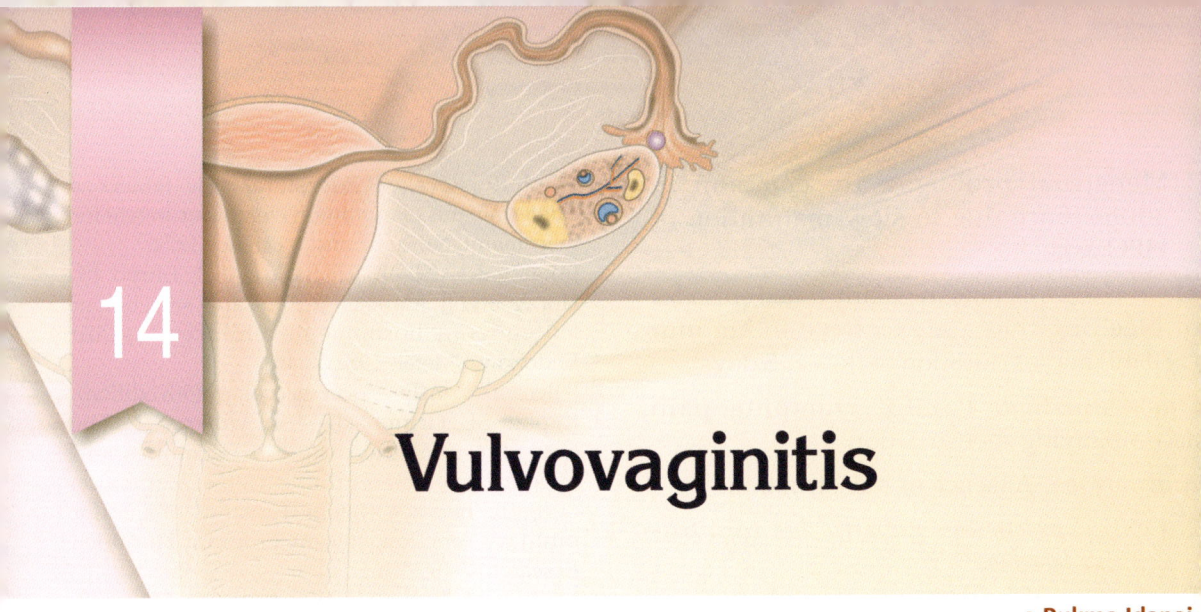

14

Vulvovaginitis

• Rukma Idanai

"Vulvovaginitis" is a medical term used to describe various conditions that cause infection or inflammation both the vagina and vulva. Vulvovaginitis is the most common of all outpatient gynecologic problems and accounts for 10% of offfice visits annually for the primary care provider. These conditions can result from a vaginal infection caused by organisms such as bacteria, yeast, or viruses, as well as by irritations from chemicals in creams, sprays, or even clothing that is in contact with this area. In some cases, vaginitis results from organisms that are sexually transmitted. The diagnostic accuracy with patients complaining of vaginal irritation and odor and discharge has been enhanced over the past several years by a greater understanding of bacterial vaginosis. By using current knowledge and simple office laboratory methods, a precise etiologic diagnosis can be made in more than 95% of patients. These patients can be divided into five diagnostic categories, each with different management strategies. In a study of vaginal infections or discharges on 20,000 consecutive patients, BV was the most common diagnosis (33%), followed by cervicitis (20–25%), fungal infection (20.5%), excessive but otherwise normal secretions (10%), Trichomonas (9.8%) and diagnosis undetermined (2–5%).

THE NATURAL DEFENCES OF THE VAGINA

A healthy vagina has natural protective mechanisms that inhibit the growth of pathogenic bacteria. Women have a natural gift to care lavishly. They nurture and protect their loved ones with lots of passion. Her intimate area protects itself with the same intensity. But the vagina needs a lot more help in its self-preservation because of its delicacy and sensitivity. The vagina takes care of itself: its walls continually produce secretions to provide lubrication, to cleanse it, and maintain its proper acidity to prevent infection.

The **vaginal defence** mechanisms include:

1. Closure by *apposition* of the anterior and posterior walls.
2. A well-developed *stratified squamous epithelium*, unbroken by entrances to glands.
3. *Vaginal acidity and flora:* A protective layer is maintained by an acidic environment produced when lactobacilli breaks down the glycogen to lactic acid. This low pH environment, in turn, allows the growth of lactobacilli and inhibits the presence of pathogenic bacteria. The normal vaginal flora consists of primarily Lactobacillus as well as streptococci, staphylococci, diphtheroids, *Gardnerella vaginalis*, *E. coli*, and several anaerobic organisms. Candida

and Mycoplasma species are also commonly found.

4. *The mucosal immune response:* Antibodies are present although titres are low. Phagocytic cells and cytokines have also been identified.

Variations in the Efficacy of Defence Mechanisms

1. *With age:* The defences are imperfect during childhood and after menopause when the vagina has thin and vulnerable epithelium, with low glycogen content and when pH approaches seven.

2. *With menstruation:* During menstruation the cervical plug is absent and vaginal acidity is lowered by the alkaline menstrual discharge. Gonococcal infection is therefore more virulent if contracted during menstruation and is more likely to ascend to the uterus and tubes at that time. *Trichomonas vaginalis* tends to occur or relapse during menstruation.

3. *During the puerperium:* The genital tract defences are weakest during and immediately after abortion or labor because of the raw placental site; epithelial breaks; bruised and devitalized tissues; wide open vulva, vagina and cervix; reduced vaginal acidity due to the discharge of liquor and lochia (both alkaline); degenerating blood clots and fragments of deciduas which offer a nidus for infection; and lowered general resistance as a result of pregnancy and possibly by anemia and malnutrition.

Is Vaginal Discharge Normal?

A woman's vagina normally produces a discharge that usually is described as **clear or slightly cloudy, non-irritating, and odor-free**.

Composition

It is a mixture of the following all of which vary in amount and character with ovarian function.

- Vulvar secretions from Bartholin's, sebaceous, sweat and apocrine glands.
- Vaginal discharge
- Cervical secretions
- Uterine secretions
- Secretions from the fallopian tube

This may also contain a contribution from peritoneal fluid.

Amount

The amount of vaginal discharge ordinarily present in the adult is such that the introitus feels comfortably moist but there is not enough to stain the under-clothing.

The amount and consistency of discharge can vary with the menstrual cycle.

At birth, the newborn female babies may have mucoid discharge for 1 to 10 days under the effect of maternal hormones. Excessive discharge can be seen in young girls during the few years before and after the menarche. Estrogen-progestogen containing oral contraceptives cause an increase in the discharge. Regular douching may cause washing away of natural secretions encouraging the cervix to secret more. It also predisposes to infection by washing away naturally protective lactobacilli (Fig. 14.1).

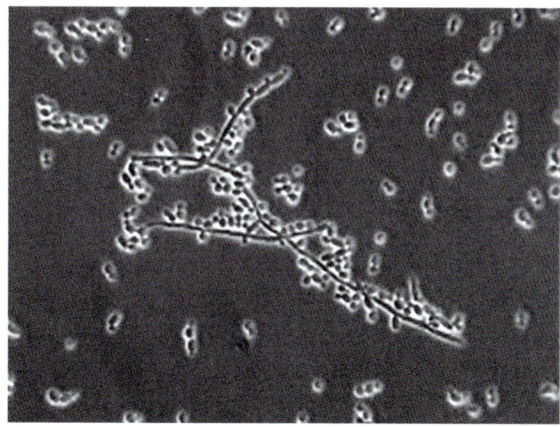

Fig. 14.1: Pseudohyphae and spores of Candida on wet smear

LEUKORRHEA

Leukorrhea means 'a running of white substance' and the term should be restricted to mean an excessive amount of the normal discharge. Leukorrhea consists mainly of the cervical component. It is characteristic of the normal discharge that, although white or cream when fresh, it dries to leave a brownish yellow stain on clothing. The patient with leukorrhea, therefore, nearly always talk of brown discharge and may deceive the medical attendant into thinking that it is blood stained. But it never causes pruritus and is never offensive.

Pathological Vaginal Discharge

- Unusual vaginal discharge especially with an unpleasant odor.
- Discharge associated with burning during urination.
- Discharge causing genital itching.
- Discomfort during intercourse
- Pruritis without abnormal discharge.

The itching may be present at any time of the day, but it often is most bothersome at night. These symptoms often are made worse by sexual intercourse.

Infectious Discharge

Discharge caused by infection is mucopurulent or frankly purulent; its color therefore varies from cream to yellow or green. It is often offensive, especially when coliform bacilli are present as primary or secondary invaders. Its chief microscopic characteristic is the presence of pus cells.

Causes of **pathologic vaginal discharge** are as follows:

- *Infectious vulvovaginitis:* Caused by *Trichomonas vaginalis, Candida albicans* or bacterial vaginosis and non-specific organisms in childhood and old age.
- *Non-infectious vaginitis:* Inflammatory vaginitis, atrophic vaginitis, chemical vulvovaginitis.
- *Cervicitis:* Chronic cervicitis, gonococcal, Chlamydia or anaerobic infection.
- *Endometritis:* Puerperal or senile.
- *Cervical or vaginal descent*
- *Neoplasms:* Benign cervical polyps or carcinoma cervix, endometrial carcinoma, vaginal malignancies. Intermittent, profuse vaginal discharge may occur in carcinoma of the fallopian tube.
- Rare causes like *vaginal adenosis, urinary and faeculent discharges, intermittent emptying of a hydrosalpinx and discharge of ascitic fluid* through the fallopian tubes and uterus.
- *Secondary infection* of wounds, abrasions, burns, chemical injuries.

Although each of these can have different symptoms, it is not always easy for a woman to figure out what problem she has? In fact, diagnosis can even be tricky for an experienced doctor. To help us better understand these entities, let us look briefly at each one of them, their identification and treatment.

Vulvovaginal candidiasis (VVC), formerly called monilial candidiasis, is a common fungal infection of the vulva and vagina caused by *Candida albicans, Candida tropicalis, Candida glabrata*, and *Candida parapsilosis*. Since the 1980s, the incidence of *non-C. albicans* infection has more than doubled and now accounts for more than 21% of cases. It has been estimated that 75% of all women will have an episode of candidal vaginitis at least once and as many as 40 to 50% will have recurrent infections. A small subpopulation, approximately 5%, will have several recurrent, often intractable episodes of VVC. Predisposing factors for VVC include: Diabetes, systemic antibiotics, pregnancy, use of oral contraceptives or corticosteroids, tight clothing, obesity, warm weather, and a decreased host immunity to Candida species.

The symptoms of VVC depend on the degree and location of tissue inflammation. In mild cases, the most common complaint is pruritus but as the disease progresses, burning, soreness, and dyspareunia occur. Dysuria is a common symptom of VVC in the urethra and must be distinguished from infection of the urinary tract to avoid the inappropriate use of antibiotics.

Vaginal discharge may not be present; however, some patients describe a characteristic white curd drainage. On examination erythema, excoriation from scratching and small red satellite lesions are present on the vulva. If present, the curd-like discharge may be localized or may coat the entire vagina. In severe cases, vulvar edema and tissue fissuring may occur.

A wet-mount preparation with saline or 10% KOH demonstrates pseudohyphae and spores in most patients. When present, the diagnosis is confirmed. They may be absent, however, in a significant number of cases because non-Albicans species may not be readily identifiable on KOH. When pseudohyphae and spores are not seen, the clinician must decide whether to treat on the basis of signs and/or symptoms or to obtain a culture. Culture media, such as Sabouraud's or Nickerson's, should be used. Growth is evident within 1 to 3 days. The presence of *C. albicans* in the absence of clinical disease is not diagnostic of candidal vaginitis.

Management

It is often helpful to classify candidiasis as uncomplicated or complicated to facilitate the selection and duration of therapy.

Uncomplicated candidal vaginitis is infection that occurs in a normal, healthy woman and involves symptoms that are sporadic and infrequent and not chronic or recurrent. In this setting, most patients do very well with a short course of therapy, regardless of whether it is topical or oral.

Complicated candidiasis represents approximately 10% of all cases and includes:
- Severe infection with severe vulvovaginal signs and symptoms including severe erythema, edema, severity pruritus, and dyspareunia.

- Recurrent disease.
- Evidence, on wet-mount KOH of budding yeast but not hyphae elements, which increases the likelihood of *C. glabrata* or *Saccharomyces cerevisiae*, species that are less likely to respond to traditional therapy.
- An abnormal host.

Pharmacologic Treatment

Local Therapies

- **Clotrimazole creams, gels or suppositories** are rapidly effective when used intravaginally at bed time. These products are now readily available. Creams directly applied over the vulva. Suppositories are given as 100 mg for 7 nights 200 mg for 3 nights, or 500 mg for 1 night only.
- **Monistat** vaginal tampons contain 100 mg of miconazole nitrate. For 5 consecutive nights, the medicated tampon is inserted and removed in the morning. There does not appear to be any difference in efficacy when compared to other methods of administration. The tampons is not available in all countries.
- **Sertaconazole** is more effective against *C. tropicalis* and *C. glabrata* strains. A single day or a 3-day suppository and 7-day cream are available.
- **Combination pessaries of clotrimazole, tinidazole, xylocaine** are also available and can be used.
- **Boric acid suppositories** as well as **gentian violet** topically are alternatives to the standard antifungal creams. These are static agents that suppress the growth of organisms and to some extent eradicate them. However, they will not sterilize the genital tract.

Oral Therapies

Imidazoles: Fluconazole is available in a 150 mg tablet taken once PO. This treatment is given with topical treatments. It offers essentially 100% compliance. It is the only

Food and Drug Administration (FDA) approved oral agent for VVC.

Itraconazole or ketoconazole 100 and 200 mg are also marketed and used as a twice daily three-day regimen.

- *Bacterial spores:* Four to six acidophilus capsules a day (especially 2–3 days before menses).
- *Vitamin C* 500 mg bid-qid to increase acidity of vaginal secretions.

Non-pharmacologic Treatment

Non-pharmacologic methods have been proposed for VVC. It is likely that the following methods simply assist in restoring acid pH to the environment so that other host factors can contribute to eradicating the infection.

- *Vinegar-in-water douching* has been considered effective if used very early in mild cases. The recommended dose is 1 to 2 tablespoons of vinegar per quart of water qid or bid for no more than 5 days.
- *Unprocessed yogurt douching* daily for 5 days has also been proposed with only anecdotal reports of its effectiveness.

Patient Education

- Excessive moisture to the vulva can be avoided by wearing loose clothing and cotton underwear which is more absorbent than nylon.
- Wiping the buttocks from front to back after bowel movements decreases the exposure of the vulva and vagina to candidial organisms.
- Diabetes should be tightly controlled.
- In most cases, general antibiotic use does not result in candidal infection with enough frequency to warrant the prophylactic use of vaginal creams. However, prophylactic treatment should be considered for those patients with a history of candidal infection from antibiotics.
- Avoid douching as it can alter the vaginal pH and wash away lactobacilli.
- Limit the use of feminine deodorant, deodorant tampons or pads.
- Changing out wet clothing, especially bathing suits, as soon as possible and avoiding frequent hot tub baths.
- Increase rest, reduce stress exposure, eat a well-balanced diet and yogurt.

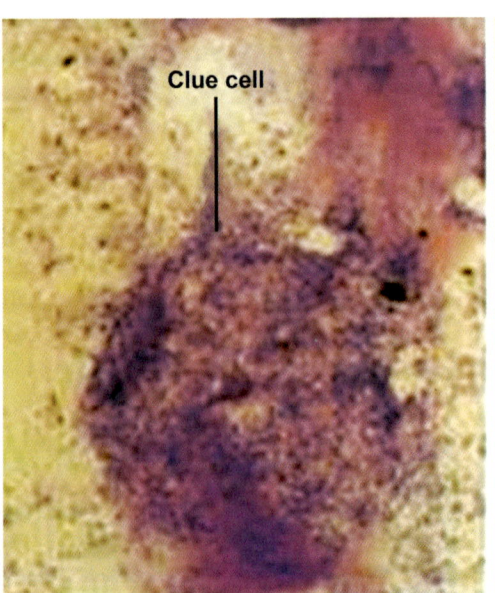 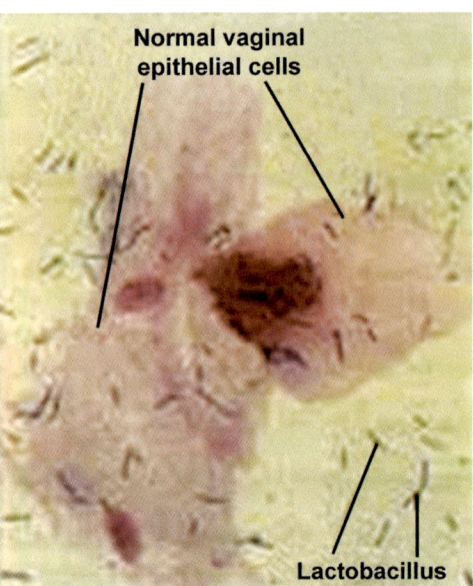

Fig. 14.2: Clue cells on wet smear

Recurrent Vulvovaginal Candidiasis

Vulvovaginal candidiasis is considered recurrent, when at least four specific episodes occur in one year, or a minimum of three episodes unrelated to antibiotic therapy occur within one year. It occurs in approximately 5% of women. Sources of infection:

- Vaginal reservoir of Candida
- Intestinal reservoir of Candida
- Sexual transmission of Candida

    Organism could be *Candida albicans* or non-albicans like: *Candida glabrata*, *Candida tropicalis*, *Candida krusei*, *Candida parapsilosis*.

Causes of Recurrence

- Non-albicans Candida is less sensitive to imidazoles.
- Non-compliance of treatment regimen.
- Frequent antibiotics use.
- Diabetes mellitus.
- Use of spermicidal jellies and creams.
- *Oral contraceptive pills users:* Candida has estrogen and progesterone receptors causing fungal proliferation.
- Genetic susceptibility.
- The first study assessing the association of host factors with susceptibility to recurrent vulvovaginal candidiasis (RVVC) dates from Sobel and coworkers in 1997, who showed that there was no difference in the ABO phenotype between RVVC patients and controls, while there was a difference between two groups regarding the Lewi's phenotype. Patients from RVVC group were more likely to have nonsecretor phenotype [Lea+b-or Le(a-b-)] rather than the secretor pheotype [Le(a-b+)].
- Epithelial cells (ECs) express various surface recognition receptors that are able to respond to *Candida albicans* components, followed by cytokine secretion and immune cell activation and differentiation. Different polymorphisms have been found for those receptors. ECs have been shown to participate in growth inhibition of Candida.

- Perspiration associated with tightly fitted clothes increase the local temperature and moisture that favours recurrent growth of Candida.
- The role of sexual transmission (controversial).

    Recurrent VVC infections may benefit from alternative strategies including prophylactic fluconazole 100 mg PO weekly or clotrimazole 500 mg suppository weekly or biweekly administration of 600 mg of boric acid or nystatin powder. Nearly all of these prophylactic regimens should be used for 3 to 6 months to be effective.

Bacterial vaginosis (Gardnerella vaginalis). This common, clinically distinct, and readily recognizable form of vaginitis was first described by Gardner and Dukes in 1955. It was not until 1978, however, when a group of researchers in Seattle reported that this infection was virtually responsible for almost all cases of nonspecific vaginitis, and then widespread understanding of this form of vaginitis and the current therapy began to emerge. The organism identified with this infection has been reclassified from *Corynebacterium vaginalis* to *Haemophilus vaginalis*, and currently, to *G. vaginalis*.

The characteristic symptoms of BV is a homogenous grayish-white discharge with fishy odor that increases in intensity after sexual intercourse. Since there is often a little tissue inflammation irritative symptoms such as itching, burning, or soreness may be absent. The pelvic examination is unremarkable except for the presence of the odorous homogenous gray-white discharge that coats the vaginal walls and the cervix. Several criteria have been described for the diagnosis.

Amsel's Criteria

1. The vaginal fluid pH is almost always greater than 4.5.
2. The saline wet-mount preparation in BV shows 20% of epithelial cells stippled with

coccobacilli, giving them a granular appearance with indistinct cell margins. There is often a paucity of leukocytes and a virtual absence of the normally appearing lactobacilli (Fig. 14.2) **(clue cells)**.

3. The fishy odor becomes much worse when a smear of the discharge is mixed with a drop of 10% KOH **(Whiff test)**.

Nugent's scoring has been used by researchers.

Culture: A culture medium for *G. vaginalis* is now readily available and can be used when the clinical and microscopic findings are equivocal.

Management

Controversy exists concerning the treatment of sexual partners. Both men and women may carry the organisms asymptomatically.

Pharmacologic Treatment

a. *Metronidazole:* The current drug of choice which can be administered
   - Orally as 250 mg tid or 500 mg bid for 7 days. The 2 g single dose of metronidazole or secnidazole given PO and repeated on day 3 has been effective. However, the 7-day regimen cures between 5% and 20% more patients than does this two-dose regimen.
   - Vaginally as 0.75% gel or in tablet form bid for 5 days.

   Patients on oral metronidazole should be instructed to avoid alcoholic beverages during the course of treatment since there may be a disulfiram-like reaction.

b. *Clindamycin* 300 mg bid PO for 7 days, or clindamycin 2% cream intravagnally for 7 nights, is equally effective. It is safer for pregnant women than metronidazole but is expensive.

c. *Ampicillin*, 500 mg PO qid for 7 days, or a **cephalosporin** (cephalexin, 500 mg PO qid for 7 days), can be used but are less effective.

BV can cause serious upper genitourinary tract infections and should be promptly treated. Women with BV undergoing a cesarean section have a six-fold increased rate of postpartum endometritis; a three-fold increased rate of post-abdominal hysterectomy cuff cellulitis; an increased premature birth rate and several studies have shown that treatment with metronidazole reduces prematurity. There is a linkage between BV and chorioamnionitis as well.

However, the screening and treatment of BV in pregnancy is controversial because some studies have failed to demonstrate any benefit to these protocols. The Centers for Disease Control and Prevention (CDC) currently recommends screening for BV early in the second trimester in women with a history of preterm delivery, followed by treatment with oral metronidazole, if appropriate.

BV Recurrence Treatment

A one-time PO or intravaginal metronidazole treatment at time of coitus may prevent recurrence for those women who have intercourse-related infections. When recurrences do not have an identifiable relation to coitus, suppression of microorganisms associated with BV while allowing lactobacilli to re-establish is the goal. Initial metronidazole treatment for a 7-day course is recommended. Then treat with either an oral or intravaginal medication every third or fourth day for an additional month.

Trichomonas Vaginalis

Trichomonas vaginalis is a flagellated protozoan for which human reservoirs are the vagina and urethra. It can be carried asymptomatically in both men and women, particularly in the postmenopausal period. The mode of transmission is almost always sexual intercourse. The infection caused by *T. vaginalis* may involve the cervix, vagina, and vulva. Symptoms vary depending on the severity of the inflammatory response. A vaginal discharge may be the only symptom. As the inflammatory response progresses, the discharge increases, and vaginal soreness, itching, dyspareunia, postcoital spotting, or a combination of these, can occur. Sometimes abnormal bleeding comes from the inflammed endocervical cells, which bleed from direct contact. Some patients complain of pelvic or lower abdominal pain. Whether this represents inflammatory involvement of the upper genital tract or referred pain from the cervix is uncertain (Fig. 14.3).

The appearance of discharge varies with the inflammatory response. Although the discharge may be minimal, most patients have a gray-white secretion. The commonly described frothy green discharge is seen in only about 10% of patients. The vulva, vagina, and cervix can become swollen and red, depending on the severity of the infection. Bleeding from the endocervix is common when touched with a cotton tipped applicator or spatula. A nonspecific discomfort with bimanual palpation of the uterus and adnexa is present in some patients.

The diagnosis is usually made by observation of the motile flagellate on a saline smear. Although this microscopic examination is highly sensitive for detecting Trichomonas infection, studies have shown that the organisms may not be visible in many patients with a symptomatic infection. Patience and diligence at the microscope are often necessary. Trichomonas cultures are available at some laboratories and can be used when the infection is suspected but not seen under the microscope, especially in the setting of a high pH. Polymerase chain reaction (PCR) is being investigated as a diagnostic method. However, it is too expensive to be practical except for patients who have a persistent purulent discharge despite treatment.

Management

The asymptomatic patient in whom *T. vaginalis* is discovered does not require treatment unless there is a concern for sexual transmission. Sometimes the presence of this organism is suggested on a Papanicolaou (Pap) smear or urinalysis report. Confirmation should be obtained by a wet smear or culture if treatment is considered

1. *Metronidazole*, as a 2-g single dose, or 250 mg PO tid for 7 days, is the treatment of choice. Both regimens are 90 to 95% effective. The sexual partner should also be treated.

   T. vaginalis has become slightly more resistant to metronidazole in recent years. When a patient has a treatment failure, not reinfection , the following regimens have been tried with varying results: Metronidazole 1 g PO bid, and metronidazole intravaginally (cream base) bid for 7 to 10 days or tinidazole 2 g PO, one-time dose.

2. *Nonoxynol-9*, 100 mg spermicidal suppositories has for 2 nights serendipitously cured a woman with trichomoniasis infection that had resisted treatment for 3 years. Another provider tried this intravaginal suppository for 1 week on two different patients; one was cured.

Cervicitis

The cause of vulvovaginitis could be actually an endocervicitis. Approximately one-third of all women with vaginal discharge have

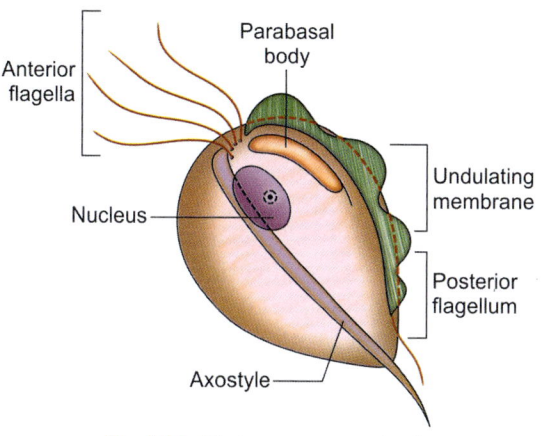

Anterior flagella

Parabasal body

Nucleus

Undulating membrane

Posterior flagellum

Axostyle

Fig. 14.3: *Trichomonas vaginalis*

endocervicitis and not a vaginal infection but it is generally overlooked as a cause. Consequently, women are treated with topical creams which do not reach the infected cervix since the inflammation extends into the underlying stroma. The cause of endocervicitis is infection with Chlamydia, gonorrhea, Trichomonas, or herpes simplex virus. Other causes have yet to be identified.

The woman generally presents with a non-irritating, non-odorous, mucoid discharge that may be yellow. Intermenstrual or postcoital spotting or both may be noted. Dyspareunia or pelvic discomfort or both may also be present. On per-speculum examination, the cervical mucosa appears inflamed with focal hemorrhages. At times, the cervix is friable and bleeds on touch. The discharge tends to be cloudy yellow or tenacious mucus from the endocervical glands. If herpes simplex virus is the etiologic agent, lesions will be seen on the vulva, vagina, or cervix. Wet-mount preparations usually show multiple WBCs and no particular pathogen unless Trichomonas is the etiologic agent. A recent study found that patients in whom a Gram's stain of a vaginal discharge showed no gram-negative intracellular diplococci and fewer than ten WBCs per oil-immersion field had a high incidence of chlamydial infections. A culture for gonorrhea and PCR for chlamydiae can be done, and testing for herpes simplex virus can be done if indicated. Management is as per the etiology or syndromic approach for cervicitis can be adopted.

Chemical Vulvovaginitis

The etiologies of chemical vulvovaginitis are different for children and adults. In children, the offending agents tend to be bubble baths, harsh soaps, and body lotions that often contain strong perfumes. In adolescents and adults, the involved agents tend to be soaps, perfumed toilet paper or pads, powders, contraceptive agents, or feminine hygiene products. A detailed history is very important.

The only necessary investigative procedure is the pelvic examination. Wet-mount preparations however rule out causes such as monilia and trichomonas. Investigations for gonorrhea and Chlamydia as indicated by history can be done.

Management is dependent on the severity of the vulvovaginitis. For mild or moderate cases, the treatment is non-fluorinated topical corticosteroids, such as 1% hydrocortisone cream, applied twice daily for 7 to 10 days to the involved perineal area. In the more severe cases, hospitalization may be necessary for pain management and bladder catheterization. Regardless of the severity, the woman must be instructed to discontinue all current and future use of the offending agent.

Molestation or abuse must be suspected in infants younger than 10 to 12 months who present with a foreign body in or trauma to the genital area. In general, this age group is not coordinated enough to insert a foreign body into the vagina. The most common foreign body in the adolescent and adult groups is the tampon. Tampons may have strings that have broken off or are difficult to reach, or they may have been forgotten until the symptoms of infection have manifested.

Atrophic vaginitis is defined as inflammation of the vaginal epithelium that is due to lack of estrogen. It is important to distinguish between atrophic vagina and vaginitis. The importance lies in the fact that atrophic vaginitis is uncommon, whereas atrophic vaginas are common. The vagina is atrophic before menarche, during breastfeeding, and postmenopausally. The physiology is thin epithelium that lacks glycogen owing to a decrease in the endogenous estrogen. The pH increases to 6.5–7.0, which can support moldering bacterial infections. However, this pH environment usually does not support candidal, trichomonal or gonorrheal infections. The vaginal walls appear thin, dry and smooth with a little or no rugations. Inflammation, petechial hemorrhages, or exudate may be present. The wet-mount preparation shows multiple WBCs with many bacteria present.

Topical estrogen (e.g. premarin) can be applied to the introitus twice daily for 2 to 4 weeks. Nonpharmacologic methods of treatment include sitz baths everyday, improved local hygiene, wearing cotton undergarments, avoidance of harsh soaps. If vulvitis is present, calamine lotion applied to the affected area provides some relief.

Inflammatory Vaginitis

Desquamative inflammatory vaginitis is a clinical syndrome characterized by diffuse exudative vaginitis, epithelial cell exfoliation, and a profuse purulent vaginal discharge. The cause of inflammatory vaginitis is unknown, but Gram stain findings reveal a relative absence of normal long gram-positive lactobacilli and their replacement with gram-positive cocci, usually streptococci. Women with this disorder have a purulent vaginal discharge, vulvovaginal burning or irritation, and dyspareunia. Initial therapy is the use of 2% clindamycin cream, one applicator full (5 g) intravaginally once daily for 7 days. Relapse occurs in about 30% of patients, who should be retreated with intravaginal 2% clindamycin cream for 2 weeks. Alternatively pessary of clindamycin can be used.

Neoplasms

Benign and malignant neoplasms of the genital tract can be a cause of vaginal discharge. Most common benign neoplasms presenting in this fashion are the polyps from the cervix or uterus.

Cervical Polyps

Cervical polyps are small pedunculated, often sessile neoplasms of the cervix. Most originate from the endocervix; a few arise from the portiovaginalis. Endocervical polyps are usually red, flame-shaped, fragile growths and may vary in size from a few millimeters in length and diameter to larger tumors 2–3 cm in diameter and several centimeters long.

Most are benign and arise as a result of focal hyperplasia of the endocervix but all should be removed and submitted for pathologic examination because malignant change may occur. Moreover, some cervical cancers present as a polypoid mass.

Asymptomatic polyps often are discovered on routine pelvic examination. Those exposed to the lumen of the genital tract can cause a continuous discharge which is at first white or cream and non-offensive. Soon, however, when the growth becomes ulcerated and infected as the necrotic tissue is exposed to the large number of organisms present in the vagina, the discharge becomes purulent, offensive and blood-stained. Often the odor is so marked that it can be appreciated as soon as the woman enters the room. Such symptoms are characteristic of a malignant neoplasm but they may also be caused by benign lesions such as a cervical polyp or a sloughing submucous leiomyoma.

Management is in office removal or hysteroscopic removal under anesthesia depending upon size, site and presence or absence of a pedicle .

Urinary and Feculent Discharges

Urinary incontinence, can be confused with a vaginal discharge. A vaginal escape of feces betokens the presence of a fistula. A urinary or feculent discharge is usually recognized easily by its smell and color but difficulty can arise in distinguishing a slight fecal escape from, say, the discharge of a senile pyometra.

Approach to a Case of Vulvovaginitis

The approach to diagnosing the patient with vulvovaginitis consists of a careful history, pelvic examination, and microscopic examination of the vaginal fluid as well as assessment of vaginal pH and amine tests. All of the parts of the evaluation contribute to, and are essential for, a precise diagnosis. The normal vaginal pH is 3.8 to 4.2.

I. *History*

A. **Current symptoms**

- Focus on changes from a patient's personal norm.
- *Discharge:* Most women have some degree of leukorrhea. "How is the current discharge different?"
- *Odor:* a. Is there any odor? b. Is the odor constant? c. Does the odor occur after coitus?
- *Pruritus:* a. Is there pattern to the itching? b. Does the itching seem to be internal, external, or both?
- *Burning:* a. Is there burning with urination? b. Does the burning occur while urinating? c. Does the burning occur as the urine touches the skin?
- How long have the symptoms been occurring? a. What makes them better? b. What makes them worse?
- *Skin irritation or lesions:* a. Is the skin irritated? (1) What areas are involved? (i) Vulva, (ii) Vagina, (iii) Rectum. b. Is there a history of sensitive skin? c. Is there a history of dry skin? d. Is there any rash or sore on any part of the body?
- Sexual activity: a. Are the sexual partners male, female, or both? b. Are the symptoms increased with sexual activity? c. In the past year, has there been more than one coitus partner? d. Is the sexual partner in a monogamous relationship with the patient? e. Is there a need for contraception?
- *Medication and contraceptives:* Medications, contraceptives have been contributory causes for vulvovaginitis, consequently, they all need to be identified.
- *Menses history:* a. Date of last menstrual period (LMP). b. Do the symptoms occur in any relationship to the menstrual cycle? c. Is the patient pregnant?
- Feminine hygiene products. Some women use over-the-counter sprays, perfume, or douches, or a combination there of, regularly.

- **Recurring vulvovaginitis** symptoms need to include the following questions:
  a. Have any medications caused itching or burning?
  b. What medications have been used for this problem? It is important to recognize that many women will have tried over-the-counter therapies or will have been prescribed a medication after a telephone consultation only. (1) miconazole, (2) setraconazole, (3) ketoconazole, (4) clotrimazole, (5) metronidazole, (6) antibiotics, (7) hydrocortisone, (8) estrogen cream, (9) acyclovir, (10) fluorouracil (5-FU) cream, (11) others including OTCs.
  c. *Systemic diseases:* Some systemic diseases can cause vulvovaginitis symptoms. A few of these include: (1) Diabetes mellitus, (2) acquired immunodeficiency syndrome (AIDS), (3) rheumatoid arthritis, (4) lupus, (5) Hodgkin's disease, (6) leukemia, (7) skin diseases such as psoriasis and eczema.

II. *Physical Examination*

Physical examination must include the vulva, vagina, and cervix. On occasion, the uterus, ovaries, and rectum also need to be evaluated. When managing difficult or recurring cases of vulvovaginitis, the goal shifts to identifying cutaneous lesions (which may need biopsy) ; obtaining vaginal secretions for further evaluation; and investigating the possibility of obscure diagnoses, such as rectovaginal fistula, vesicovaginal fistula, bladder leakage, and urethral diverticulum.

III. *Laboratory Procedures*

a. Saline and potassium hydroxide (KOH) preparations generally take less than 3 minutes yet are invaluable in identifying what is or is not causing the vulvovaginitis complaint. If there is an excess of white blood cells (WBCs), a mixed infection must be considered.

b. Cultures of the vaginal fluids or cervix may be necessary to clarify the diagnosis.

c. The pH of the normal vaginal discharge is 3.8 to 4.2. An alkaline pH suggests BV or *T. vaginalis*.

Syndromic Approach to Vaginal Discharge

The importance of reproductive tract infections (RTIs) in causing morbidity and long-term sequelae has been recognized by the World Health Organization (WHO), which has recommended the syndromic approach to RTIs at the community level. In most cases, several different infections are found to coexist with RTIs; the availability of facilities for accurate laboratory diagnosis in peripheral centres is lacking. Patients are thus denied the benefit of prompt therapy leading to sequelae.

The management of a patient presenting with vaginal discharge depends on the availability of a speculum and/or laboratory facilities. If a woman presents with a complaint of vaginal discharge to a health facility where even a speculum is not available, she and her partner are treated empirically for gonorrhea, Chlamydia, candidiasis, trichomoniasis and bacterial vaginosis if her partner has a genital ulcer or discharge. In the absence of a lesion in the partner, treatment for gonorrhea is omitted from the above protocol. If speculum examination is feasible, treatment is given according to the nature of discharge:

- *Mucopus:* Treat for gonorrhea and chlamydia.

- *Profuse discharge:* Treat for trichomoniasis and bacterial vaginosis.

- *Clumped discharge:* Treat for candidiasis. If the partner has a lesion, the couple are given treatment for gonorrhea and Chlamydia as well. If a microscope is available, a wet mount examination (with saline and KOH) is carried out to look for trichomonads, yeast cells and clue cells, and treatment given accordingly. If the problem persists after this primary management, the patient is referred to a higher care center.

However, due to the magnitude of the problem and the reasons cited above, evaluation and validation of this strategy as a public health measure is currently underway and requires further evaluation.

Bibliography

1. Akhtar S, et al. J Pak Med Assoc. 2012;62(10): 1049–52.
2. Burns FM, et al. Diagnosis of bacterial vaginosis in a routine diagnostic laboratory. *Med Lab Sci* 1992;49:8.
3. CDC 2010 STD treatment guidelines.
4. Jeffcoate N. Vaginal Discharge. Jeffcoate's Principles of Gynaecology. 2008;656–661.
5. Sobel JD, et al. Vulvovaginal candidiasis: Epidemiologic, diagnostic and therapeutic considerations. *Am J Obstet Gynaecol* 1998; 178:203–11.
6. Ramsay S, et al. Practical management of recurrent vulvovaginal candidiasis. Trends in Uro Gyn and sexual health. Nov/Dec 2009.
7. United Kingdom National Guidelines on the management of vulvovaginal candidiasis.

15

Abnormal Uterine Bleeding

• **Kiran Pandey**

Abnormal uterine bleeding (AUB) is defined as bleeding from uterine corpus that is abnormal in regularity, volume, frequency or duration and occurs in absence of pregnancy. It may be **acute or chronic.**

It is a major gynecological problem responsible for as many as one third of all out patients. The prevalence of AUB in reproductive age group ranges from 9 to 30%.

It is a debilitating disorder both medically and socially. In addition, it is the commonest cause of iron deficiency anemia in the developed world and of chronic illness in the developing world.

AUB is a revised terminology which has been introduced by Fig. 15.1, 2011. It includes the existing terminology of dysfunctional uterine bleeding along with menstrual abnormalities from other causes according to**PALM-COEIN classification system**. According to bleeding pattern, it uses the term **"Heavy menstrual bleeding" or "Intermenstrual bleeding"**.

Pathophysiology

The pathophysiology of abnormal uterine bleeding and DUB has been thoroughly reviewed. The cyclical hormonal stimulation of endometrial growth by estrogen during the follicular phase of the menstrual cycle, followed by estrogen and progesterone after ovulation, is the mainstay of normal

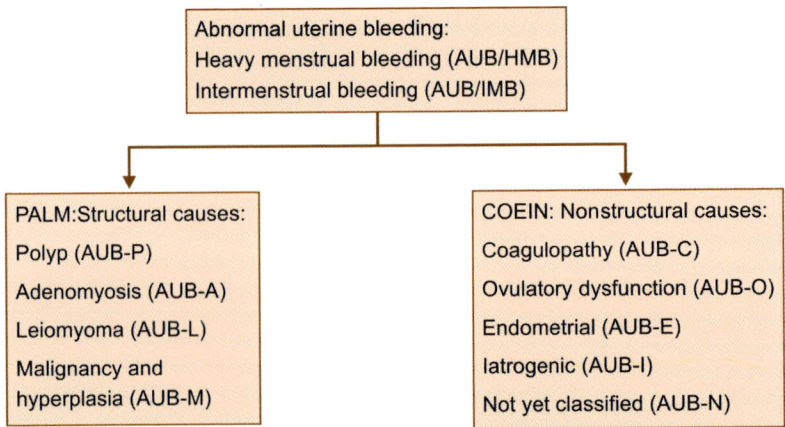

Fig. 15.1: Classification for AUB

development of the proliferative and secretory endometrium respectively.**Withdrawl of both of these hormones following degeneration of the corpus luteum** is believed to result in the menstrual blood flow.

- DUB is believed to occur as a result of the **derangement of the cyclical sex hormonal stimulation** orchestrated by follicular development, followed by ovulation and formation of corpus luteum and its degeneration when pregnancy does not occur.

- Menstrual bleeding occurs mostly from the upper two-thirds of the uterine cavity following **tissue necrosis of the endometrium associated with disruption of microvasculature**and the **release of tissue necrosis factors released from migratory leukocytes with deposition of platelets/fibrin thrombi in small blood vessels.** The molecular events underlying the endometrial tissue and vascular breakdown are related to the **release of proteolytic enzymes from lysosomes of the endometrial inflammatory cells.**

- In DUB, endometrial tissue breakdown located in the superficial layer (subsurface) of the endometrium occurs either focally in scattered areas of the endometrium (resulting in breakthrough spotting) or diffusely throughout the endometrial cavity (resulting in heavier withdrawl bleeding). Such derangement of the endometrial tissue necrosis is believed to occur due to vascular alterations that are **associated with continuous estrogen stimulation unopposed by progesterone (anovulatory DUB) or irregular progesterone stimulation due to dysfunctional corpus luteum (ovulatory DUB)** while **proliferative endometrium is encountered in anovulatory** DUB, ovulatory DUB is not appreciated histologically. It is supposed that in ovulatory DUB **there is increase in prostaglandins causing vasodilatation like PGE_2 and PGI_2 in comparison to** vasoconstrictors like **$PGF_{2\alpha}$ and thromboxane A_2 which is a platelet aggregator**.

Polyp (AUB-P): There seems to be a little controversy regarding the inclusion of endometrial and endocervical polyps. These epithelial proliferation comprise a variable vascular, glandular, fibromuscular and connective tissue component and are often asymptomatic. But it is generally accepted that at least some polyp contribute to the genesis of AUB. The lesions are usually benign but a small minority may have malignant features. For the basic classification system, polyps are categorized as being either present or absent, as defined by one or a combination of ultrasound and hysteroscopic imaging with or without histopathology. Although there is no distinction regarding the size or no of polyps, it is probably important to exclude polypoidal appearing endometrium from this category because such an appearance may be a normal variant (Fig. 15.1).

Adenomyosis (AUB-A)

Adenomyosis is a disorder characterized by the extension of endometrial glands and stroma into the myometrium. Estimates of the prevalence of adenomyosis vary widely, ranging from 5%. Heavy menstrual bleeding and painful menstruation are the major symptoms of adenomyosis, occurring in approximately 50–60% and 25–30% of women respectively. Diagnosed by ultrasound or MRI (Fig. 15.2).

Leiomyomas (AUB-L)

It is a benign tumor of smooth muscles of the uterus and is commonly known as fibroid. It is the most common benign tumor of the genital tract. Age is most common risk factor with lifetime risk in women over 45 yrs of age is more than 60%. Higher association of AUB is observed with submucosal lesion, compared to intramural and subserosal leiomyomas (Fig. 15.3).

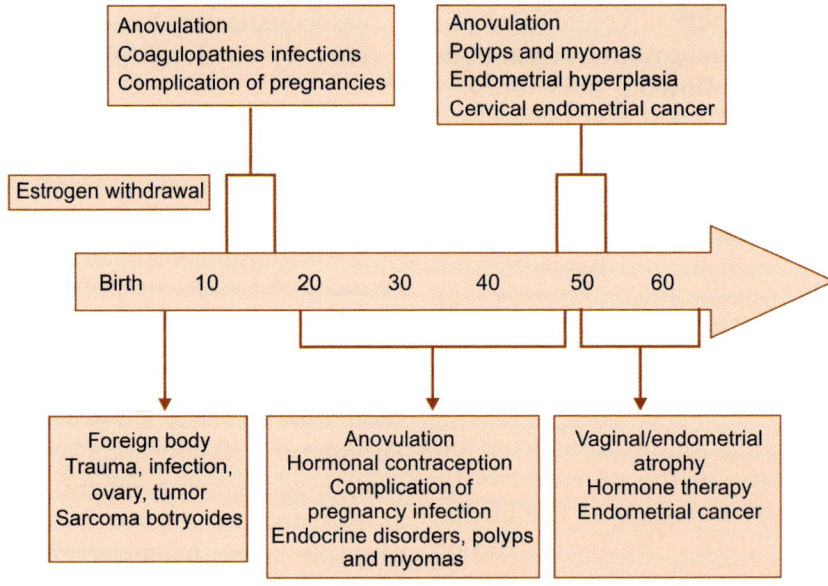

Fig. 15.2: Usual causes of abnormal bleeding by age

Malignancy (AUB-M)

AUB-M includes both malignant and non malignant lesions (Fig. 15.4), usually it is the primary symptom of endometrial neoplasia. In perimenopausal age 70% have benign lesions, 15% have hyperplasias and 15% have endometrial cancer. Approximately 50% of the women diagnosed with endometrial hyperplasia also have concurrent endometrial carcinoma.

Coagulopathy (AUB-C)

10–20% of women with HMB have a disorder of hemostasis that may be overlooked during the differential diagnosis. Bleeding from anticoagulation therapy is listed under AUB-C.

Ovulatory Dysfunction (AUB-O)

Patients with unpredictable menses with variable flow are usually associated with endocrinopathies, such as polycystic ovary syndrome or hypothyroidism. AUB-O suggests dysfunction of ovulation and therefore is synonymous with anovulatory AUB. It should not be confused with ovulatory AUB which is described as AUB-E. Because AUB-O is an endocrinologic abnormality the underlying disorder should be treated medically rather than surgically.

Endometrial Causes (AUB-E)

Most patients in this category will have regular cycles, normal ovulation and no definable cause of AUB (ovulatory). Usually present with HMB, which may indicate a disorder of endometrial hemostasis. Others may present with IMB, which may be secondary to inflammation, infection, or abnormal inflammatory responses.

Iatrogenic (AUB–I)

Causes include IUD, exogenous gonadal steroids and other systemic agents that effect blood coagulation or ovulation.

Not Yet Classified (AUB-N)

Reserved for entities that are poorly defined and/or not well-examined, such as arteriovenous malformation and myometrial hypertrophy. With more evidence, entities such as these will likely be placed into a new or existing category.

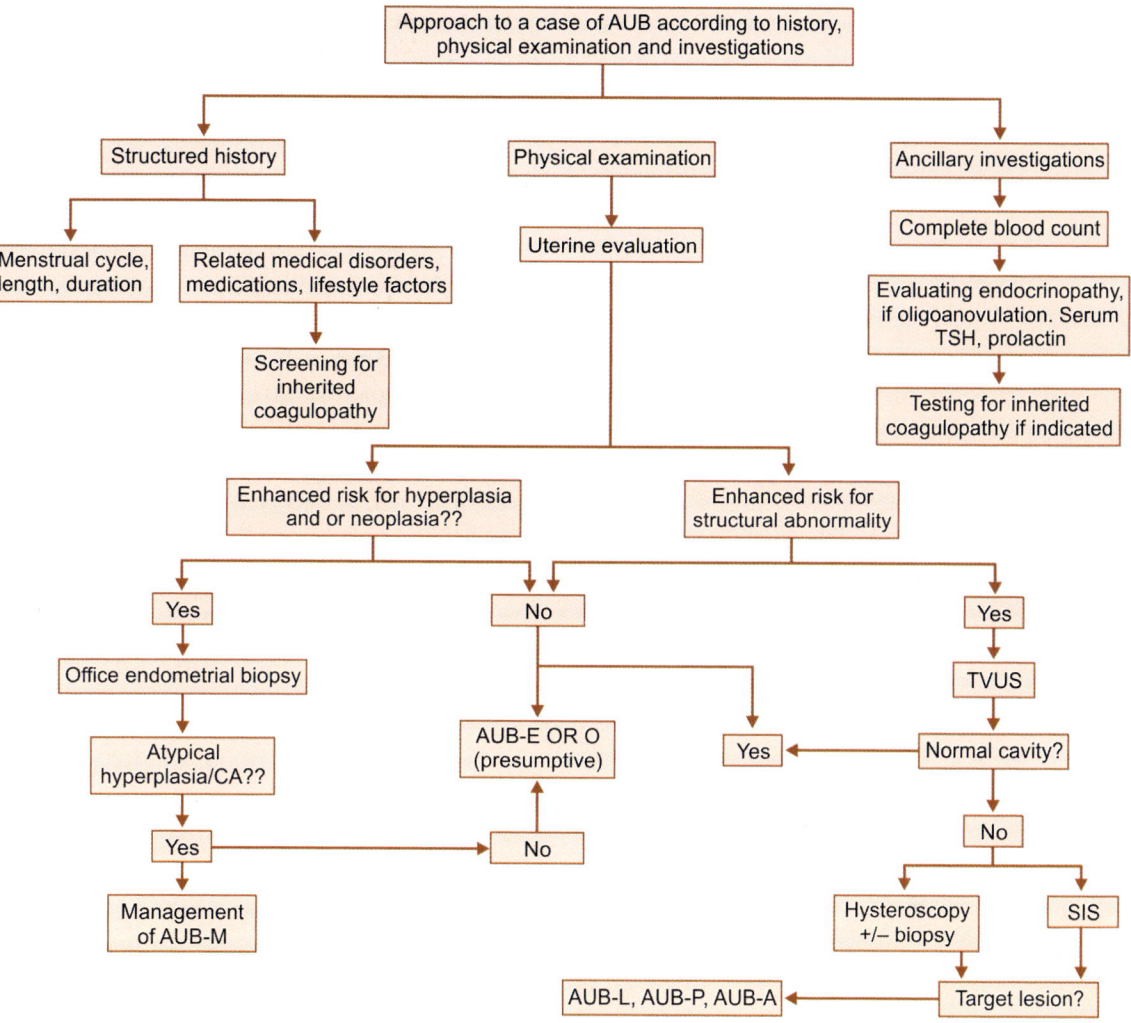

Fig. 15.3: Diagnosis of AUB

Notation

Following appropriate investigation, an individual may be found to have, one or more potential causes of, or contributors to, their AUB symptoms. Consequently, the system has been designed to enable categorization and notation in a fashion that allows for this circumstance. It is recognized that this increased level of complexity will be of most value to specialists and researchers.

The formal approach follows the example of the WHO TNM staging of malignant tumors, with each component addressed for all patients. For example, **if it were determined that an individual had a disorder of ovulation, a leiomyoma, and no other abnormalities**, they would be categorized as follows in the context of a complete evaluation:

AUB P0 A0 L1 M0 C0 O1 E0 I0 N0

Recognizing that, in clinical practice, the full notation might be considered to be cumbersome, an abbreviation option has been developed. The patient previously described would be categorized **AUB-L;O** (Fig. 15.5).

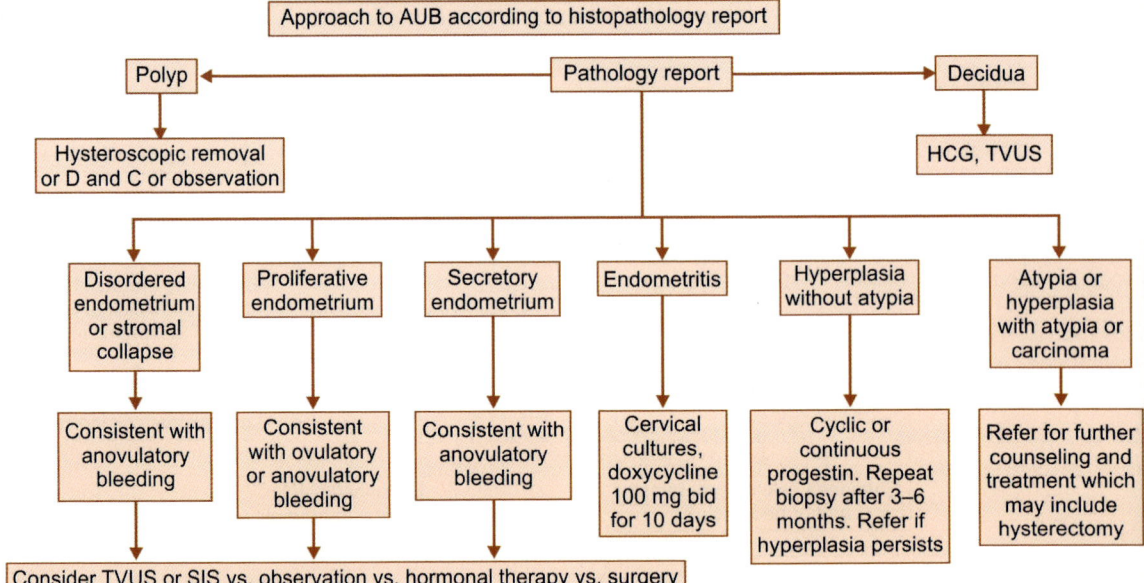

Fig. 15.4: Management options for AUB

Diagnosis and Management

Structured history is very important in a case of AUB so as to identify the cause and treat accordingly. Essential points of history are:

- Age of the women
- Amount, frequency, regularity of bleeding, presence of postcoital or intermenstrual bleeding and any dysmenorrhea or premenstrual symptoms which can help to distinguish anovulatory from ovulatory bleeding.

- Symptoms of anemia.
- Reproductive history
- Impact on social, sexual functioning and quality of life.
- Symptoms suggestive of systemic causes of bleeding such as hypothyroidism, hyperprolactinemia, coagulation disorders, PCOS, adrenal or hypothalamic disorders.
- Symptoms that may indicate underlying pathology:
  - Persistent post-coital bleeding

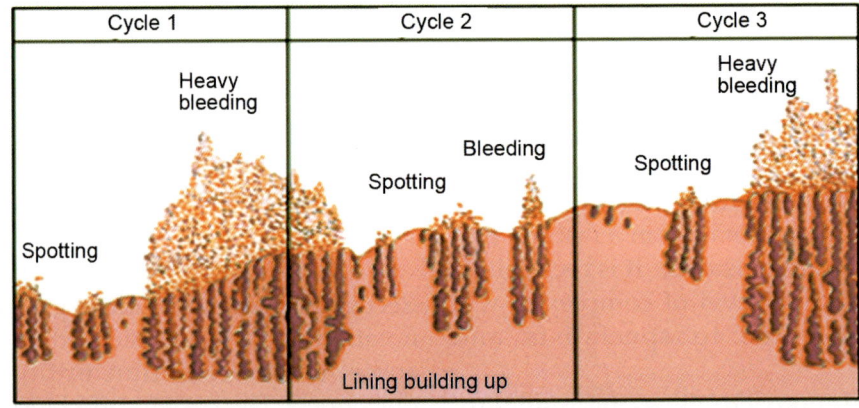

Fig. 15.5: Dysfunctional uterine bleeding

– Persistent intermenstrual bleeding
– Dyspareunia
– Dysmenorrhea
– Pelvic pain and or pressure symptoms
– Vaginal discharge
- A family history of inherited coagulation disorders, PCOS, or endometrial or colon cancers.
- Drug history of warfarin, heparin, NSAIDS, hormonal contraceptives.
- History of blood transfusion.
- Risk factors for endometrial carcinoma age, obesity, nulliparity, PCOS, diabetes, HNPCC.

Physical Examination

i. *General assessment* for vital signs, weight/BMI, thyroid examination, skin examination (pallor, bruising, striae, hirsutism, petechiae.
ii. *Abdominal examination* for any mass and hepatosplenomegaly.
iii. *Gynecological examination* includes inspection of vulva, vagina, cervix, anus and urethra, **bimanual examination of uterus and adnexal structures**.

Investigations

- *Pregnancy test:* To exclude abnormal bleeding related to complications of pregnancy.
- *Complete blood count:* To exclude anemia and thrombocytopenia.
- *Serum progesterone:* To document ovulation and anovulation.
- **Pap smear**
- *Serum TSH:* To exclude thyroid disorder.
- *LFT and KFT:* To exclude medical disorders.
- *Coagulation profile:* To exclude coagulopathies.
- *Endometrial sampling/endometrial biopsy:* To rule out chronic endometritis, hyperplasia and adenocarcinoma. Presently hysteroscopic guided biopsy is the gold standard.

Imaging

i. TVS
ii. SIS (saline infusion sonography)
iii. Hysteroscopy
iv. MRI

Treatment

The primary objective of treatment in women with anovulatory bleeding is to induce or restore the normal menstruation. Hospitalization is indicated for women with active hemorrhage who are hemodynamically unstable and those with symptomatic anemia or a serious underlying medical illness.

Progestin Therapy

- Commonly used norethindrone or medroxyprogesterone.
- Cyclic vs continuous—orally or via IUD
- Growing evidence indicates that LNG-IUS can be very effective in providing relief from both menorrhagia and dysmenorrhea in women with adenomyosis. Mirena— very well tolerated, reduce bleeding 79–94% best of all treatment options.
- In oligomenorrheic anovulatory women with episodic abnormal bleeding self-limited progestogen withdrawal bleeding can be induced by cyclic treatment with orally active progestin (medroxyprogesterone acetate 5–10 mg daily for 12–14 days each month). Failed progestin treatment suggests strongly that other pathology is responsible for the problem and needs further evaluation.

Estrogen-progestin Therapy

- Women with anovulatory bleeding who are sexually active and not immediately prepared to persue pregnancy generally are best managed by estrogen-progestin therapy.
- Acute prolonged episodes of heavy anovulatory bleeding also can be treated effectively with high dose estrogen-

progestin therapy, provided endometrial thickness is normal or increased.

- Any monophasic combination oral contraceptive can be used, beginning with one pill twice daily and decreasing to one pill daily thereafter. Treatment should continue for a total of at least 2 weeks, even when bleeding markedly slows or stops, which can be expected within 24–48 hrs.
- Regulates cycle especially with anovulatory bleeding.

Estrogen Therapy

- When acute, heavy bleeding results in a thin, denuded endometrium, high dose estrogen therapy is the best initial treatment: Progestin or estrogen-progestin therapy is unlikely to succeed and may aggravate the problem.
- IV conjugated equine estrogen 25 mg every 4 hrs until bleeding slows. Causes nausea, breast tenderness, given slowly or can cause vasovagal reaction and may increase the risk of thromboembolism.

GnRH Agonist

- Very effective at achieving amenorrhea. Limited by side effects of hot flushes, depression, osteopenia and cost.
- In women with severe anemia resulting from menorrhagia, preoperative GnRH induced amenorrhea can provide temporary relief from further bleeding, which allows hemoglobin levels to normalize, decreasing the rate of transfusion before surgery and also the size of myomas allowing vaginal surgery.

Tranexamic Acid

Antifibrinolytic agent reversibly blocks lysine binding sites on plasminogen. Thereby preventing fibrin degradation. Dose is 1–1.5 gm 3–4 times daily for 4–7 days during menses.

Nonsteroidal Anti-inflammatory Drugs

- Might be considered the first line therapy for ovulatory women with heavy menstrual bleeding and no demonstrable pathology.
- NSAID treatment reduces blood loss by 20–40%.

Surgical Treatment

Curettage

- In women with acute bleeding, dilatation and curettage can be performed as both a diagnostic and therapeutic procedure.
- Surgical denudation of basal endometrial layer is presumed to acutely stimulate all of the normal process involved in cessation of normal menstrual bleeding—local clotting mechanisms, vasoconstriction of basal arterioles and re-epithelialization.

Hysteroscopy

- Good for structural causes, myomectomy, polypectomy, etc.
- Hysteroscopic myomectomy is a logical choice for a single small submucous myomas.
- For endometrial polyp it is a simple and highly effective remedy.

Endometrial Ablation

- Hysteroscopic ablation includes laser, rollerball coagulation, loop resection, and vaporization.
- Nonhysteroscopic ablation includes thermal balloon, cryoablation, radiofrequency probe, unipolar or bipolar electrodes, diodes laser, photodynamic therapy.
- Submucous fibroids less than 3 cm microwave ablation may be ideal.

Hysterectomy is a definitive procedure (abdominal, vaginal, laparoscopic or laparoscopically assisted vaginal). Indications of hysterectomy are:

- Uterine fibroids/other benign lesions that do not respond to conservative treatment option.
- Atypical hyperplasia on histopathology.

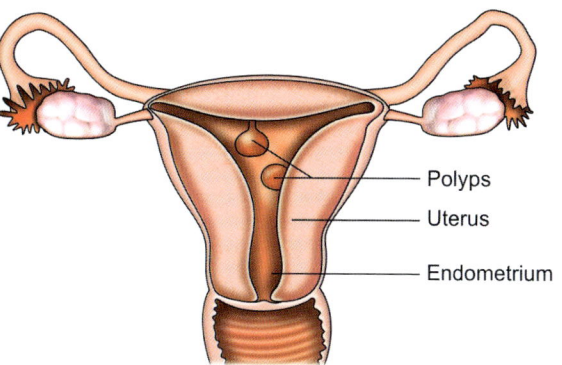

Fig. 15.6: Endometrial polyp

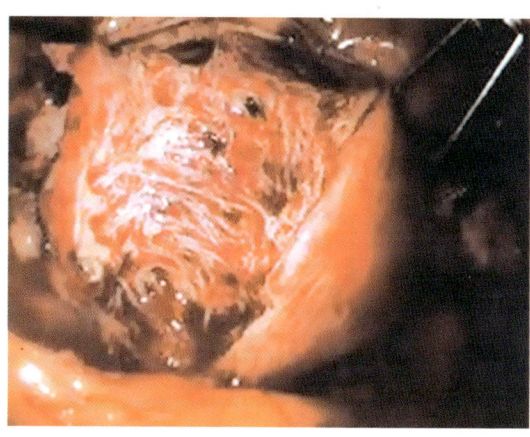

Fig. 15.7: Cut-section of uterus showing adenomyosis

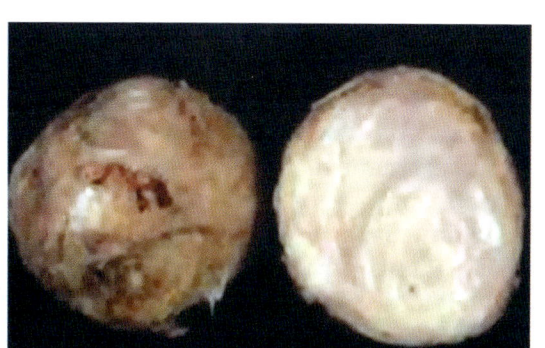

Fig. 15.8: Leiomyoma uterus

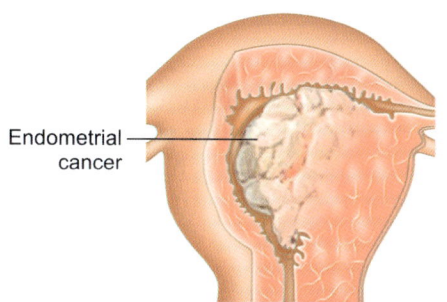

Fig. 15.9: Endometrial cancer

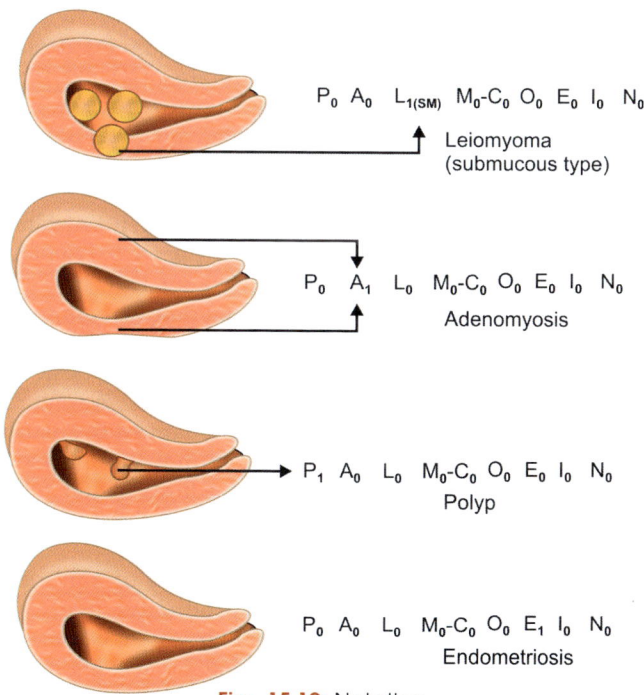

P_0 A_0 $L_{1(SM)}$ M_0-C_0 O_0 E_0 I_0 N_0

Leiomyoma
(submucous type)

P_0 A_1 L_0 M_0-C_0 O_0 E_0 I_0 N_0

Adenomyosis

P_1 A_0 L_0 M_0-C_0 O_0 E_0 I_0 N_0

Polyp

P_0 A_0 L_0 M_0-C_0 O_0 E_1 I_0 N_0

Endometriosis

Fig . 15.10: Notation

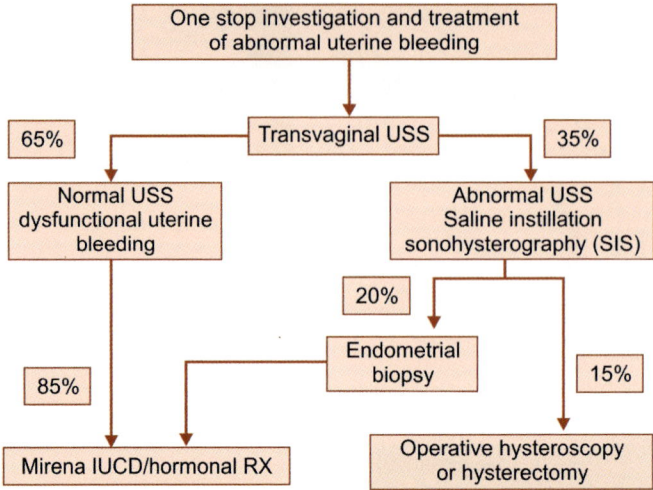

Fig . 15.11: Treatment for AUB

- Severe and intractable endometriosis and/or adenomyosis, after pharmaceutical or other surgical options have failed.
- Certain types of reproductive system cancers (uterine, cervical, ovarian, endometrium).

Key Points

- Menstrual disorders are the most prevalent gynecologic health problem and heavy menstrual bleeding affects up to 30% of women at some time during their reproductive years.
- The societal and personal burden of AUB lies in its major impact on quality of life, productivity, and health care utilization and cost.
- There is a requirement for the development of the classification system, on several levels, for the causes of AUB, which can be used by clinicians, investigators and even patients to facilitate communication, clinical care, and research.
- The manuscript PALM-COEIN (polyp; adenomyosis; leiomyoma;malignancy and hyperplasia; coagulopathy; ovulatory dysfunction; endometrial; iatrogenic and not yet classified.) has been approved by international federation of Gynecology and Obstetrics (FIGO).

- Medical management should be the initial treatment for most patients if appropriate. Surgical management should be considered for patients who are not clinically stable, or fail to respond to medical management.

Bibliography

1. 44 NCG. Heavy menstrual bleeding,United Kingdom: national institute of health and clinical excellence, 2007.
2. Anastasiadis PG, Koutalki NG, Skaphida PG, Galazios GC, Tsikouras PN, Liberis VA Endometrial polyps; prevalence, detection, and malignant potential in women with abnormal uterine bleeding. Eur J Gynaecol Oncol 2000 21(2); 180–3.
3. Ash SJ, Farell SA, Flowerdew G. Endometrial biopsy in DUB. J Reprod Med 1996:41(12):892–6
4. Breitkopf DM, Frederickson RA, Synder RR Detection of benign endometrial masses by endometrial stripe measurement in postmenopausal women. Obstet Gynaecol 2004;104(1).
5. Critchley HO, Warner P, Lee AJ, Brechin S, Guise J, Graham B. Evaluation of abnormal uterine bleeding: comparison of three outpatient procedures within cohorts defined by age and menopausal status. Health Technol Assess 2004 8(34):1–139.
6. Diagnosis of abnormal uterine bleeding in reproductive age women. Practice bulletin no.128. ACOG Obstet Gynaecol 2012;120:197–206
7. Dueholm M, Lundorf E, Hansen ES, Ledertoug S, Olesen F. Evaluation of uterine cavity with

magnetic resonance imaging, transvaginal sonography, hysterosonographic examination, and diagnostic hysteroscopy. Fertil Steril 2001: 76(2):350–7.

8. Farquhar CM, Lethaby A, Sowter M, Verry J, Baranyai J. An evaluation of risk factors for endometrial hyperplasia in premenopausal women with abnormal menstrual bleeding. Am J Obstet Gynaecol 1999;181(3):525–9.

9. Kadir RA, Economides DL, Sabin CA, Owens D, Lee CA. Frequency of inherited bleeding disorder in women with menorrhagia. Lancet 1998; 351(9101):485–9.

10. Kouides PA, Conard J, Peyvandi F, Lukes A, Qadir R. Hemostasis and menstruation: appro-priate investigation for underlying disorders of hemostasis in women with excessive menstrual bleeding. Fertil Steril 2005:84(5): 1345–51.

11. Lieng M, Istre O, Sandvik L,Qvigstad E. Prevalence, 1-year regression rate, and clinical significance of asymptomatic endometrial polyps; cross-sectional study.J Minim Invasive Gynaecol 2009;16(4);465 71.

12. Lu KH, Broaddus RR. Gynaecological tumours in hereditary nonpolyposis colorectal cancer: we know they are common now what? Gynaecol Oncol 2001;82(2):221–2.

13. Malcolm CE, Cumming DC. Does anovulation exist in eumenorrheic women? Obstet Gynaecol 2003;102(2):317–8.

14. Metcalf MG. Incidence of ovulation from menarche to menopause; observations of 622 New Zealand women. NZ Med J 1983;96(738): 645–8.

15. Munro MG, Critchley HO, Border MS, Fraser IS, FIGO classification system (PALM-COEIN) for causes of abnormal uterine bleeding in non gravid women of reproductive age. Int J Gynaecol Obstet 2011;113:3–13

16. Saheta Astha, Hariharan C, Sharma Urvashi; IOSR Journal of Dental and Medical Sciences; e-ISSN: 2279-0853, p-ISSN 2279-0861. Volume 13 , Issue 11 Ver. II (nov 2014), pp 63–67.

17. Speroff Leon, Fritz Marc A. Clinical Gynecologic Endocrinology and Infertility, 8th edn, 2012 (15); 591–617.

18. Srivastava A, Mansel RE, Arvind N, Prasad K, Dhar A, Chabra A. Evidence-based management of mastalgia. A meta-analysis of randomized trials breast 2007:16(5):503–12.

19. Sushan A, Revel A , Rojansky N. How often are endometrial polyps malignant? GynaecolObstet Invest 2004;58(4);212–5.

20. Weiss G, Maseelall P, Schott LL, Brockwell SE, Schocken M, Johnston JM. Adenomyosis a variant, not a disease? Evidence from hysterecto-mised postmenopausal women in the study of Women's Health Across the Nation. (SWAN). Fertil Steril 2009;91(1):2016.

16

Etiopathogenesis and Symptomatology of Endometriosis

• Nutan Jain

Endometriosis is a benign pathological condition characterized by presence of endometrial glands and stroma outside the endometrial cavity and uterine musculature. Pelvic viscera and peritoneum are the most common sites for implantation of ectopic endometrium. However, endometriosis has been described in extra pelvic sites, including anterior abdominal wall, surgical scars, diaphragm, omentum, small intestine, appendix, lung, urinary tract, musculoskeletal and nervous systems.[1–5] Endometriosis presents with subfertility and pelvic pain both adversely affecting the quality of life.

Prevalence and Epidemiology of Endometriosis

The prevalence of endometriosis in general population is difficult to assess due to selection bias as only the patients undergoing surgery are definitively diagnosed. Even the method of surgery, i.e. laparotomy versus laparoscopy and the skill of the surgeon in assessing the lesions, affect the likelihood of diagnosis of endometriosis. However, the overall prevalence of endometriosis in reproductive age women is between 3 and 10%.[6–7] The prevalence is 40–50% in women complaining of pelvic pain, 9–50% in infertile women and 1–7% in asymptomatic women undergoing tubal ligation.

Endometriosis is a disease of reproductive age group (25–35 years). It is rare before menarche and regresses after menopause. The prevalence of asymptomatic endometriosis is higher in Asians than in white women and much lower in blacks. Early menarche, short menstrual cycles with heavy menstrual bleeding, low parity, higher social class, lower body mass index, dioxins or polychlorinated biphenyles (PCB), increase intake of alcohol, fat, red meat, and caffeine increase the risk of endometriosis.[8]

Pregnancy, multiparity, prolonged periods of lactation, regular exercises and diet rich in vegetables and fruits are protective against the development of endometriosis.[8] Young girls under age 17 years presenting with endometriosis, are mostly found to have associated Mullerian obstructive anomalies. Prenatal exposure of diethylstilbestrol is also associated with increased risk of endometriosis.

Pathogenesis of Endometriosis

The pathogenetic mechanism of endometriosis has proven to be elusive and many theories have been proposed. However, a single mechanism has not been able to explain the spectrum of this multifactorial disease with multifaceted features. The various proposed theories are:

1. Retrograde menstruation theory
2. Coelomic metaplasia theory
3. Induction theory
4. Venous and lymphatic dissemination
5. Immunological theory
6. Genetic predisposition
7. Environmental effects

Retrograde Menstruation Theory

It is known that 70 to 90% of women have retrograde menstruation especially those who have endometriosis. Endometrial cells have been reported to be seen in 59–79% of women and endometriosis is more common in women with obstructive Mullerian anomalies and in those who have short and heavy menstrual cycles. Endometriotic lesions are more common in dependent portions of the pelvis. Based on these observations Sampson in 1927 proposed the most widely accepted theory called the retrograde menstruation and implantation theory.[9,10] According to the theory the endometrial tissue shed during menstruation is transported via the fallopian tubes into the peritoneal cavity where it gets implanted on the surfaces of pelvic organs. However, this theory falls short in explaining the occurrence of disease in locations remote from the peritoneal cavity such as lungs, skin, lymph nodes and breast. It also does not explain the mechanism of endometriosis in early puberty and in newborns.

Coelomic Metaplasia Theory

Based on the fact that the ovarian surface epithelial could be experimentally transformed into a metaplastic endometriotic tissue in mice by genetic activation of K-ras oncogene, Meyer has proposed a similar mechanism for endometriosis especially to explain the occurrence of this disease in premenarcheal girls and in unusual locations such as pleura or lungs.[11]

Induction Theory

This theory is rather an extension of the Coelomic Metaplasia theory which elucidates the likely endogenous biochemical factors that can transform the undifferentiated peritoneal epithelium into endometrial tissue. However, this theory has not been demonstrated in primates.[12,13]

Vascular and Lymphatic Dissemination Theory

Appearance of endometriotic tissue in far away locations such as umbilicus, digestive tract, thoracic cavity, lung etc has also been explained by vascular and lymphatc carriage of the endometriotic tissue.

Immunological Theory

It has been observed that though retrograde menstruation occurs in majority of patients, not all women with retrograde menstruation develop endometriosis. Thus endometriosis has been proposed to be a disease of immunological surveillance failure.[14] Patients with endometriosis have been found to have impaired immune function with defective macrophages and NK cells that have impaired recognition and clearance of endometrial debris in the peritoneal fluid. Rather than acting as scavengers of the endometrial cells these macrophages and monocytes produce growth factors and cytokines conducive to growth of endometriotic cells. A possible association between endometriosis and other autoimmune diseases has also been noted.

Inflammatory Mediators Produced in Ectopic Endometrium

Prostaglandins	Inflammation
Cytokines	Peritoneal adhesion
Matrix metalloproteinases (mmp)	Invasion
VEGF-A	Growth
Estrogen	Proliferative changes

Genetic Factors

Endometriosis has been found to have polygenic inheritance with first degree relatives having 7 times more prevalence of endometriosis. Disease is more severe and occurs at an earlier age in women with a history of disease in first degree relative.[15–17]

Molecular Defects

Molecular biological evidence suggests that ectopic endometrium of endometriosis has been found to have higher local estrogen and prostaglandins (PGE_2) production as well as resistance to progesterone as compared to eutopic endometrium. This has been explained by epigenetic hypomethylation of promoters of SF-1 and ERβ genes. This further leads to a vicious self-perpetuating cycle of chronic inflammation.

However, there is no stand alone theory and all these theories are supposed to explain the pathogenesis of endometriosis in a complementary manner as shown in Fig. 16.1.

Classification

Endometriosis may be pelvic or extra pelvic. Pelvic endometriosis is classified into three types:

Superficial Peritoneal Endometriosis

The lesions are usually seen in the dependent portion of the pelvis, usually the surface of the ovaries, pelvic peritoneum over the anterior and posterior surfaces of uterus, pouch of Douglas, uterosacral ligaments and broad ligaments. Such lesions may also be seen on cervix, vagina and rarely even on the vulva.

Ectopic endometrium irritates the surrounding tissue and causes an inflammatory reaction leading to increased presence of macrophages and neovascularization. Later a fibrotic tissue is formed around the endometriotic tissue thus encapsulating it. The endometriotic tissues grow into the surrounding tissue without any regards to the tissue boundaries. Gross appearance of superficial peritoneal endometriosis includes early, subtle lesions which are papular or vescicular with a diameter of <5 mm. Such lesions may occur singly or in clusters. Hemorrhagic lesions appear red and flame-shaped because of increased local vascularity with newly formed radiating vessels. These lesions represent the most active type of lesions (Fig. 16.1). Powder burn lesions which appear puckered and blue black (Fig. 16.2) are formed due to bleeding into the endometriotic tissue and breakdown into various hemoglobin degradation products such as hemosiderin. These lesions are flat or show slight elevations over the peritoneal surface. Eventually, these lesions fibrose into white or black pigmented lesions. Peritoneal pockets or Allen Masters pockets (Fig. 16.3) may also harbor endometriotic tissue.[18,19]

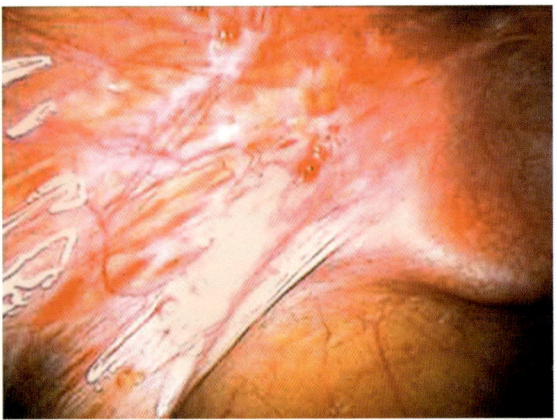

Fig. 16.1: Red, brown endometriotic implants noted

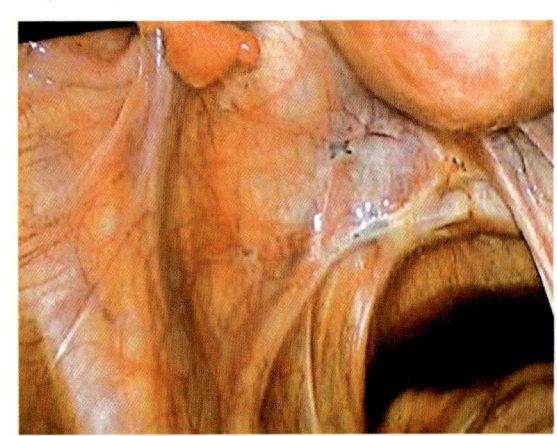

Fig. 16.2: Blue, black lesion

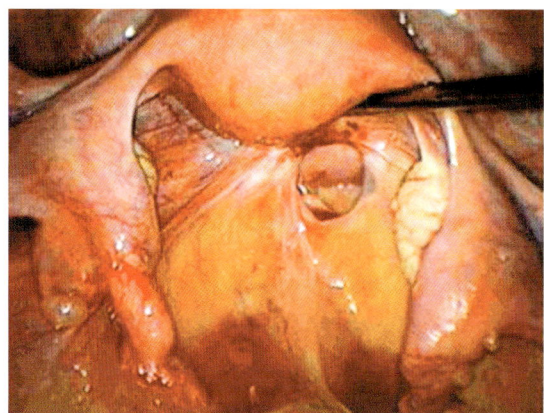

Fig. 16.3: Peritoneal defects

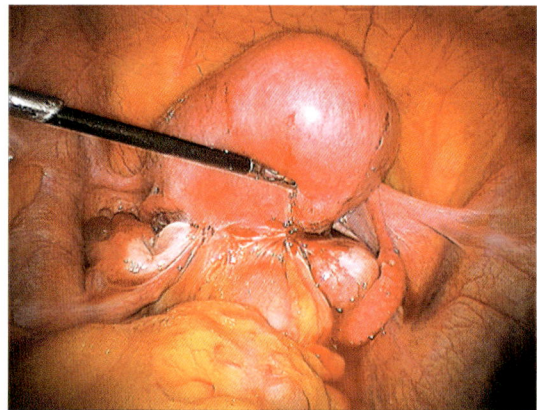

Fig. 16.5: The rectosigmoid is clearly attached to the posterior part of the cervix

Deep Infiltrating Endometriosis

This is also called posterior pelvic endo-metriosis. It is the most severe form of disease described by Donnez et al[20] as adenomyosis of rectovaginal septum. Novak and Woodruff[21] verified the lesion as a combination of fibromuscular tissue with endometriotic glands and stroma. These lesions extend more than 5 mm beneath the peritoneum mostly localized to the posterior to the posterior cul de sac, uterosacral ligaments and also to the uterovesical fold (Figs 16.4 and 16.5).

Three types of lesions have been described (Fig. 16.6).

• Type 1 lesions are those involving large pelvic area and are typical or subtle and surrounded by white sclerotic tissue.

• Type 2 lesion is associated with retraction of bowel and on excision usually reveals a nodule.

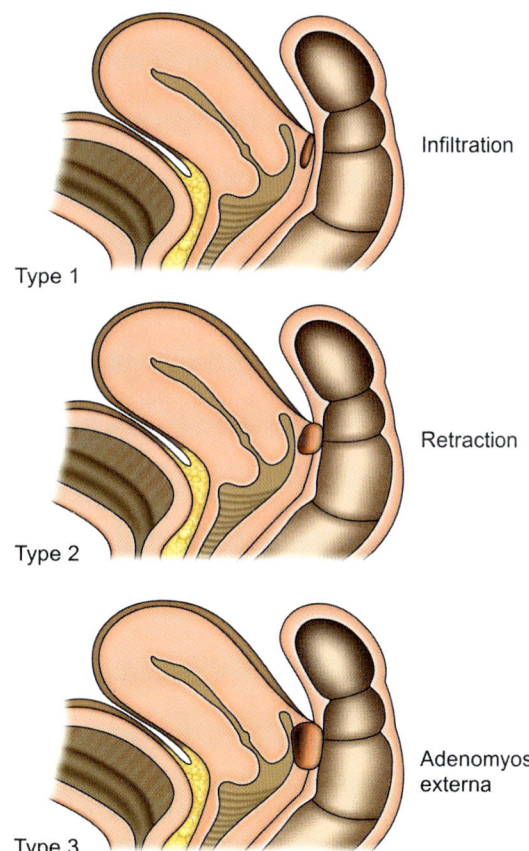

Fig. 16.6: Deep infiltrating endometriosis (Koninckx PR, Martin CD. Fertil Steril 1992;58:1924/8)

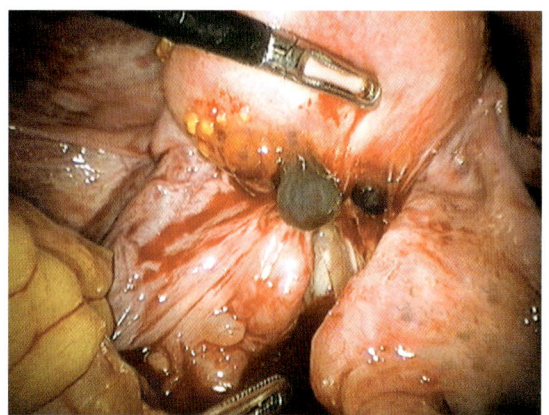

Fig. 16.4: Deep infiltrating endometriosis

Symptoms of endometriosis				
Pain	*Menstrual problems*	*Bladder symptoms*	*Infertility*	*Bowel symptoms*
• Triple dysmenorrhea	• Heavy menstrual flow	• Suprapubic pain		• Painful defecation
• Chronic pelvic pain	• Premenstrual spotting	• Frequency		• Feeling of incomplete
• Deep dyspareunia		• Dysuria		evacuation
• Ovulation pain		• Urgency		• Bleeding per rectum
		• Hematuria		during menstrual cycle

- Type 3 lesions are nodular and involve the rectovaginal septum. Such nodules can be clinically felt during rectovaginal examination and are tender. Type 3 lesions that may appear as blue nodules in the vaginal fornices and represent the most severe form of the disease.

OVARIAN ENDOMETRIOSIS

Ovarian endometriosis is confined to the surface of the ovary and is said to be caused by inversion and invagination of the ovarian cortex along with the endometriotic deposits. Such lesions are usually up to 12 cm in diameter located on the anti-mesenteric surface and adherent to pelvic side wall, posterior surface of broad ligament and uterus. They appear as red, blue or black spots on ovaries and are filled with tarry thick, chocolate-colored material thus called 'Chocolate cysts'. Usually patients with ovarian endometriosis also have accompanying deep infiltrating endometriosis (Figs 16.7a and b).

Extra pelvic endometriosis constitutes less than 12% of all cases and involves variety of organs such as urinary tract, GI tract, pulmonary and thoracic cavities as well as surgical scars.

Histological confirmation of endometriotic lesion is by presence of endometrial glands and stroma with varying degree of fibrosis and hemorrhage. Presence of stroma is more characteristic of endometriosis than glands. Often, histologic confirmation of endometriosis is not achieved after surgical excision.[22] This is the result of a loss of histologic detail from repetitive intraluminal hemorrhages. A

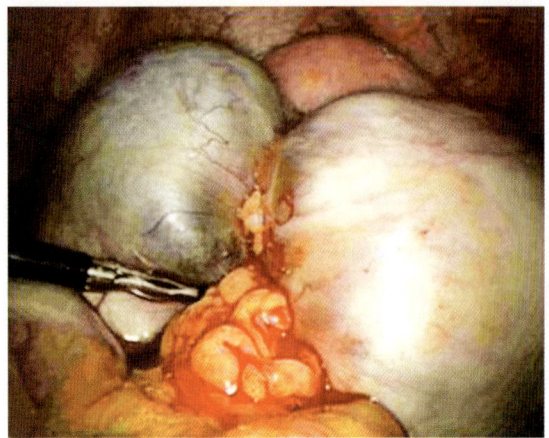

Fig. 16.7a: Chocolate cyst

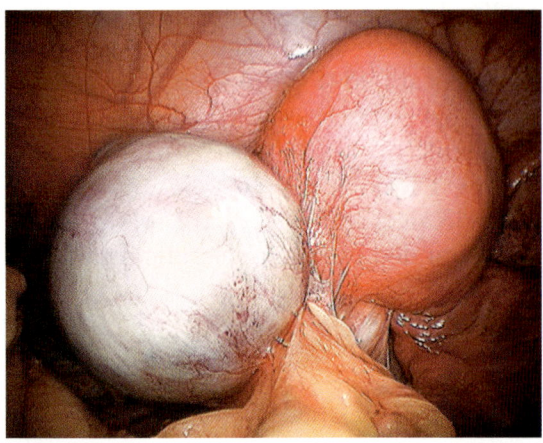

Fig. 16.7b: Ovarian endometrioma adherent to posterior surface of uterus and obliterated POD

presumptive diagnosis can be made based on the gross findings in combination with hemosiderin-laden macrophages and fibrous tissue around a hemorrhagic cyst. Microscopic endometriosis is defined as a presence of endometrial glands and stroma in macroscopically normal peritoneum, however, macroscopically normal appearing peritoneum rarely contains microscopic endometriosis.

Clinical Presentation

Endometriosis can present with a spectrum of symptoms none of which are pathognomonic for the disease. Most common symptoms are pelvic pain, infertility and dysfunctional uterine bleeding. Other less common symptoms such as, dyschezia-feeling of incomplete evacuation and pelvic pain after defecation, rectal bleeding and obstruction in bowel endometriosis. Suprapubic pain with hematuria, frequency and urgency in cases of urinary bladder involvement while back and flank pain in cases of ureteric involvement. Pulmonary lesions may cause cough hemoptysis, pleural effusion. Sciatica may be caused by involvement of the retroperitoneal space. Rarely cyclical headaches or seizures may indicate brain lesions.[23–26] Scar endometriosis is diagnosed as cases of painful, swollen scar during menstrual cycle.

Pelvic Pain

Pelvic pain affects up to 80% of the patients and is the most common symptom of endometriosis.[25] Dysmenorrhea, deep dyspareunia; pain on defecation (dyschezia) and chronic pelvic pain are commonly associated with endometriosis. Dysmenorrhea which is termed as triple Dysmenorrhea, starts before the onset of bleeding, continues through the menstrual period and persists in postmenstrual phase. It is diffuse, located deep in pelvis, severe and worsens progressively. Deep dyspareunia is associated with endometriotic implants involving the uterosacral ligament, rectovaginal septum, upper vagina, or posterior cul-de-sac and is usually more intense during menstruation. Endometriosis implants on or near the rectum may present as dyschezia though because of associated chronic deep seated pelvic pain in endometriosis, patients may overlook this symptom. Thus, a specific inquiry with regard to the cyclic occurrence of painful bowel movements may be necessary.

Mechanisms to explain pain symptoms have been proposed but remain speculative. Scarring and retraction from fibrosis result in anatomical distortion and fixation of pelvic structures. Fibrosis and adhesions that cause nerve damage, tissue destruction, and devitalization of tissues from the disruption of blood supply explain the severe pain associated with deep infiltrating endometriosis.[27] Prostaglandin and histamine release due to inflammation resulting from cyclic focal bleeding in peritoneal implants in mild and minimal disease causes pain. Evidence also suggests that persistent neural input from endometriotic tissues results in central sensitization of nociceptive inputs leading to somatic hyperalgesia. Severity of disease has no relationship with severity of pain, as women with advanced disease have few or no symptoms and those with mild disease have incapacitating pain.[28]

Infertility

Infertility is frequently the only presenting symptom in patients with endometriosis. Because of limitations from selection bias, the incidence of infertility in women with endometriosis is unknown. The incidence of endometriosis in infertile women, however, ranges from 4.5 to 33% (mean 14%).[29]

The mechanistic explanation for infertility may involve either an anatomical distortion of the tubes due to adhesions or functional abnormalities like oocyte pickup and transport dysfunction, altered tubal peristalsis and implantation failure. Various theories have blamed reduced fecundity on altered folliculogenesis, ovulatory dysfunction, sperm phagocytosis, impaired fertilization and defective implantation, inhibition of early embryo development, luteal phase defects, and immunologic alterations.[30–39]

The environment of chronic inflammation also leads to increased peritoneal fluid volume and increased number, concentration, and activity of macrophages. These macrophages may also affect the gamete function or embryo growth by exerting direct cytotoxic effects or by releasing cytokines and proteolytic enzymes into the pelvic milieu.[40–43]

Dysfunctional Uterine Bleeding

DUB can be associated with endometriosis. Though anovulation is a cause of DUB, in endometriosis studies have demonstrated the two to be associated with endometriosis rather than anovulation being the cause of DUB.[44,45]

Physical Examination

Physical examination may fail to reveal any abnormality in cases of minimal superficial endometriosis. Abdominal examination in large ovarian endometriomas may reveal a large tender mass located in the iliac fossa that is found to be arising from the pelvis and not freely mobile. On pelvic examination, advanced diseases may present with fixed retroverted uterus, tender and nodular thickening of the uterosacral ligaments, nodular thickening posterior to uterus, and in cul-de-sac. Bluish nodules in vaginal fornices may be seen on per speculum examination in cases of vaginal infiltration (Fig. 16.8a). All these features are usually more

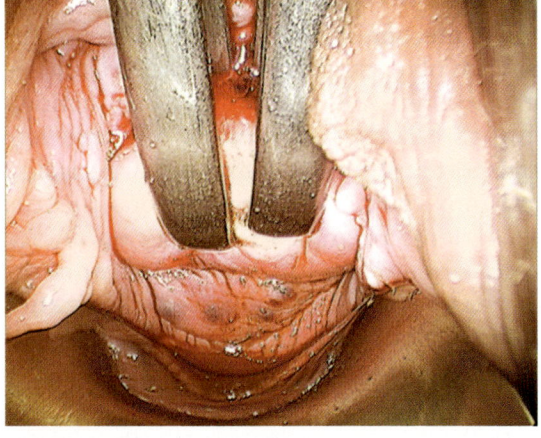

Fig. 16.8a: Bluish nodules seen in vaginal fornices during per speculum examination

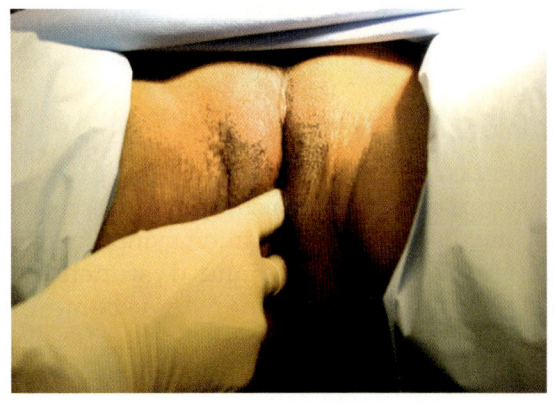

Fig. 16.8b: Bimanual examination

pronounced at the time of menstruation. Bimanual pelvic examination with a gloved index finger in vagina and a lubricated middle finger in rectum may reveal a tender rectovaginal nodule (Fig. 16.8b).

Diagnosis

Diagnosis of endometriosis requires direct visualization and histological evidence of endometrial glands and stroma. The clinical assessment identifies the patient at risk for endometriosis and further evaluation includes diagnostic imaging, laboratory tests and laparoscopy.

Imaging

Ultrasonography and magnetic resonance imaging may be a useful adjunct in identification of patients with endometriosis. Transvaginal ultrasonography detects ovarian endometriomas with 83% and 98% sensitivity and specificity respectively. However, diagnosis of non-ovarian superficial peritoneal foci of disease and pelvic adhesions is poor with a sensitivity of as low as 11% with imaging.[46]

Indirect signs as adherent ovary behind the uterus which is also tender on probe movement are suggestive of endometriosis. We have very routinely identified endometriosis of grade I and grade II, to III severity without ovarian endometriomas just by tender, adherent ovaries sign, rather than PID. Endometriosis is much more common and should be considered strongly, more so in cases of infertility and chronic pelvic pain. Ovarian endometriomas can have varying ultrasonographic features but appear typically as a round homogenous hypoechoic low level echo cyst (ground glass appearance) with or without septations surrounded by echogenic capsule. There might be no or poor vascularization of capsule and septa (Fig. 16.9a). Some cyst may have internal heterogeneous trabeculations or a non-vascularized echogenic portion (Fig. 16.9b).[47] Recent development of high frequency transducers, enable the diagnosis of rectovaginal nodules. Transrectal sonography (TRUS) identifies vaginal and rectal wall infiltration with a sensitivity and specificity of 97% and 96% respectively. The diagnostic accuracy can be improved by Doppler flow studies, useful in differentiating endometriomas from malignant lesions. The

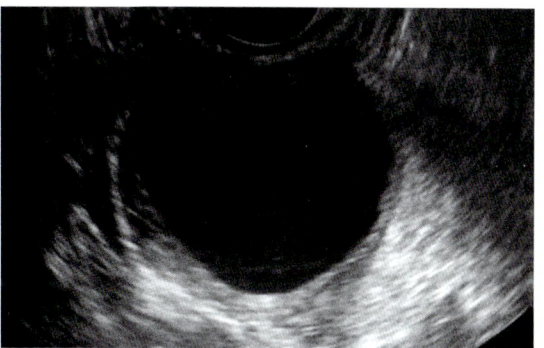

Fig. 16.9a: Homogenous, hypoechoeic low level echo cyst with this internal heterogeneous trabeculations

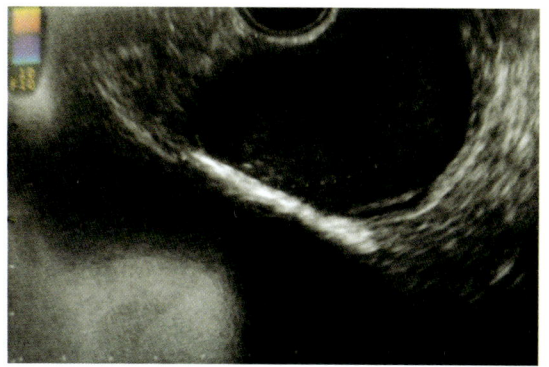

Fig. 16.9b: Rounded, homogeneous, hypoechoeic low level echo cyst with internal septa

presence of fixed retroverted uterus, adherent ovaries without the presence of big endometriomas, and extreme tenderness on maneuvering the vaginal probe indicates involvement of rectovaginal septum, rectal and vaginal wall infiltration.

Magnetic resonance imaging (MRI) is useful when further characterization of adnexa is required. MRI is superior in differentiating an ovarian endometrioma from other adnexal masses and can detect ovarian adhesions, extraperitoneal endometriotic masses and rectovaginal disease. The diagnostic sensitivity, specificity and predictive accuracy for MRI diagnosis of endometriomas are 90%, 98% and 96% respectively.[48] Serial ultrasonography and MRI may be also useful in monitoring the therapeutic response to treatment of endometriosis and to detect recurrence after medical or surgical treatment.

Barium studies and intravenous urography may be helpful in cases with suspected GI tract and ureteric involvement respectively and should be carried out systematically to evaluate extragenital endometriosis. Treatment strategies are planned with colorectal surgeon and urologist prior to taking up a patient of deep infiltrating endometriosis (DIE) for complete extirpation of disease.

LAPAROSCOPY

Visualization of lesions by laparoscopy and histological examination of excised tissue is gold standard for diagnosis of endometriosis. The optimal time to perform a diagnostic laparoscopy is not clear but it is better avoided during or within 3 months of hormonal medical treatment lest lesions may be suppressed and thus miss being diagnosed. A careful and systemic examination is essential to identify and document all endometriotic lesions.

Classical peritoneal implant is blue black "powder burned" or "gunshot" with varying degree of fibrosis all around, seen on ovaries, ovarian fossa and dependent areas of pelvis including cul-de-sac, and uterosacral ligaments. Endometriotic implants can also appear as atypical red flame like, petechial, vesicular, polypoidal and white opaque lesions. It may also be found as yellow-brown patches in ovarian adhesions or in peritoneal defects (Allen-Master windows).

Ovarian endometrioma are located on anterior surface with associated retraction, pigmentation and peritoneal adhesions of ovary. These cysts are filled with dark brown, thick, viscous fluid "chocolate fluid" and thus called chocolate cysts. Visual inspection is highly reliable for diagnosis but biopsy of suspicious areas and endometriomas of size more than 3 cm in diameter to confirm diagnosis and to exclude possibility of malignancy is needed. Ovarian endometriosis is mostly co-occurs with extensive deep infiltrating endometriosis.

The extent of deep infiltrating endometriosis is difficult to determine. It may give a false impression of minimal disease, resulting in under estimation. It is characterized by partial or complete obliteration of cul-de-sac. Tethering of the surrounding tissue to non-pliable tissue suggests contraction and scarring. However, the exact depth of penetration can only be identified at the time of excision.

Laboratory Tests

Serum CA-125 is a cell surface antigen (glycoprotein) expressed by derivatives of coelomic epithelium including endometrium. Levels of CA-125 are elevated in endometriosis, epithelial ovarian cancers, acute pelvic inflammatory disease, leiomyomata, early pregnancy and during normal menstruation. The sensitivity of CA-125 as a screening test for endometriosis is poor (20–50%). Compared to laparoscopy, CA-125 has no value as a diagnostic tool.[49] However, serial CA-125 determinations may be useful in predicting the recurrence after medical or surgical treatment of endometriosis.

PP14 a serum protein has been evaluated as a marker for diagnosis endometriosis with 59% sensitivity and 96% specificity. PP14 level correlates with severity of endometriosis.[50,51]

Elevated serum antibodies are observed against endometrial antigens, tropomyosin 3 (TPM3), stomatin-like protein 2 (SLP2) and tropomodulin 3 (TMOD3) in endometriosis patients.[52] These antibodies are found with 83% and 79% sensitivity and specificity respectively.[53]

Cyclically increased concentrations of cytokeratin 19 (CYFRA 21-1), a structural protein specific for epithelia, in urine during luteal phase could serve as a valuable non-invasive diagnostic parameter in the workup of clinically manifesting endometriosis.[54]

Classification and Staging of Endometriosis

In 1979, American fertility society introduced a classification system based on surgical finding at laparoscopy or laparotomy, assigning a point score based on size, depth, location and associated adhesions of lesions. The classification was revised in 1985 and re-revised in 1996 to improve consistency in scoring and prognostic value for women with infertility and pain. The current ASRM, American Society for Reproductive Medicine is the most widely accepted classification tool despite its limitations (Fig. 16.10). It has a poor correlation with pregnancy outcome, and also has a considerable interobserver and intra-observer variability. The ASRM classification also fails in predicting disease progression, rate of recurrence or severity of symptoms. The biggest drawback is failure to include deep infiltrating endometriosis which is being increasingly recognized.

A more descriptive and relatively simple classification used in clinical practice which is as follows:

1. Minimal endometriosis includes isolated superficial peritoneal disease with no significant associated adhesions.

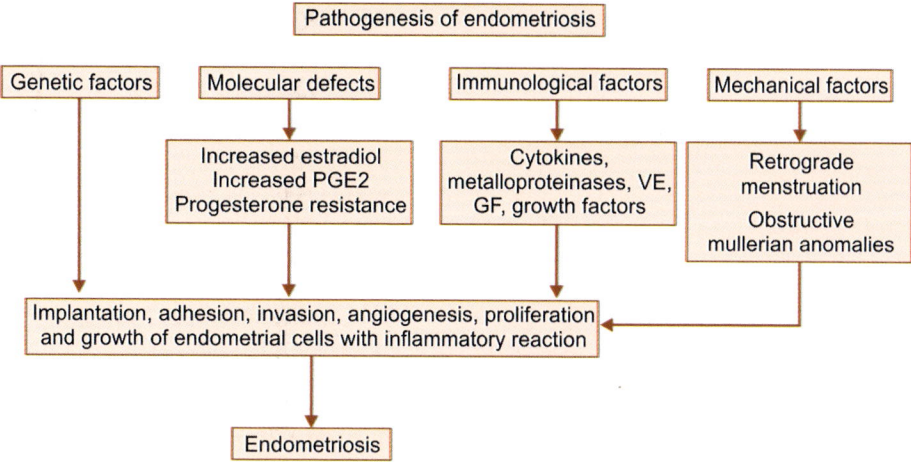

Fig. 16.10: ASRM classification

2. Mild endometriosis has scattered superficial peritoneal and ovarian lesions, totaling less than 5 cm, with no significant adhesions.

3. Moderate endometriosis is a multifocal disease both superficial and deep, with associated tubal and/or ovarian adhesions.

4. Severe endometriosis is a multifocal disease both superficial and invasive, including big ovarian endometriomas, associated with tubal, ovarian and cul-de-sac adhesions.

A new staging system was proposed in 2009, known as endometriosis fertility index (EFI). The EFI score (0-10, with 0 representing the poorest and 10 the best prognosis) predicts cumulative pregnancy rates (without IVF) over 3 years after surgery, with a range of 10% (EFI 0-3) to 75% (EFI 9-10). It is a promising tool in developing treatment plans in patient surgically diagnosed as endometriosis.[55]

Conclusion

Endometriosis is a benign, chronic and progressive pathological condition of reproductive age group with involvement of pelvic and extrapelvic sites which presents with pelvic pain and infertility. It is a multi-factorial disease with multi-faceted features. Diagnosis of endometriosis is established by direct inspection and histological verification.

Laparoscopy is the gold standard for diagnosis of endometriosis.

Acknowledgement: I would like to pay sincere thanks to my OT staff Mr Vishram, Ms Anamika and Mr Saurabh who helped a lot to accomplish this work.

References

1. Cowart CL, London SN. Extrapelvic endometriosis. Infertil Reprod Med Clin North Am 1992;3:731.
2. 4. Koger KE, Shatney CH, Hodge K, McClenathan JH: Surgical scar endometrioma. Surg Gynecol Obstet 1993;177:243.
3. Schenken RS. Pathogenesis in Endometriosis: Contemporary Concepts in Clinical Management. p 1. Philadelphia: JB Lippincott, 1989.
4. Markham SM. Extrapelvic endometriosis. In Thomas E, Rock J (eds). Modern Approaches to Endometriosis, p 151. Boston: Kluwer Academic, 1991.
5. Carta F, Guiducci G, Fulcheri E, et al. Radicular compression by extradural spinal endometriosis: case report. Acta Neurochir 1992;114:68.
6. Cramer D W. Epidemiology of endometriosis in adolescents. In: Wilson EA (ed): Endometriosis. Alan Liss (1987), New York pp 5–8.
7. Kuohung W, Jones GL, Vitonis AF et al. Characteristics of patients with endometriosis in the United States and the United Kingdom. Fertil Steril 2002; 78:767–72.
8. McLeod BS, Retzloff MG. Epidemiology of endometriosis: an assessment of risk factors. Clin Obstet Gynecol 2010;53:389–96.

9. Sampson JA. Heterotopic or misplaced endometrial tissue. Am J Obstet Gynecol 1925;10:649.

10. Sampson JA. Peritoneal endometriosis due to menstrual dissemination of endometrial tissue into peritoneal cavity. Am J Obstet Gynecol 1927;14:422.

11. Dinulescu DM, Ince AT, Quad BJ, et al. Role of K-ras and Pten in development of mouse models of endometriosis and endometroid ovarian cancer. Nat Med 2005;11:63–70.

12. Levander G, Normann P. The pathogenesis of endometriosis: an experimental study. Acta Obstet Gynecol Scand 1995;34:366–98.

13. Merrill JA. Endometrial induction of endometriosis across milipore filters. Am J Obstet Gynecol 1966;94:780–89.

14. Dmowski WP, Steele RW, Baker GF. Deficient cellular immunity in endometriosis. Am J Obstet Gynecol 1981;141:377.

15. Simpson JL, Elias S, Malinak LR et al: Heritable aspects of endometriosis. I. Genetic studies. Am J Obstet Gynecol 1980;137:327.

16. Coxhead D, Thomas EJ. Familial inheritance of endometriosis in a British population. A case control study. J Obstet Gynaecol 1993;13:42.

17. Moen MH, Magnus P: The familial risk of endometriosis. Acta Obstet Gynecol Scand 1993;72:560.

18. Chatman DL, Zbella EA. Pelvic peritoneal defects and endometriosis: further observations. Fertil Steril 1986;46:711.

19. Redwine DB. Peritoneal pockets and endometriosis: confirmation of an important relationship, with further observations. J Reprod Med 1989;34:270.

20. Donnez J, Nisolle M, Gillenot S, et al. Recto-vaginal septum adenomyotic nodules: a series of 500 cases. Br J Obstet Gynaecol 1991;104:1009–13.

21. Novak ER, Woodruff JD. Pelvic endometriosis. Novak's Gynecologic and Obstetrics Pathology. 1974;506.

22. Metzger DA, Olive DL, Haney AF. Limited hormonal responsiveness of ectopic endometrium: histologic correlation with intrauterine endometrium. Hum Pathol 1988;19:1417.

23. Foster DC, Stern JL, Buscema J, et al. Pleural and parenchymal pulmonary endometriosis. Obstet Gynecol 1981;58:552.

24. Nezhat C, Seidman D, Nezhat F, Nezhat C. Laparoscopic surgical management of diaphragmatic endometriosis. Fertil Steril 1998;69:1048.

25. Thibodeau LL, Prioleau GR, Manuelidis EE, et al. Cerebral endometriosis: case report. J Neurosurg 1987;66:609.

26. Denton RO, Sherrill JD. Sciatic syndrome due to endometriosis of sciatic nerve. South Med J 1955;48:1027.

27. Pittaway DE. Diagnosis of endometriosis. Infertil Reprod Med Clin North Am 1992;3:619.

28. Vercellini P, Trespidi L, De Giorgi O, et al. Endometriosis and pelvic pain: relation to disease stage and localization. Fertil Steril 1996;65:299.

29. Pauerstein C: Clinical presentation and diagnosis. In Schenken RS (ed): Endometriosis: Contemporary Concepts in Clinical Management. Philadelphia: JB Lippincott, 1989.

30. Dmowski WP, Radwanska E, Binor Z, Rana N. Mild endometriosis and ovulatory dysfunction: effect of danazol treatment on success of ovulation induction. Fertil Steril 1986;46:784.

31. Tummon IS, Maclin VM, Radwanska E, et al. Occult ovulatory dysfunction in women with minimal endometriosis or unexplained infertility. Fertil Steril 1988;50:716.

32. Muscato JJ, Haney AJ, Weinberg JB. Sperm phagocytosis by human peritoneal macrophages: a possible cause of infertility in endometriosis. Am J Obstet Gynecol 1982;144:503.

33. Mahadevan MM, Trounson AO, Leeton JF. The relationship of tubal blockage, infertility of unknown cause, suspected male infertility, and endometriosis to success of in vitro fertilization and embryo transfer. Fertil Steril 1983;40:755.

34. Yovich JL, Yovich JM, Tuvik AI, et al. In vitro fertilization for endometriosis. Lancet ii: 1985;552.

35. Grant A. Additional sterility factors in endometriosis. Fertil Steril 1966;17:514.

36. Damewood MD, Hesla JS, Schlaff WD, et al. Effect of serum from patients with minimal to mild endometriosis on mouse embryo development *in vitro*. Fertil Steril 1990;54:917.

37. Taketani Y, Kuo T-M, Mizuno M: Tumor necrosis factor inhibits the development of mouse embryos co-cultured with oviducts: possible relevance to infertility associated with endometriosis. J Mamm Ovar Res 1991;8:175.

38. Pittaway DE, Maxson W, Daniell J, et al: Luteal phase defects in infertility patients with endometriosis. Fertil Steril 1983;39:712.

39. Gilmore SM, Aksel S, Hoff C, et al. In vitro lymphocyte activity in women with endometriosis-an altered immune response? Fertil Steril 1992;58:1148.

40. Drake TS, Metz SA, Grunert GM, O'Brien WF. Peritoneal fluid volume in endometriosis. Fertil Steril 1980;34:280.

41. Dunselman G, Hendrix M, Bouckaert P, Evers J. Functional aspects of peritoneal macrophages in endometriosis of women. J Reprod Fertil 1988;82: 707.

42. Haney A, Muscato J, Weinberg J. Peritoneal fluid cell populations in infertility patients. Fertil Steril 1981;35:696.

43. Halme J, Becker S, Hammond M, Raj S: Pelvic macrophages in normal and infertile women: the role of patent tubes. Am J Obstet Gynecol 1982; 142:890.

44. Scott RB, Te Linde RW: External endometriosis-the scourge of the private patient. Ann Surg 1950; 131: 697.

45. Soules MR, Malinak LR, Bury R, Poindexter A: Endometriosis and anovulation: a coexisting problem in the infertile female. Am J Obstet Gynecol 1976;125:412.

46. Friedman H, Vogelzang RL, Mendelson EB, et al. Endometriosis detection by US with laparoscopic correlation. Radiology 1985;157: 217.

47. Athey PA, Diment DD: The spectrum of sonographic findings in endometriomas. J Ultrasound Med 1989;8:487.

48. Togashi K, Nishimura K, Kimura I, et al. Endometrial cysts: diagnosis with MR imaging. Radiology 1991;180:73.

49. Mol BWJ, Bayram N, Lijmer JG, et al. The performance of CA-125 measurement in the detection of endometriosis: a meta-analysis. Fertil Steril 1998;70:1101.

50. Koninckx PR, Riittinen L, Seppala M, et al. CA-125 and placental protein 14 concentrations in plasma and peritoneal fluid of women with deeply infiltrating pelvic endometriosis. Fertil Steril 1992;57:523.

51. Telimaa S, Kauppila A, Rönnberg L, et al. Elevated serum levels of endometrial secretory protein PP14 in patients with advanced endometriosis: suppression by treatment with danazol and high-dose medroxyprogesterone. Am J Obstet Gynecol 1989;161: 866.

52. Gajbhiye R, Sonawani A, Khan S, Suryawanshi A, Kadam S, Warty N, et al. Identification and validation of novel serum markers for early diagnosis of endometriosis. Human Rerprod.2012 Feb; 27(2):408–17.

53. Wild RA, Hirisave V, Bianco A, et al. Endometrial antibodies versus CA-125 for the detection of endometriosis. Fertil Steril 1991;55:90.

54. Risto Gjavotchanoff. CYFRA 21-1 in urine: a diagnostic marker for endometriosis? Int J Womens Health. 2015;7:205–211.

55. Adamson GD1, Pasta DJ Fertil Steril. Endometriosis fertility index: the new, validated endometriosis staging system. 2010 Oct;94(5): 1609–15.

17

Medical and Surgical Treatment of Endometriosis

• Nutan Jain

Endometriosis is a multi-faceted disease that requires the gynecologist to call up on the art and science of medicine and customize the treatment depending on presentation in an individual patient. Endometriosis patients can be treated with analgesics, hormones, surgery, assisted reproduction or a combination of all these modalities. The goal is to eliminate the disease, provide symptomatic relief for pain and infertility and prevent recurrence.

Treatment of endometriosis should be individualized. As women with endometriosis are mostly of reproductive age group presenting with pain and subfertility, preservation of reproductive function is desirable. Women should be involved in decision making about treatment options. Endometriosis is a chronic disease and with a high recurrence rate after both medical and surgical treatment which often provides only temporary relief. WHO recently defined endometriosis surgery as "all surgical procedures carried out to diagnose, conserve, correct and/or improve reproductive function". Endometriosis surgery should be considered a reproductive surgery.

Prevention

To prevent endometriosis no strategies are uniformly successful. Women engaged in aerobic activities at an early age have a reduced incidence of endometriosis. Oral contraceptives by inhibiting ovulation and reducing the volume of menstrual flow may offer protection against endometriosis, but the hypothesis regarding OCPs for primary prevention of endometriosis is not sufficiently substantiated.

Medical Treatment

Women with pelvic pain with suspected endometriosis in the absence of definitive diagnosis and no other indication for surgery can be managed empirically with counselling, analgesics, nutritional therapy, progestins, combined oral contraceptives and GnRH analogues. Pain symptoms may improve in most of the patients but medical therapies have no measurable effect on fertility and are not effective in ovarian endometriomas and pelvic adhesions.

Ectopic endometrium and uterine endo-metrium responds similarly to ovarian estrogen and progesterone. Cyclical hormonal changes are responsible for symptoms of endometriosis. All medical therapies act by suppressing the ovarian steroidogenesis, there by inducing atrophy of ectopic endometrial implants, interrupting the cycle of stimulation and bleeding. Hence medical treatment is not given in women in whom fertility is immediately desired.

Evidence suggests that combined oral contraceptives, progesterone, GnRH agonists and danazol are all equally effective in relieving pain and have similar recurrence rate. However, they differ in cost and side effect profile. After discontinuation of treatment symptoms recur in 5–15% of cases in first year and 40–50% cases in five-year.

Drugs Used in Medical Management

Nonsteroidal Anti-inflammatory Drugs

Endometriosis is a chronic inflammatory disease; NSAIDs are effective in reducing endometriosis associated pain. NSAIDs act not only through central inhibition of prostaglandin synthesis, but it also activates endogenous opioids and serotonins. It acts by local anti-nociceptive effect and also by reducing central sensitization, hence effective in reducing chronic pain in endometriosis patients.

NSAIDs cause gastric ulceration and also inhibit ovulation by inhibiting prostaglandin synthesis, as prostaglandins mediate follicle rupture at ovulation. A recent Cochrane review contraindicates use of NSAIDs for pain in endometriosis as there is inconclusive evidence to show their effectiveness.[1]

Progestagens

Progestagens are the first choice for treatment of pain associated with endometriosis. They have anti-proliferative effect resulting in decidualization of endometrial tissue which further leads to atrophy. Progestagens have lower cost and lower incidence of side effects as compared to danazol or GnRH analogues. Several different progestins have been used effectively for treatment of pain. There is no evidence that any single agent or dose is preferable to another. Medroxyprogesterone acetate orally (20–100 mg daily) or 150 mg intramuscular every three months can be given. Norethindrone acetate (5–15 mg daily)

or magesterol acetate (40 mg daily) have been used and have similar efficacy and side effects to those of medroxyprogesterone acetate. Levonorgestrel releasing intrauterine device have particular value in reducing dyspareunia, dysmenorrhea, pelvic pain, and significant reduction in size of rectovaginal nodules in patients with deep infiltrating endometriosis.

Side effects include nausea, weight gain, fluid retention, and breakthrough bleeding. Rarely depression and mood disorders are significant problem. At higher doses, progestins have suppressive effects on hypothalamic pituitary ovarian axis and may induce hypogonadal state leading to bone mineral depletion but recovery is rapid after discontinuation of treatment.

Combined Oral Contraceptives

Estrogen-progestin contraceptive, taken in continuous or cyclical fashion, induce a state of "pseudopregnancy" resulting in amenorrhea due to decidualization of endometrial tissue and enhanced apoptosis of endometrium. Hormonal therapy has been designed to suppress estrogen synthesis, there by inducing the atrophy of ectopic endometrial implants or interrupting the cycle of stimulation or bleeding.[2,3] Combined contraceptives are first choice in women with mild symptoms who also need contraception. Symptomatic relief of dysmenorrhea and pelvic pain is reported in 60–95% of patients, with a 5–10% of annual reoccurrence rate. Combined contraceptives help to prevent progression of endometriosis they are less expensive and side effects are minimal.

Gonadotropin Releasing Hormone Agonists

The GnRH analogues are synthetic long-acting decapeptides. Pulsatile release of GnRH from hypothalamus stimulates the release of FSH and LH from pituitary gland while sustained effect of long acting GnRH analogues induces a hypogonadotrophic-hyogonadal state akin to "pseudomenopause or medical oophorectomy".[4] Ovarian steroid production is suppressed and the lesions undergo atrophy.

GnRH agonists can be administered intramuscularly, subcutaneously or intra-nasally. All GnRH agonists are equally efficacious in relieving pain in women with endometriosis. Within 4 weeks, 75% of women on treatment are rendered hypogonadal and by 8 weeks the effect is 100%. Side effects include symptoms of hypoestrogenism (hot flushes, progressive vaginal dryness, decreased libido, depression, irritability). Primary concern with prolonged use of GnRH is bone demineralization because of hypoestrogenism.[5] Bone loss appears in both trabecular and cortical bone with standard treatment regimens (6 months) and can approach or even exceed 1% per month. Bone loss slowly reverses after discontinuation of treatment, but not completely in all women. Add-back therapy by adding estrogen (conjugated equine estrogen 0.625 mg to 1.25 mg) and progesterone (norethindrone acetate 5 mg) with GnRH agonists minimizes the short term and long term complications of hypoestronism and preserve bone mineral density.[6] Calcium 1000 mg daily is also beneficial with long-term GnRH agonist therapy. Generally long-term patients tend to undergo annual dexa scan to appraise bone density.

DANAZOL

Danazol has been used as a first-line medication in treatment of endometriosis.[7] It is a derivative of 17α-ethinyltestosterone given orally and it acts by suppressing mid cycle follicle stimulating hormone and luteinizing hormone surge, which results in a chronic anovulation and amenorrhea. Danazol also inhibits steriodogenesis and increases free testosterone by displacing it from sex hormone-binding globulin.[8–12]

Danazol treatment is effective in reducing pain in 90% of women with endometriosis.

Studies have shown a 60% disease regression in danazol treated women as compared to 18% in women who received placebo.[13] Median time to recurrence of pain is 6 months after discontinuation of treatment. Danazol is usually started with lower doses 400 mg daily and slowly titrated to desired effect to minimize the side effects. Treatment with danazol is to be avoided in pregnancy as it results in virilization of female fetus.

Side Effects of Danazol Treatment[14]

Side effects	Incidence (%)	Side effects	Incidence (%)
Weight gain	85	Acne	27
Muscle cramps	52	Fatigue	25
Decreased breast size	48	Hirsutism	21
Flushing	42	Decreased libido	20
Mood change	38	Nausea	17
Oily skin and hair	37	Headache	17
Depression	32	Dizziness	10
Sweating	32	Insomnia	10
Edema	28	Increased libido	8
Change in appetite	28	Deepening of voice	7

GESTRINONE

Gestrinone is a 19-testosterone derivative that acts as an androgen receptor and progesterone receptor agonist, resulting in amenorrhea and endometrial atrophy similar to danazol. Studies showed a significant reduction in endometriotic implants and associated pain in patients with endometriosis on treatment with gestrinone as compared to placebo.[15]

Drug is administered orally 5–10 mg weekly in two- or three-divided doses. Compared to danazol, incidence of side effects is less with gestrinone.

DIENOGEST

Dienogest is a 19-norprogestin that lacks androgenic effects while having beneficial antiandrogenic properties that are usually found in progesterone derivatives. It has minimal effect on lipid and carbohydrate levels. Dienogest is almost completely absorbed, and has a high bioavailability after oral administration, similar to other 19-norprogestins. It is relatively short half-life of 10 hours means there is no risk of accumulation after repeated dosing. At doses of 2 mg and 3 mg of continuous use, Dienogest induces a hypoestrogenic and hypergestagenic local endocrine environment, causing a decidualization of endometrial tissue followed by atrophy of the endometriotic lesions.[15,16] During its use the ovarian activity is effectively suppressed by the doses, with a rapid return to ovulation after cessation of dienogest administration. Dienogest also demonstrates antiproliferative, anti-inflammatory and antiangiogenic effects. Dienogest has an efficacy, safety, and tolerability profile that is favorable for long-term use. At present it is supposed to be the wonder drug for medical management of endometriosis.

Surgical Treatment for Endometriosis

The goal of surgical treatment is to restore normal anatomical relationship, restore fertility, excise or destroy all visible lesions and to prevent or delay the recurrence of endometriosis. Although treatment of endometriosis can be performed via laparotomy or laparoscopy, with improvements in instrumentation and operative technique, laparoscopy is the treatment of choice. Laparoscopy provides better visualization, less tissue trauma, less adhesion formation, faster postoperative recovery and a lower complication rate. However, this comes at a cost of loss of three-dimensional perspective as well as inability to palpate structures, more operator fatigue and requirement for expensive instrumentation.[17,18] In present scenario laparotomy is still preferred over laparoscopy in situations requiring extensive enterolysis, bowel resections and similar difficult manipulations depending on the surgeon's skills.[19] While doing laparotomy patient should be placed in lithotomy position so that rectal and vaginal manipulations with rectal probe and vaginal sponge can be performed by an assistant. This helps to create cleavage plane between rectum and vagina. The results obtained with laparoscopy are equivalent or better than laparotomy.

A meta-analysis of all trials published in English literature from 1977-1995 as well as evidence based reviews have concluded that surgical treatment for all stages of endometriosis results in improved fertility.[20] Fecundity of infertile women with mild to moderate endometriosis was studied by Milingos et al of 151 laparoscopically diagnosed patients with stages 1 and 2 endometriosis, 49 were treated surgically, 59 with medical treatment and 43 were kept on expectant management. Cumulative pregnancy rates were found to be 36.7%, 30.5% and 20.9% respectively.[21] The effects of surgery on fertility in women with mild to moderate endometriosis have been studied in two randomized control trials. One was a multi-centric Canadian trial[22] and second a small Italian trial.[23] A Cochrane review attempted to reconcile these conflicting studies with a meta-analysis and concluded that laparoscopic surgical treatment improved fertility.[24]

Newer durgs in treatment of endometriosis
Selective progestrone receptor modulators
• Mifepristone
• Mesoprogestins
Aromatase inhibitors
• Letrozole
• Anastrozole
GnRH antagonists
Angiogenesis inhibitors
Matrix metalloproteinase inhibitors
Immunomodulators
• Pentoxyphylline
Selective estrogen receptor modulator
• Raloxifene

Because of anatomical distortion associated with moderate to severe endometriosis, surgery is treatment of choice for endometriosis associated infertility. It has been demonstrated that invasive, adhesive, or endometriotic disease is best dealt with surgically compared with the nonsurgical approach. During surgery the techniques are directed toward removing all endometrial implants under magnification in a minimally invasive fashion while maintaining hemostasis. Adhesions are excised rather than simply lysed because of possibility of presence of endometriotic tissue within adhesions. Rate of success correlates with meticulous surgical technique that maintains serosal integrity and decrease the risk of *de novo* adhesion formation.

PERITONEAL ENDOMETRIOSIS

Peritoneal implants of endometriosis in mild to minimal disease can be ablated with unipolar or bipolar electrosurgical instruments or lasers, or excised by sharp dissection (Figs 17.1a and b). A technique popularized by Nezhat et al[25] employs the use of hydrodissection and high power superpulse or ultra pulse CO_2 laser. This technique offers greater safety margin as lactated Ringer solution is injected beneath the lesion which does not allow the laser energy to penetrate and reach underlying ureter or bowel. Superiority of one method over the other has not been substantiated.

OVARIAN ENDOMETRIOMA

Ovarian endometriomas involve into excision of the cyst wall (Figs 17.2a and b) as this minimizes the thermal injury to ovary, ensures complete removal of disease and allows obtaining specimen for histopathological examination. Small endometriomas of <3 cm diameter can be treated by drainage and electrocoagulation or laser (CO_2 laser, potassium titanyl-phosphate laser, or argon laser). A meta-analysis of data from four comparative trials showed a recurrence of endometriomas in 18% in women treated with coagulation or laser vaporization, compared with 6% who had cyst enucleation.[26,27] Two retrospective studies showed 50% and 52% pregnancy rates in laparoscopically treated endometriomas in infertile patients. A prospective cohort study showed cumulative pregnancy rates of 52% and 46% over a period of 3 years after treatment of endometriomas by laparoscopy and laparotomy respectively. Recurrence rate is less than 10% with associated 20% recurrence of *de novo* adhesion formation.[28,29] The use of adhesion barriers reduces adhesion formation but there is no convincing evidence that they improve pregnancy rates. The risk of ovarian failure after bilateral ovarian cyst enucleation is approximately 2.5%.

Surgical technique involves careful adhesiolysis with use of sharp dissection to

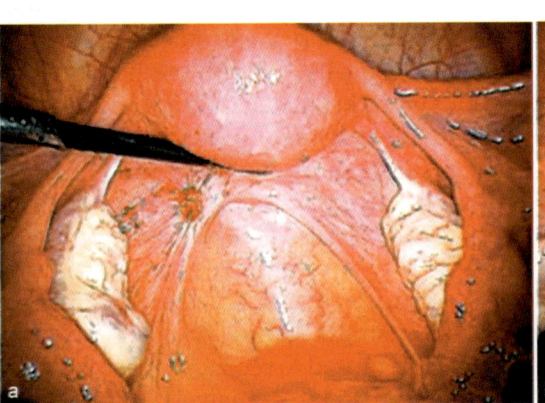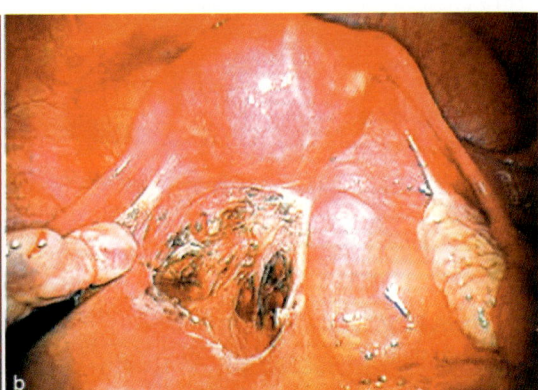

Figs 17.1a and b: a. Minimal endometriotic implants noted; b. all endometriotic implants fulgurated, laid open and excised

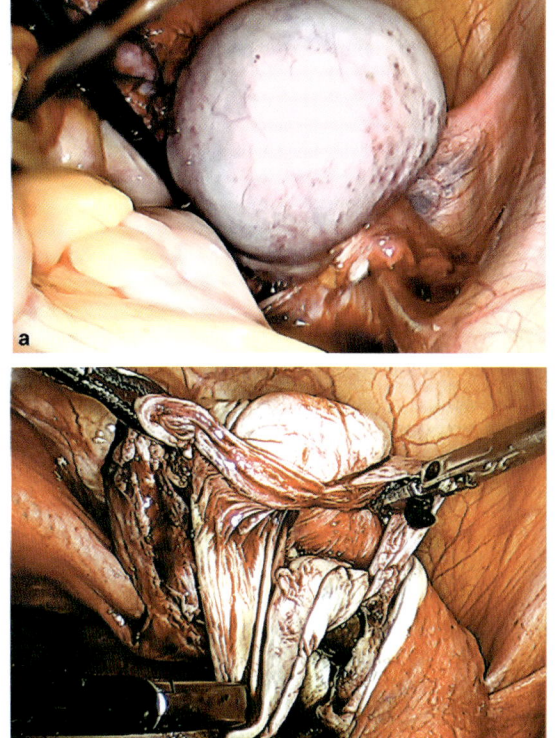

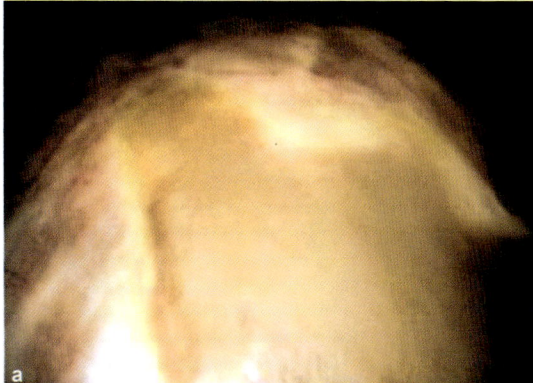

Figs 17.2a and b: a. Endometriotic cyst; b. Enucleation of cyst lining

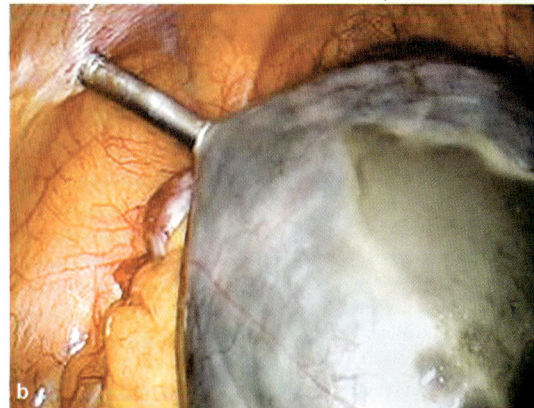

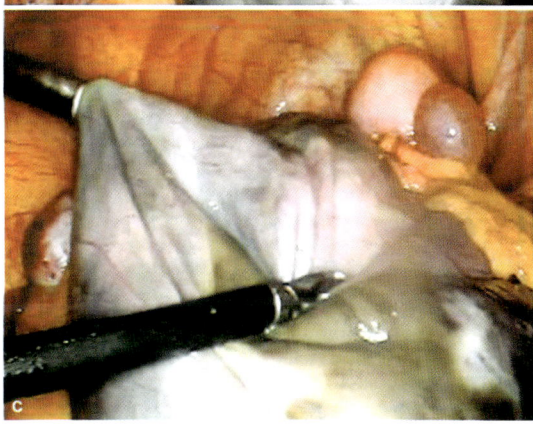

Figs 17.3a to c: a. Huge, big endometriotic cyst; b. cyst decompressed using direct suction irrigation system; c. cyst totally decompressed

mobilize the ovaries. Second step is to incise the surface of ovary in zone of maximum relaxation, possibly on antimesenteric border at farthest distance from fimbria. Cyst is decompressed using suction drainage and its contents are carefully washed (Figs 17.3a to c). Cyst is inspected laparoscopically all the while looking for vegetations or neovascularization suggesting a neoplastic pathology. Correct plane of cleavage is identified among the cyst wall and ovarian tissue; with bimanual opposite traction using atraumatic graspers the inner lining of cyst wall is stripped from normal ovarian tissue. Following that a careful inspection of cyst bed is done to look for any bleeding zones in order to coagulate them with bipolar forceps. The enucleated cyst lining is removed and sent for histopathological analysis. Endo bag can also be used for cyst wall removal when size is too large.

In cases of big cyst for anatomical reconstruction and to prevent adhesion the ovary is suspended to anterior abdominal wall (Fig. 17.4a) or to round ligament (Fig. 17.4b) using a non-absorbable nylon suture on a straight needle. Suture is removed after 2–3 weeks on the patients follow-up visit.

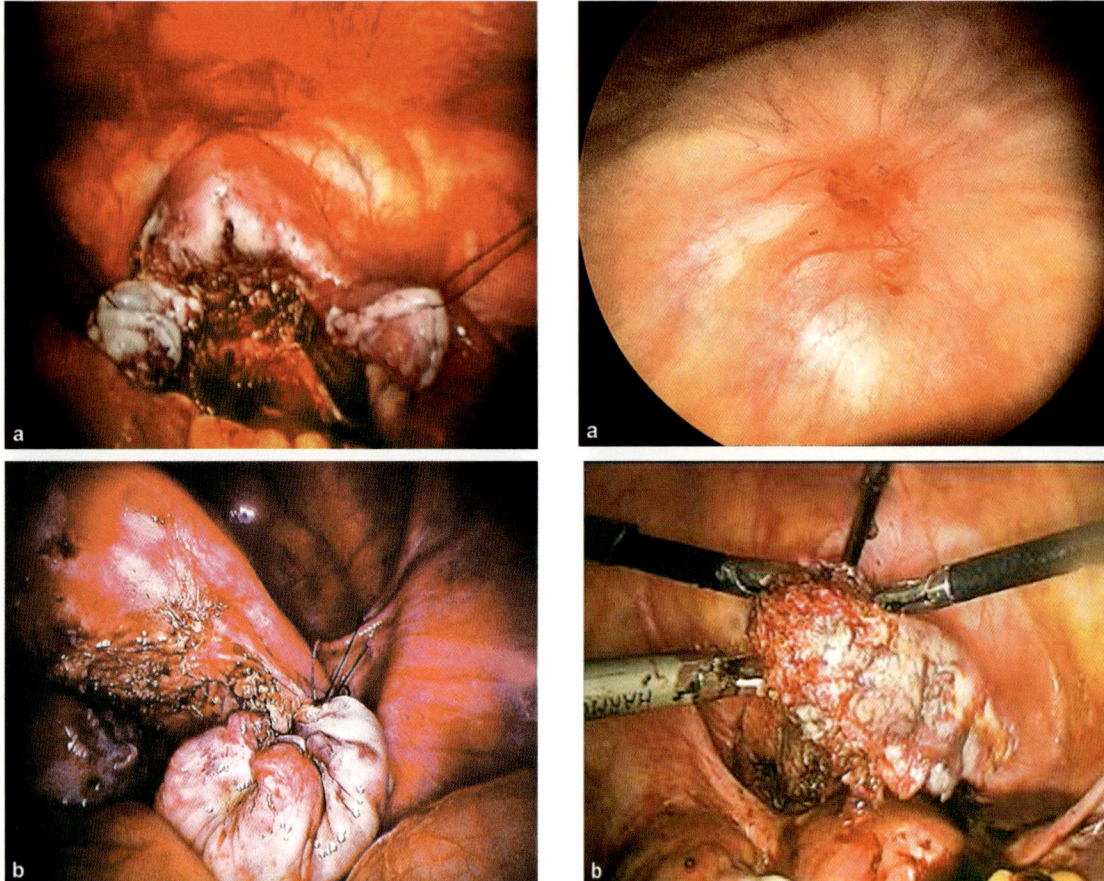

Figs 17.4a and b: a. Both ovaries suspended to anterior abdominal wall; b. ovary suspended to round ligament

Figs 17.5a and b: a. Large endometriotic lesion seen inside the urinary bladder; b. lesion totally excised with reconstruction of bladder in 3 layers

Surgical treatment of pelvic pain associated with endometriosis, appears to be useful, especially in women where pain is not relieved by medical treatment or when associated with deep infiltrating endometriosis.

DEEP INFILTRATING ENDOMETRIOSIS

Deep infiltrating endometriosis is a multifocal disease and complete excision must be performed in one step to avoid repeat surgeries. Surgery is done at specialized center as it requires a multidisciplinary approach involving pain clinic and counseling. A more advanced disease involving gastrointestinal or urinary tract (Figs 17.5a and b) requires a proper preoperative preparation and a team

approach. A thorough bowel preparation including peglac enema is needed pre-operatively. During surgery anesthetist should try not to use nitrous oxide as it bloats the bowel and makes dissection in rectovaginal space difficult. At the vaginal end, uterus needs to be elevated with a strong uterine elevator like RUMI, rectal probe is used for rectal manipulation and a sponge on a ring forceps is placed in the posterior vagina. (Figs 17.6a and b) All this helps to create a cleavage plane between back surface of uterus and rectum, allows delineation of vagina from rectum and helps in complete rectal mobilization. Complete excision of disease requires excision of nodular tissue from posterior vagina, rectum, posterior cervix and

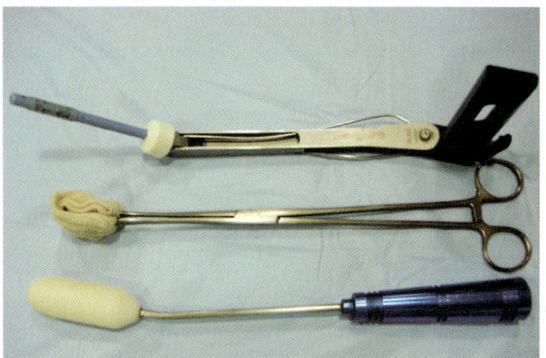

Fig. 17.6a: Uterine elevator, vaginal probe and rectal probe

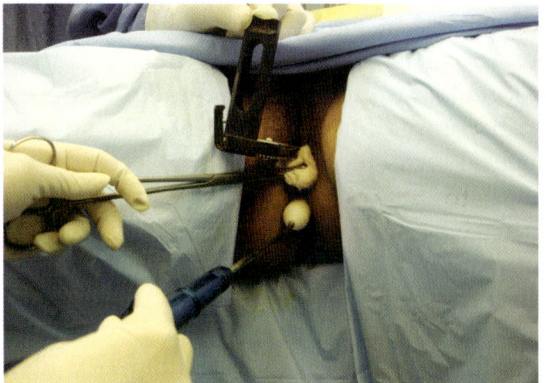

Fig. 17.6b: Placing the rectal probe, vaginal probe and uterine elevator

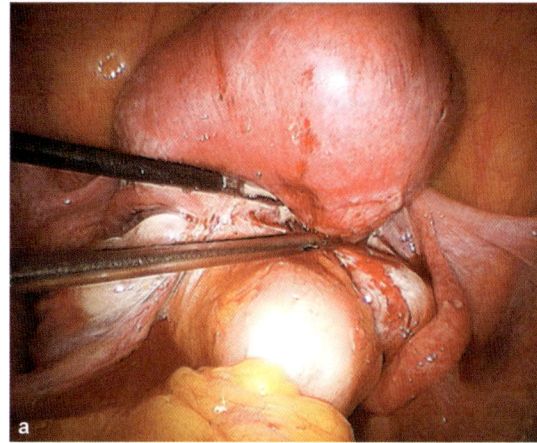

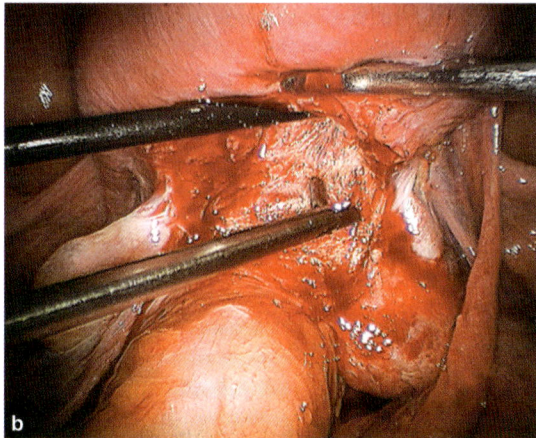

Figs 17.7a and b: Using scissors to expose the plane of cleavage between the rectum and cervix till the rectum is completely freed and identifiable below the lesion

uterosacral ligaments. First step is to open the peritoneum covering the cul de sac between endometriotic lesion and rectum, thus mobilizing rectum from loose areolar tissue of rectovaginal septum. This is followed by lateral clearing between rectum and uterosacral ligaments; this not only clears the disease but also plays an important role in pain relief. Excision of nodular uterosacral should be performed after checking course of pelvic ureters (Figs 17.7a to e). Vaginal involvement necessitates excision of involved vagina with a 0.5 cm disease free margin. Healthy margins of vagina are re-approximated by suturing. Vaporization of all endometriotic implants is done after rectal mobilization, lateral clearing and excision of endometriotic

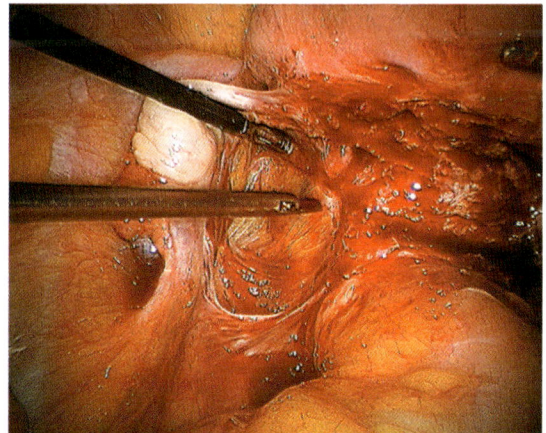

Fig. 17.7c: Dissection in lateral pelvic side wall and section of uterosacral ligament lateral to the rectum

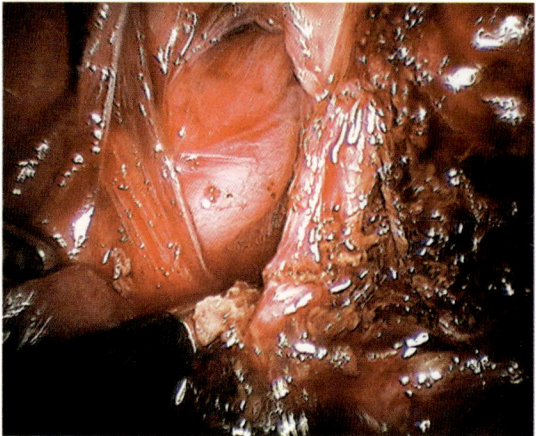

Fig. 17.7d: Lateral pelvic sidewall dissection to explore the ureter before transecting the uterosacral ligament

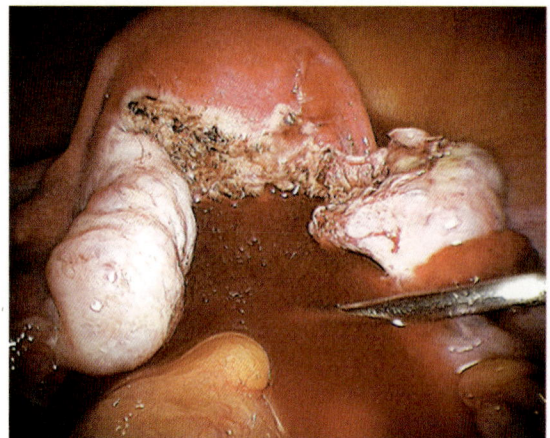

Fig. 17.8: Under water examination

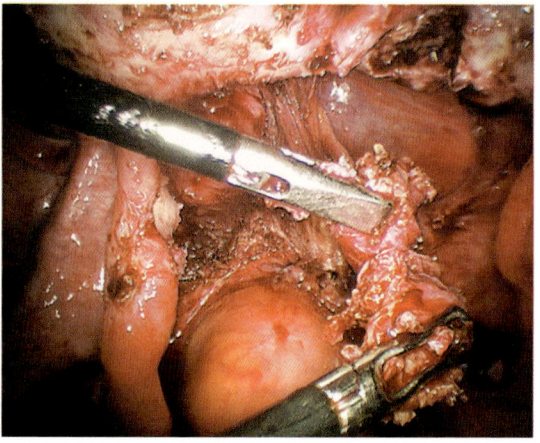

Fig. 17.7e: Pararectal space cleared and uterosacral ligament excised

nodule. Thorough suction lavage is done and hemostasis is secured. At the end, rectum is checked by methylene blue dye or insufflating air through rectum and doing under water examination (Fig. 17.8).

Rectal excision partial or full thickness is still debatable. It is unnecessary except in cases of rectal bleeding caused by full thickness penetration of rectal mucosa by endometriotic lesion and bowel obstruction. Rectal excision as part of treatment for pelvic pain is not commonly practiced. In Indian scenario it is difficult to take consent and explain the need of colostomy, if at all arises. In the Western

world end to end anastomosis with rectal resection is done in conjunction with a colorectal surgeon in patients who present with complaints of severe rectal pain and cyclical rectal bleeding.

Postoperative adhesion after such an extensive surgery is a concern. Adhesion can be prevented by using surface adhesion barrier like interceed. Fluid barriers like icodextrin 4% or Ringer lactate are used for uniform application. Approximately 3 liters of Ringer lactate is left in abdomen after surgery. Hydrofloatation prevents the opposing surfaces to adhere to each other by a film of fluid which gradually gets absorbed over next 4–5 days which is the time of maximum fibroblastic reaction/formation.

Postoperatively patients are discharged next day. In case of vaginal excision, antibiotics are given for 7 days. If bowel resection and anastomosis is done patient is kept nil orally for four days and a suction drain is kept in situ.

Open surgery for endometriosis: All the above procedures done by laparoscopic route can be replicated by open laparotomic approach by using high frequency generators and hand probe of ultrasonic harmonic ACE (Johnson & Johnson) for ablation, fulguration and resection of endometriosis. The biggest benefit in my opinion, the generalist can learn from laparoscopic surgery, is to place the patient in lithotomy position so that they can use vaginal probe and rectal probe for manipulation. In laparotomic approach visualization is compromised, so we can get extra benefit by making the rectum and uterus actually participate in the surgery by putting the rectal probe and vaginal probe. On moving the probe in divergent direction, uterus will move anteriorly and rectum will move posteriorly. Thus dissection planes can be made easier with use of high frequency generator and harmonic ace and we can try to replicate the laparoscopic approach in open surgery.

For treatment of pelvic pain associated with endometriosis not responsive to medical treatment laparoscopic uterosacral nerve ablation (LUNA) and presacral neurectomy (PSN) (Figs 17.9a to c) can be done.[30,31] Presacral neurectomy involves interrupting the sympathetic innervation to uterus at the level of superior hypogastric plexus. LUNA involves the ablation of parasympathetic nerves passing through the uterosacral ligaments.

Definitive surgery consisting of hysterectomy and salpingo-oophorectomy is considered for patients who fails medical or conservative treatment and have completed childbearing hence they can accept loss of fertility. 90% of patients are relieved of pain after the radical treatment.[32] But at least one ovary should be conserved in pre-menopausal women.

Hormone replacement therapy with progestin instead of estrogen after bilateral salpingo-oophorectomy reduces the risk of renewed growth of residual endometriosis and also reduces the development of adenocarcinoma, presumed to arise from residual endometriotic lesions in women treated with unopposed estrogen.

Management of Recurrence

The rate of recurrence increases with the stage of the disease, duration of follow-up and the occurrence of previous surgery. The younger

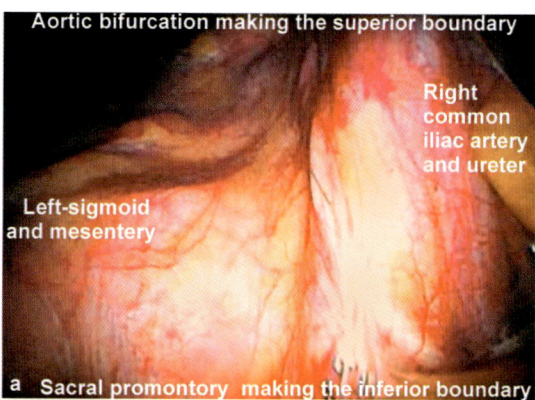

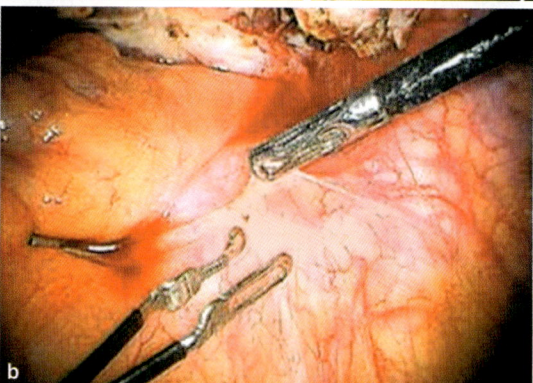

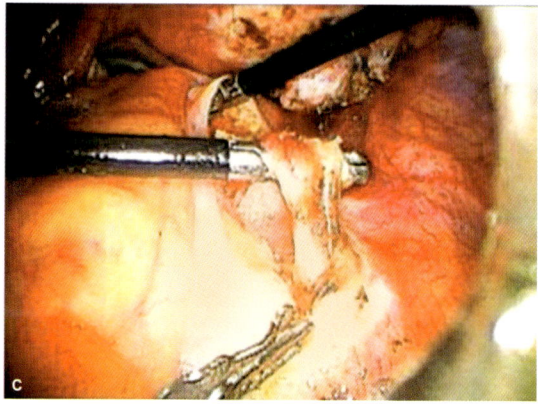

Figs 17.9a to c: a. Presacral space; b. grasping the peritoneum over sacral promontory and applying bipolar forceps for initial coagulation; c. fully exposed presacral nerve after removing the loose areolar fibrofatty tissue

the patient at the time of diagnosis is, the higher the risk of recurrence will be. The first-line of management to prevent recurrence is to allow the women to conceive as soon as possible as postoperatively the most conducive period is 6 to 12 months. In case immediate pregnancy is not desired regular use of cyclical or continuous OCPs in the postoperative period prevents recurrence of endometriosis like in young, unmarried girl, use of OCP till the time of marriage and child-bearing. For reproductive age group patient, levonorgestrel IUCD and depot MPA have been found to alleviate pain symptoms associated with menstruation and to reduce recurrence as compared to surgery alone. Surgical treatment of recurrence should be based on the desire of conception as well as on the psychological profile of the patient as it is known that in 20–40% patients pain may recur after surgery and the patient may still require additional surgical procedures in 15–20% cases.

Assisted Reproductive Technologies in Endometriosis

In addition to surgically restoring the anatomy and removing the disease, patients may benefit from medical assisted reproduction including controlled ovarian hyperstimulation with intrauterine insemination, and *in vitro* fertilization. Due to adverse environment for the oocyte a step wise graduated intervention beginning with hyperstimulation with clomifene citrate or gonadotropins followed by IUI to IVF techniques in more resistant cases provide better results.

Holistic Interventions for Endometriosis

Besides surgical and medical management of endometriosis patients have been found to benefit from a gamut of alternative therapies such as TENS (transcutaneous electrical nerve stimulation), acupuncture, homeopathy, reflexology, traditional Chinese medicine. Also use of vitamin B_1 and magnesium have been found to relieve pain. Though no conclusive evidence has been found in their support, the patient should not be discouraged from using them in case she finds relief. Exercise and yoga specially started in teenage help in preventing disease occurrence and progression.

Conclusion

Endometriosis is a significant cause of morbidity in fertile age group. However, the disease can be very recalcitrant and require the surgeon to employ a whole range of treatment options ranging from medical treatment to surgery to advanced ART. Customization of the treatment depending on patients' psychological status, her pain threshold and need for fertility, is the key stone of management of endometriosis. Need for fertility may dictate surgical restoration of anatomy aggressively followed by efforts to get the patient to conceive using hyper-stimulation with IUI or with ART while patients in whom pain is the only concern may benefit more with medical therapy.

Acknowledgements: I would like to pay sincere thanks to my OT staff Mr Vishram, Ms Anamika and Mr Saurabh who helped a lot to accomplish this work.

References

1. Allen C, Hopewell S, Prentice A. Nonsteroidal anti-inflammatory drugs for pain in women with endometriosis. Cochrane Database Syst Rev. 2005 Oct19;(4):CD004753.
2. Andrews MC, Andrews WC, Strauss AF. Effects of progestin-induced pseudopregnancy on endometriosis: clinical and microscopic studies. Am J Obstet Gynecol 1959;78:776.
3. Kistner RW. The treatment of endometriosis by inducing pseudopregnancy with ovarian hormones: a report of 58 cases. Fertil Steril 1959; 10:539.
4. Meldrum DR, Chang RJ, Lu J, Vale W. Medical oophorectomy using a long-acting GnRH agonist—a possible new approach to the treatment of endometriosis. J Clin Endocrinol Metab 1982;51:1081.
5. Johansen JS, Riis BJ, Hassager C, et al. The effect of a gonadotropin-releasing hormone agonist analog (nafarelin) on bone metabolism. J Clin Endocrinol Metab 1988;67:701.
6. Surrey ES. Add-Back Consensus Working Group. Add-back therapy and gonadotropin-releasing hormone agonists in the treatment of patients with endometriosis. Can a consensus be reached? Fertil Steril 1999;71:420.

7. American Fertility Society. Revised American Fertility Society classification for endometriosis. Fertil Steril 1986;43:351.

8. Barbieri RL, Canich JA, Makris A, Todd RB. Danazol inhibits steroidogenesis. Fertil Steril 1977;28:809.

9. McGinley R, Casey JH. Analysis of progesterone in unextracted serum: a method using danazol—a blocker of steroid binding to proteins. Steroids 1979;33:127.

10. Chamness GC, Asch RH, Pauerstein CJ. Danazol binding and translocation of steroid receptors. Am J Obstet Gynecol 1980;136:426.

11. Jenkin G, Cookson CI, Thorburn GD. The interaction of human endometrial and myometrial steroid receptors with danazol. Clin Endocrinol 1983;19:377.

12. Tamaya T, Murakami T, Yamada T, et al. Serum hormone and steroid hormone receptor levels during luteal phase and long-term treatment with danazol. Fertil Steril 1983;40:585.

13. Telimaa S, Puolakka J, Ronnberg L, Kaupilla A. Placebo-controlled comparison of danazol and high-dose medroxyprogesterone acetate in the treatment of endometriosis. Gynecol Endocrinol 1987;1:13.

14. Buttram VC Jr, Belue JB, Reiter R. Interim report of a study of danazol for the treatment of endometriosis. Fertil Steril 1982;37:478.

15. Herkert O, Kuhl H, Sandow J, Busse R, Schini-Kerth VB. Sex steroids used in hormonal treatment increase vascular procoagulant activity by inducing thrombin receptor (PAR-1) expression: role of the glucocorticoid receptor. Circulation. 2001;104(23):2826–31.

16. Köhler G, Faustmann TA, Gerlinger C, Seitz C, Mueck AO. A dose-ranging study to determine the efficacy and safety of 1, 2, and 4 mg of dienogest daily for endometriosis. Int J Gynaecol Obstet 2010;108(1):21–25.

17. Bruhat MA, Mage C, Chapron C, et al. Present-day endoscopic surgery in gynecology. Eur J Obstet Gynecol Reprod Biol 1991;41:4.

18. Carbon Dioxide Laser Laparoscopy Study Group. Initial report of the carbon dioxide laser laparoscopy study group. Complications J Gynecol Surg 1989;5:269.

19. Luciano AA, Manzi D: Treatment options for endometriosis. Surgical therapies, Infertil Reprod Med Clin North Am 1992;3:657.

20. Adamson GD, Pasta DJ. Surgical treatment of endometriosis-associated infertility. meta-analysis compared with survival analysis. Am J Obstet Gynecol 1994;171:1488.

21. Milingos S, Mavrommatis C, Elsheikh A, Kallipolitis G, Loutradis D, Diakamanolis E. Fecundity of infertile women with minimal or mild endometriosis. A clinical study. Arch Gynecol Obstet 2002;267:37–40.

22. Marcoux S, Maheux R, Berube S. Laparoscopic surgery in infertile women with minimal or mild endometriosis. Canadian Collaborative Group on Endometriosis. N Engl J Med 1997 Jul 24;337(4):217–22.

23. Parazzini F. Ablation of lesions or no treatment in minimal-mild endometriosis in infertile women: a randomized trial. Gruppo Italiano per lo Studio dell'Endometriosi. Hum Reprod. May 1999; 14(5):1332–1334.

24. Jacobson TZ, Duffy JM, Barlow D, Farquhar C, Koninckx PR, Olive D. Laparoscopic surgery for subfertility associated with endometriosis. Cochrane Database Syst Rev 2010;(1):CD001398.

25. Nezhat C, Nezhat F, Pennington E. Laparoscopic treatment of infiltrative rectosigmoid colon and rectovaginal septum endometriosis by the technique of videolaparoscopy and the CO_2 laser. Br J Obstet Gynaecol Aug 1992;99(8):664–7.

26. Kojima E, Morita M, Otaka K, et al. Nd: YAG laser laparoscopy for ovarian endometriomas. J Reprod Med 1990;35:592.

27. Marrs RP. The use of potassium-titanyl-phosphate laser for laparoscopic removal of ovarian endometriomas. Am J Obstet Gynecol 1991;164:1622.

28. Wood C, Mabler P, Hill D. Diagnosis and surgical management of endometriomas. Aust N Z J Obstet Gynaecol 1992;32:161.

29. Canis M, Mage G, Wattiez A, et al. Second-look laparoscopy after laparoscopic cystectomy of large ovarian endometriomas. Fertil Steril 1992;58:617.

30. Tjaden B, Schlaff WD, Kimball A, et al. The efficacy of presacral neurectomy for the relief of midline dysmenorrhea. Obstet Gynecol 1990; 76:89.

31. Lichten EM, Bombard J. Surgical treatment of primary dysmenorrhea with laparoscopic uterine nerve ablation. J Reprod Med 1987;32:37.

32. Reich H, et al. Hysterectomy for advanced endometriosis and bowel resection anastomosis. state of the art atlas of endoscopic surgery in Infertility and Gynaecology. 2nd edition 2010; 26:266.

18

Male Infertility

• Kuldeep Jain

Prevalence of infertility in India is 15–20% of which male factor infertility is seen in 20–40%.[1] However, in recent times varying factors have led to increase in this infertility. Apart from being the only factor responsible for infertility, a large number of couples have both male and female factors. To treat male infertility anatomy, physiology, and endocrinology of spermatogenesis should be understood. Also since semen quality is used as measure of male fecundity, importance of semen parameters for appropriate treatment should be known.

Male infertility is defined as the failure of a couple to conceive due to male factor after cohabitation for >1 year (<35 years) and >6 months (>35 years) as per WHO 2010 guideline.[2]

REVIEW OF ANATOMICAL, PHYSIOLOGICAL AND ENDOCRANIAL ASPECTS OF MALE FERTILITY

It requires millions of sperms to travel from testis via the ejaculatory duct through urethra into the female genital tract to reach the ampulla of fallopian tubes. Thereafter a single sperm enters the ova resulting into fertilization and development of embryo. This developing embryo has to subsequently implant in the uterus to result in pregnancy.

Stained with hematoxylin and eosin
1. Seminiferous tubule

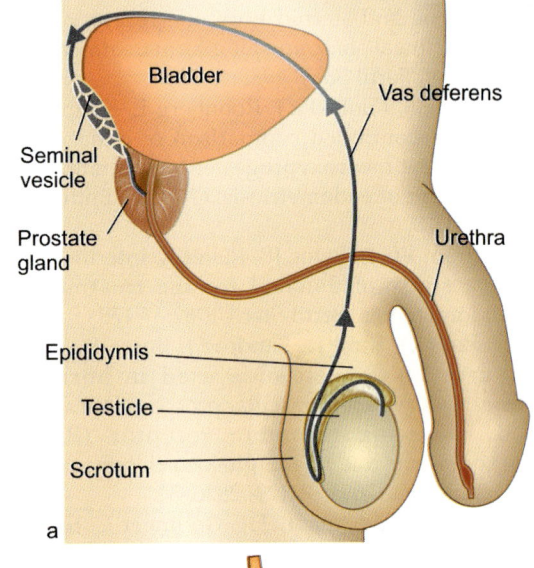

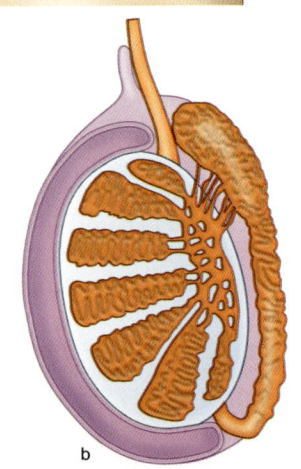

Figs 18.1a and b: Male genital tract

2. Spermatogonia
3. Primary spermatocytes
4. Secondary spermatocytes
5. Spermatids
6. Interstitial connective tissue
7. Leydig cells

Microscopic Picture of Testis

All components in the testis have specific functions. Function of basement membrane is to form blood testis barrier to serve as an immunological barrier of testis and its contents. Disruption of this barrier produces antisperm antibody. Diploid germ cells are precursor cells for mature sperms. Sertoli cells—nurse cells to control the development of sperms and Leydig cells—secrete androgens essential for normal testicular descent and sperm maturation.

Microscopic Picture of Sperm

The sperm in course of its maturation sheds its organelles and cytoplasmic fluid and the mature sperm becomes the smallest cell of human body. Mitochondria ensheath around the proximal end of tail fibrils in the mid piece to focus energy where it is needed. The DNA condenses and becomes inactive. Golgi body

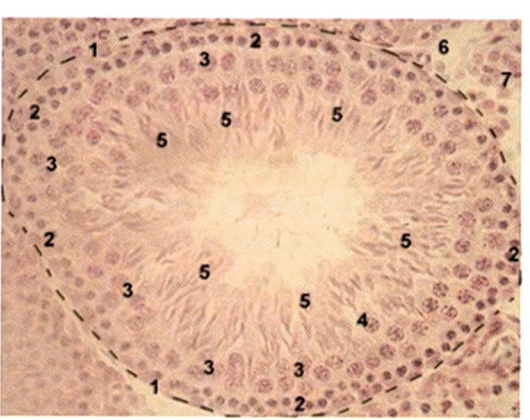

Fig. 18.2: Illustration of microscopic aspect of testis and physiological correlation. Stained with hematoxylin and eosin. (1) seminiferous tubule, (2) spermatogonia, (3) primary spermatocytes, (4) secondary spermatocytes, (5) spermatids, (6) interstitial connective tissue, (7) Leydig cells

forms acrosome and lies in front of the nucleus. It contains acrosin and hyaluronidase which help the sperms to penetrate the granulosa layer surrounding the oocyte.

Endocrinology of Spermatogenesis

GnRH acts on anterior pituitary to secrete FSH and LH. FSH acts on germ cells and Sertoli cells to produce sperms and their maturation while LH acts on Leydig cells which produce testosterone and androstenedione. They are responsible for secondary sex characters and sperm maturation. Spermatogenesis requires very high intratubular testosterone. Pharmacotherapy with testosterone cannot achieve these levels and paradoxically leads to depression of spermatogenesis. High FSH indicates seminiferous tubule damage and high LH Leydig cell damage.

Etiopathogenesis

Causes of male infertility can be divided into:
1. Pre-testicular
2. Testicular
3. Post-testicular

Pre-testicular and post-testicular causes are correctable. Primary testicular failure causes irreversible damage expect in cases associated with varicocele.

Pre-testicular azoospermia can be caused by endocrine abnormalities that are characterized by low levels of sex steroids and abnormal gonadotropin levels. These abnormalities can be hypogonadotropic hypogonadism congenital (e.g., Kallmann syndrome, Prader-Willi syndrome, Laurence-Moon-Biedl syndrome), acquired (e.g. hypothalamic or pituitary disorders: tumors, trauma or effect of chemotherapy or radiotherapy) or secondary to adverse effect from a medication.[2] hypergonadotropic hypogonadism[3] excess of steroids or androgens seen in pituitary, adrenal or testicular tumors.[3–7]

Testicular causes include congenital, acquired or idiopathic disorders that lead to spermatogenic failure. Congenital testicular

Seminiferous tubule (cross section)
Epididymis
Testis
Seminiferous tubule
Primordial germ cell
Spermatogonium (diploid)
Mitotic division
Primary spermatocyte (diploid) (in prophase of meiosis)
First meiotic division
Secondary spermatocyte (haploid)
Second meiotic division
Spermatids (haploid)
Spermatids (at two stages of differentiation)
Sertoli cell
Sperm cells (haploid)

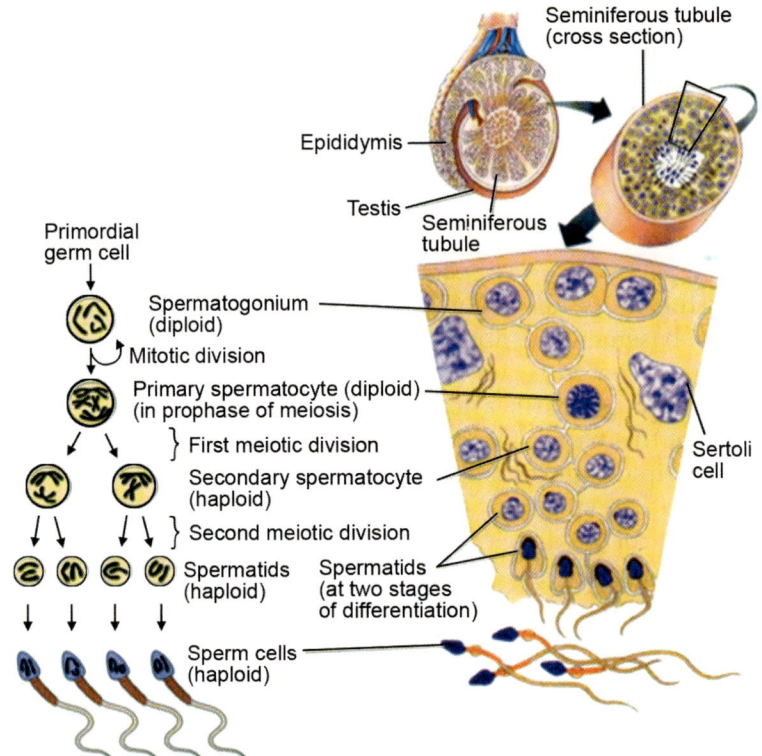

Fig. 18.3: Illustration of spermatogenesis

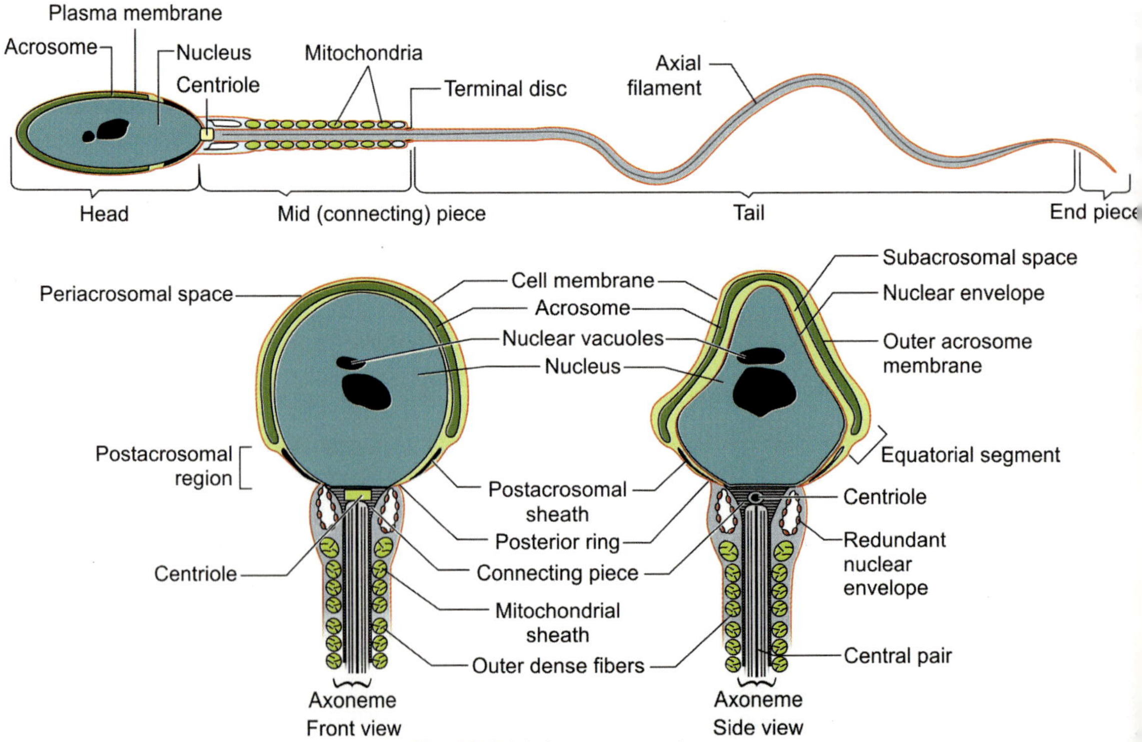

Plasma membrane
Acrosome
Nucleus
Centriole
Mitochondria
Terminal disc
Axial filament
Head
Mid (connecting) piece
Tail
End piece
Periacrosomal space
Cell membrane
Acrosome
Nuclear vacuoles
Nucleus
Subacrosomal space
Nuclear envelope
Outer acrosome membrane
Equatorial segment
Postacrosomal region
Postacrosomal sheath
Posterior ring
Connecting piece
Mitochondrial sheath
Outer dense fibers
Centriole
Centriole
Redundant nuclear envelope
Central pair
Axoneme
Front view
Axoneme
Side view

Fig. 18.4: Mature spermatozoa

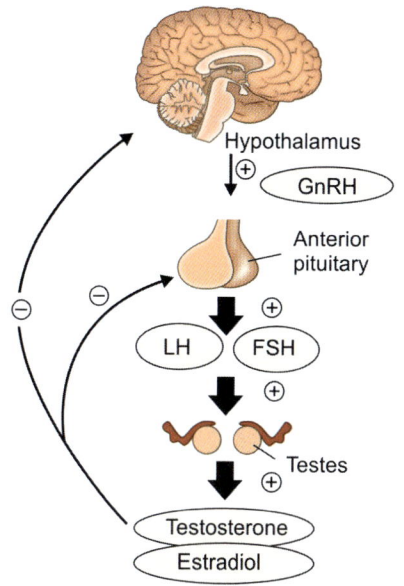

Fig. 18.5: Hypothalamo–pituitary–gonadal axis

These obstructions can also be congenital, caused by a bilateral absence of the vas deferens (CBAVD), or acquired because of infection or surgery (vasectomy or an iatrogenic injury). Obstructive azoospermia (OA) is also classified according to the localization of the obstruction: epididymal (postinfection), vasal (vasectomy, CBAVD) or ductal (müllerian cysts).[9]

Azoospermia may also be clinically classified as obstructive (post-testicular) and non-obstructive (pretesticular or testicular). Obstructive azoospermia (OA) is less common than non-obstructiveazoospermia (NOA) and occurs in 15 to 20% of men with azoospermia. Although NOA indicates impaired sperm production of the entire testis by definition, it has been observed that focal normal spermatogenesis can be observed in 50 to 60% of men with NOA[9].

causes consist of anorchia, testicular dysgenesis (cryptorchidism), genetic abnormalities (Y chromosome deletions), germ cell aplasia (Sertoli cell—only syndrome) and spermatogenic arrest (maturation arrest). Acquired testicular causes include trauma, torsion, infection (mumps/orchitis), testicular tumors, medications, irradiation, surgery (compromising vascularization of testis), systemic diseases (cirrhosis, renal failure) and varicocele.[8]

Post-testicular causes include ejaculatory disorders or obstructions, which impair the transport of spermatozoa from the testis.

Difference between obstructive azoospermia (OA) and non-obstructive azoospermia (NOA)	
Obstructive azoospermia	Non-obstructive azoospermia
Normal volume testis	Small and soft testis
Indurated epididymis	Epididymis flat and soft

Diagnostic Protocol

Diagnosis of male fertility requires thorough evaluation which includes:

1. History
2. Physical examination

Medical history	Physical examination	Hormone measurement
1. Prior fertility	1. Testis size (normal testis volume >14 Ml)	1. FSH
2. Viral orchitis or cryptorchidism	2. Testicular consistency	2. LH
3. Genital trauma/surgery	3. Sec. sexual characters: Body hair distribution, gynecomastia	3. Testosterone
4. Infections such as epididymitis or urethritis	4. Vas/epididymis consistency	
5. Gonadotoxin exposes such as prior radiation therapy/chemotherapy, recent fever or heat exposure and current medications	5. Varicocele	
	6. Digital rectal examination (DRE) for masses	
	7. Testis epididymis vas deferens: Size, consistency to differentiate between obstructive and non-obstructive azoospermia	
6. Family history of birth defects, mental retardation, reproductive failure or cystic		

3. Detailed semen analysis—WHO and strict Kruger's criteria.
4. Blood tests—routine: Hemogram, blood sugar, HIV, VDRL, HCV, HbsAg endocrinological (as per requirement)—only in cases of severe OAT/azoospermia, FSH, LH, testosterone prolactin, TSH.
5. *USG:* KUB for associated renal anomalies USG.
6. *Scrotal USG/TRUS:* Vas, testis, epididymis, varicocele, ejaculatory duct cyst.
7. Special tests—sperm function tests, pituitary imaging.
8. Karyotyping, genetic study, Y microdeletion.

A description of all the relevant steps is detailed as under:

Imaging in Male Infertility

Scrotal ultrasonography (US), transrectal US (TRUS), TRUS-guided seminal vesiculography, vasography, abdominal US and cranial imaging are all imaging studies that can be used to evaluate males with azoospermia and abnormal seminal parameters. Role of imaging in routine evaluation is limited however in specific circumstances, it serves as an important tool.

TRUS is also able to identify other known and potentially correctable OA causes, such as müllerian (utricular) or Wolffian (ejaculatory duct) cysts, ejaculatory duct calcifications, congenital unilateral or bilateral absence of the vas deferens, and obstructing seminal vesicle cysts.[10]

Abdominal US imaging should be considered if there is a unilateral or bilateral congenital absence of the vas deferens. Because of the embryologic origins of the vas deferens and the kidney, anomalies in these organs tend to coexist. One study has demonstrated that 26% and 11% of men with unilateral or bilateral congenital absence of vas deferens, respectively also exhibit renal agenesis.

Hormonal Analysis

Hormonal analysis helps to differentiate pretesticular, testicular and post-testicular etiologies of azoospermia.

Genetic Investigation

Genetic factors occupy an important place in the evaluation and management of the azoospermic male. Such factors can be pretesticular (e.g. Kallmann syndrome), testicular (e.g. Klinefelter's syndrome or Y chromosome microdeletions) or post-testicular (CBAVD). Genetic counseling provides couples with information about the nature, inheritance pattern, and implications of genetic disorders to help them make informed medical and personal decisions.

Semen Analysis

Semen analysis is of paramount importance as it is a reliable measure of male fecundity. It should be done at least 48 hours after last ejaculation. Over the period, the values of normal semen has changed drastically thus changing the definition of male infertility. Current normal values (as per WHO 2010 manual) has been a subject of debate and controversy and due to these controversies

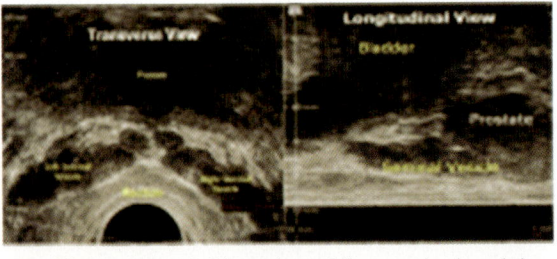

Fig. 18.6: Transrectal imaging of the seminal vesicles

Table 18.1: Normal male hormone range	
Hormones	*Values*
Total testosterone	300–1,000 ng/dl
Free testosterone	4–20 ng/dl (1–4% of total test)
LH	1.6–8 IU/L
FSH	1.3–8.4 IU/L
Prolactin	4.2–15 ng/ml

many people continue to use old values as normal (Table 18.2).

Fructose Level

Regarding the level of fructose in the semen, WHO specifies a normal level of 13 µmol per sample. Absence of fructose may indicate a problem with the seminal vesicles.

pH

WHO criteria specify normal pH as 7.2–7.8. Acidic ejaculate (lower pH value) may indicate one or both of the seminal vesicles are blocked. An ejaculate with (higher pH value) may indicate an infection, pH value outside of the normal range is harmful to sperm.

Liquefaction

The liquefaction is the process when the gel formed by proteins from the seminal vesicles is broken up and the semen becomes more liquid. It normally takes less than 20 minutes for the sample to change from a thick gel into a liquid. In the NICE guidelines, a liquefaction time within 60 minutes is regarded as within normal ranges. Increased liquefaction time is suggestive of prostatic/seminal vesicle abnormality and is associated with low fertility potential.

Morphology

Regarding sperm morphology, the WHO criteria as described in 2010 state that a sample is normal (samples from men whose partners had a pregnancy in the last 12 months) if 4% (or 5th centile) or more of the observed sperm have normal morphology.

WHO morphological critaria and more stringent criteria, the so-called Tygerbergor strict Kruger's criteria enhances objectivity and decreases intra-laboratory variability. According to WHO criteria, a morphologically normal spermatozoon has an oval head and an acrosome covering 40–70% of the head area. A normal spermatozoon has no neck, midpiece, tail abnormalities nor cytoplasmic droplets larger than 50% of the sperm head.

In strict criteria spermatozoon is normal if it has an oval head, 4.0–5.0 µm long and 2.5–3.5 µm wide, measured with an ocular micrometer. The length-to-width ratio should be 1.50–1.75. A normal spermatozoon has a well-defined acrosome that covers 40–70% of the head. The midpiece is thin, less than 1 µm wide, about 1.5 times longer than the head. Cytoplasmic droplets, if present, should not be larger than half of the head width. The tail is thin, uniform, uncoiled and about 45 µm long. According to this classification system, all borderline forms are considered as abnormal.[11]

Morphology is the best predictor of success in fertilizing oocytes during *in vitro* fertilization and is best correlated with outcome.

Abnormalities of Semen

- *Aspermia:* Absence of semen

Table 18.2: Cut-off reference values for semen characteristics as published in consecutive WHO manuals					
Semen characteristics	*WHO 1980*	*WHO 1987*	*WHO 1992*	*WHO 1999*	*WHO 2010*
Volume (ml)	ND	≥2	≥2	≥ 2	≥1.5
Sperm count (10^5/ml)	20–200	≥20	20	≥ 20	≥15
Total sperm count (10^6)	ND	≥40	40	≥ 40	≥39
Total motility (%)	≥60	≥50	50	≥ 50	≥40
Progressive motility	≥2	≥25%	25%	≥ 25% (a)	≥32% (a + b)
Vitality (%)	ND	≥50	75	≥ 75	≥58
Morphology (%)	80.5	≥50	30	(14)	≥4
Leukocyte count (10^6/ml)	<4.7	<1.0	<1.0	<1.0	<1.0

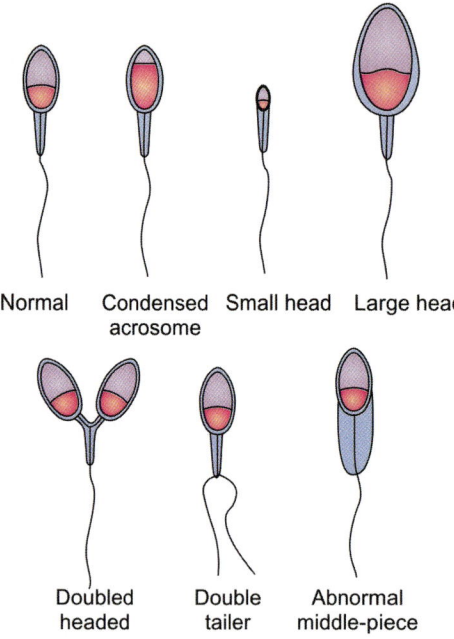

Fig. 18.7: Types of sperms

- *Azoospermia:* Absence of sperm
- *Hypospermia:* Low semen volume
- *Hyperspermia:* High semen volume
- *Oligozoospermia:* Low sperm count
- *Asthenozoospermia:* Poor sperm motility
- *Teratozoospermia:* Sperm carry more morphological defects than usual
- *Necrozoospermia:* All sperm in the ejaculate are dead
- *Leucospermia:* A high level of white blood cells in semen
- *Oligo-astheno-teratozoospermia (OAT):* Low sperm count, low motility and high abnormal sperm count.

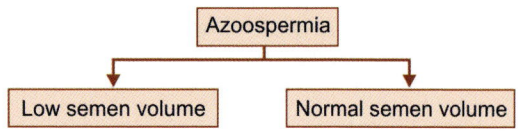

Workup for Azoospermic Patients

To enforce standardization worldwide, WHO definition is recommended. As per WHO azoospermia is defined as inability to identify any mature sperm on high power on at least two occasion (examination requires and examination after pelleting).

Testicular Biopsy/Fine Needle Aspiration Cytology (FNAC)

In order to distinguish between obstructive and nonobstructive causes of azoospermia, diagnostic testicular biopsy is indicated for patients with normal testicular size, at least one palpable vas deferens and a normal serum FSH level. Biopsy can be done by needle under local anesthesia or open biopsy.

It is advisable to be done in a tertiary care centre, where there is expertise to assess testicular histology and facilities for sperm recovery and cryopreservation are available.

Management of Male Infertility

Management of male infertility can be medical, surgical, ART or combined .In clinical practice, semen parameters reflect male fecundity and guide the planning and management in male infertility.

Medical treatment has limitations and are applicable to a select group of patients only.

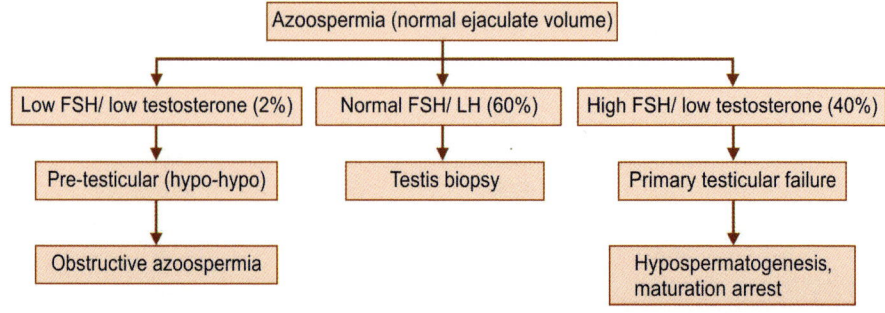

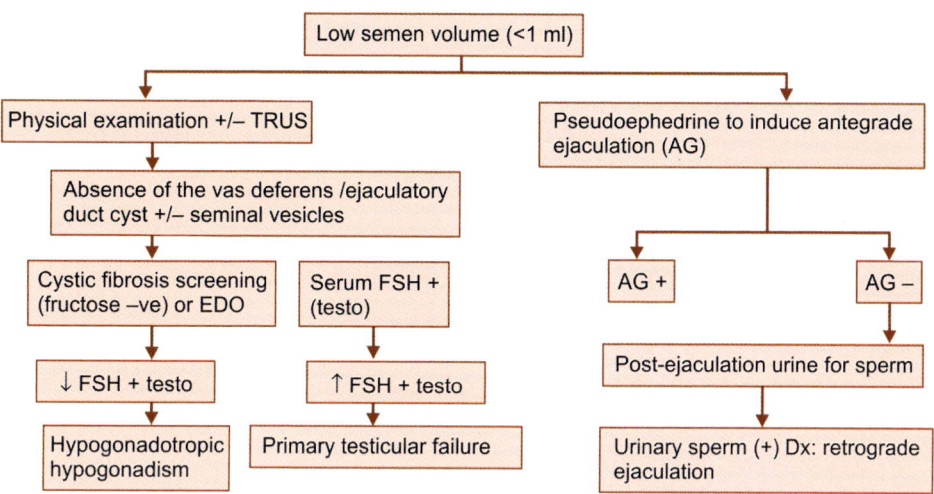

ART has revolutionized the management of male infertility. In mild idiopathic oligo-astheno-teratozoospermia (OAT), intrauterine insemination (IUI) is preferred and should be offered for at least 3 cycles before moving on to more advanced procedure like IVF or ICSI. In severe OAT, IVF/ICSI are indicated. In NOA (non-obstructive azoospermia), medical/surgical sperm recovery treatment followed by ICSI and in OA, surgical treatment followed by ICSI should be the management of choice. Donor IUI can be offered to patients with severe OAT and azoospermia if there are financial constraints. Details of relevant medical and surgical treatment is described as under.

Medical Management of Male Infertility

Conventionally, most of the patients are prescribed some form of medical therapy once abnormal seminal parameters are reported However, medical management is definitive

To summarize				
Condition	Serum FSH	Testes size	Semen volume	Feature
Hypogonadotropic Hypogonadism	Lower undetectable FSH, LH, testosterone, prolactin normal	Small soft	Normal	Hyposmia/anosmia may be present
Seminiferous tubular failure	High	Small soft	Normal	--
Boderline azoospermia	Normal to mild elevation	Normal to slightly small	Normal	Biopsy hypospermato-genesis or maturation arrest
Condition	Serum FSH	Testes size	Semen volume	Fructose
Ejaculatory duct obstruction	Normal	Normal	Very low	Absent
Vasal aplasia	Normal	Normal	Very low	Absent
Vasal obstruction	Normal	Normal	Normal	Present
Epididymal obstruction	Normal	Normal	Normal	Present
Intratesticular obstruction	Normal	Normal	Normal	Present

and is beneficial in a select number of patients. In others, medical treatment offers only empirical treatment. Most of the medical therapy requires continuation of drugs for at least two consecutive spermatogenic cycles to get optimal response except antibiotic therapy. The aim of medical treatment is:

1. To stimulate and restore normal spermatogenesis
2. Maintain cellular concentration of androgen in normal range to develop and establish androgenization.

Indications of Definitive Medical Treatment

- Hypogonadotropic hypogonadism
- Hyperprolactinemia
- Genital tract infection
- Sexual dysfunction
- Retrograde ejaculation

Hypogonadotropic Hypogonadism

Hypogonadotropic hypogonadism is characterized by low FSH, LH and testosterone and shows consistent response to medical treatment.

To induce spermatogenesis, initiation is done by INJ. HCG which has intrinsic LH like activity or LH. Completion of spermatogenesis is done by gonadotropins (HMG). In partial gonadotropic deficiency or those in which prepubertal HCG stimulation has been given and in post-pubertal acquired hypogonadotropic hypogonadism, initiation and maintenance of spermatogenesis can be done with HCG alone. Patients should be counselled in detail for long drawn treatment and cost involved.

In hypogonadotropic hypogonadism various regimens are advocated—IM injection of hCG 2000 IU/twice a week or inj hCG 5000 IU for 3 months to 1 year is given. If after 6 months of hCG no spermatozoon is seen in the ejaculate, hCG is substituted with HMG at 75 IU thrice a week for 6 months to 1 year. Alternatively inj hCG is given every week for 4–6 weeks then inj. HMG 75 IU thrice a week is also added and continued for 6–12 months.[12]

Also GnRH pulsatile administration can induce spermatogenesis but it is not pratical.

For androgenization, testosterone orally or parental can be given.

Testosterone undecanoate—40 mg bd or mesterolone 25 mg tds or qid or deep IM testosterone 250 mg/once a month enhance gonadal function.

Hyperprolactinemia causes decreased libido and impaired erectile function. For sexual dysfunction, along with testosterone oral bromocriptine 1.2 mg/day HS, increase dose each week till the patient becomes euprotactinenic. Alternatively Cabergoline-0.5 mg once/twice a week can be given. Dose can be increased to 1 mg.

Advantage—better tolerated, longer half life. Hypothyroidism and hyperthyroidism also leads to defective spermatogenesis resulting into oligo and asthenospermia and is correctable by appropriate medication.

Genital Tract Infection

As per WHO manual 2010, presence of >5 million/ml round cells or pus cells in semen sample can be termed as leukocytospermia and should be treated. Identification of white cells in semen require staining with eosin-nigrosin, and requires treatment. It is ideal to culture semen for identification of presence of infection and prescribing the appropriate antibiotics as per culture sensitivity for at least 2–4 weeks however it is difficult to get a positive culture most of the time and in these cases, doxycycline 100 mg twice a day should be given for 3–4 weeks to eliminate infection.

Role of Antioxidants

There is now a little doubt that oxidative stress causes damage to the function of sperm causing structural damage to DNA and accelerating cell apoptosis, which consequently lead to the inability to achieve conception or lack of development of the embryo.

Reviewing the current literature revealed that carnitines and vitamin C and E have been clearly shown to be effective by many well-conducted studies and may be considered as a first-line treatment. The efficacy of anti-oxidants, such as glutathione, selenium and coenzyme Q10 has been demonstrated by a few, but well-performed studies, and may be considered second line.

Issue of concern is the dose of antioxidant preparations. It appears that in the case of oxidative stress, doses of antioxidants should be higher than usual daily dose and used for at least three months, because the development of a mature sperm from spermatogonia is 72 ±4 days.[13]

Surgical Management

In obstructive azoospermia the mainstay of treatment is surgical correction as under. Surgery in obstructive azoospermia varies with site of obstruction. In clinical practice, there is limited indication of vasography and that is to identify site of obstruction only if reconstructive surgery is to be done.

- *Repair of varicocele:* Varicocele is a common finding in fertile as well as infertile man and may be an important cause of OAT. However neither all men with varicocele require surgery nor all varicolectomy result in significant improvement in fecundity.

Surgery should be offered to select a few who fulfill all of the following criteria:
- Couple has known infertility
- The female partner has normal fertility or potentially a treatable cause of infertility
- The varicocele is clinically palpable (subclinical varicocele detected on ultrasound should not be operated)
- The male partner has abnormal semen parameter or sperm function tests.[14]

Assisted reproduction techniques (ART) in male infertility: In current clinical pracitise when specific treatment improves the sperm quantity or quality to a limited degree but not enough for natural conception, ART offers treatment to alleviate male factor subfertility. ART aims at increasing the probability of fertilization by bringing the spermatozoa closer to [intrauterine insemination (IUI) or *in-vitro* fertilization (IVF)] or even within [intracytoplasmic sperm injection (ICSI)] the oocyte(s), thereby bypassing some functional deficits of the male gametes. In the latter, the rate of fertilization is enhanced by micro-injecting one single spermatozoon directly into the oocyte's cytoplasm, i.e. ICSI. ICSI allows the successful use of ejaculated, epididymal or testicular spermatozoa to obtain fertilization *in vitro*.

IUI in male infertility: Intrauterine insemination (IUI) is used to treat the mild to moderate

Procedure	Indication success	Rate	Complication
Microsurgical vasovasal anastomosis (VVA)	Postvasectomy infection/ vas obstruction due to infection	Sperm return: 70–90% Pregnancy: 30–74%	Failure, stricture (depends upon duration of vasectomy and length of tube preserved
Microsurgical vaso-epididymal anastomosis (VEA), side to side/ vasotubular	Obstructions limited to cauda epididymis sparing the caput and body of the epididymis	Sperm return: 70% Pregnancy: 20–40%	Spontaneous closure of anastomosis, scarring of epididymis
Transurethral resection of ejaculatory ducts (TURED)	Ejaculatory duct obstruc-tion. Duct enters the distal prostatic urethra near the verumontanum	Sperm return: 50–70% Pregnancy: 20%	Including hematuria, hemato-spermia, urinary tract infection, epididymitis, and a watery ejaculate due to reflux of urine

forms. It is reasonable to offer IUI as first-line treatment if total motile sperm concentration (TMSC) is greater than 10 million when balancing the risk and cost of alternate treatments. A meta-analysis authored by Boomsma et al[15] shows that, while gradient techniques yield the highest recovery rates, no semen preparation technique appears superior when compared to others that are also in common use. According to retrospective cohort studies, most pregnancies achieved with IUI in women under 37 years of age will occur during the first 3–4 treatment cycles.[16]

IVF or ICSI for male factor infertility: If pregnancy is not achieved after 3–4 cycles of IUI then the next reasonable step to circumvent male subfertility is IVF or ICSI. Contemporary strategies for deciding between IVF and ICSI are either formulated using experience-based preset cut-off values or created with the assumption that ICSI is the more robust insemination technique. Various studies have proposed a minimum motile count of at least one million spermatozoa

in the native semen sample, the motile progressive count after sperm preparation one million to 0.5 million progressive motile spermatozoa or even 0.2 million motile progressive spermatozoa and 5% normal forms below which poor fertilization after conventional IVF is anticipated. However, in this era of ICSI, should all male factor patients be offered ICSI remains a subject of debate as fertilization failure seen in 50% of IVF cases and is the main limiting factor of IVF as compared to ICSI. However, world over, more and more centers have shifted to practice ICSI for all male factor infertility.[17]

Absolute indications for ICSI in male factor infertility
- TMSC (total motile sperm concentration) <1 million
- TMSC >10 million in previous two IVF with no or poor fertilization
- Sperms aspirated from epididymis or testis
- TMSC <5 million with <4% normal forms
- Frozen thawed sperms with poor survival

Table 18.3: Comparison of various sperm retrieval techniques

Procedure	Technique	Success rate	Drawback	Complication
From epididymis				
PESA	Simple/quick	Sperm recovery: 78–83% Pregnancy: 35–40%	Blind procedure	Epididymal injury, bleeding post-surgery fibrosis
MESA	Microsurgical Procedure under operating	Preferred method, sperm recovery 80–85%	Requires surgical expertise and setup	Minimal fibrosis
From testies				
TEFNA	Simple, noninvasive	Sperm recovery 90–93%	Blind technique	Testicular vessel injury, architectural defect, hematoma
TESE	Surgical expertise required	Preferred method, sperm recovery: 94–98%	Requires surgical expertise and setup, time consuming	-Do-
Modified TESE	Surgical expertise required	Sperm recovery: 94–98%	Requires surgical expertise and setup, time consuming	-Do- (but minimal chances of injury and inflammation)

Abbreviations: PESA—percutaneous epididymal sperm aspiration; MESA—microsurgical epididymal sperm aspiration; TEFNA, testicular fine needle aspiration cytology; TESE—testicular sperm extraction; Modified TESE, microdissection testicular sperm extraction.

Sperm retrieval methods for ICSI

All methods provide sufficient number of viable sperms for ICSI and cryopreservation. As long as viable sperms can be aspirated, neither duration of obstruction nor mobility of sperms affects the outcome of ICSI. Repeated sperm aspiration can be performed successfully, minimal interval recommended between sperm retrieval procedures is 3–6 months.[18]

Conclusion

A thorough knowledge of the etiopatho-physiology of the various cause of male infertility is very important for right approach to just management of infertile couple. medical management has a limited but definitive role in specific conditions. ART has changed scenario completely as most of primary testicular dysfunctions are difficult to treat medically and only hope for these patients is ICSI combined with surgical retrieval donor insemination is to be offered to those patients who cannot afford these procedures or no sperm is available for ICSI. Proper evaluation and counselling is needed before treatment.

References

1. Hirsh A "Male subfertility". BMJ (2003);327 (7416): 669–72.
2. Cooper TG, Noonan E, von Eckardstein S, Auger J, Baker HW, Behre HM, Haugen TB, Kruger T, Wang C, Mbizvo MT, Vogelsong KM. World Health Organization reference values for human semen characteristics. Hum Reprod Update 2010 May-Jun;16(3):231–45.
3. Agarwal A, Prabakaran SA, Said TM. "Prevention of Oxidative Stress Injury to Sperm". Journal of Andrology 20005;26(6):654–60.
4. Robbins WA, Elashoff DA, Xun L, Jia J, Li N, Wu G, Wei F. "Effect of lifestyle exposures on sperm aneuploidy". Cytogenetic and Genome Research 2005;111 (3-4): 371–7.
5. Emsley J. Nature's building blocks: an A-Z guide to the elements. Oxford [Oxfordshire]: Oxford University Press 2001;p. 76.
6. Ji G, Long Y, Zhou Y, Huang C, Gu A, Wang X. Common variants in mismatch repair genes associated with increased risk of sperm DNA damage and male infertility. BMC Med 2012; 10:49.
7. Silva LF, Oliveira JB, Petersen CG, Mauri AL, Massaro FC, Cavagna M, Baruffi RL, Franco JG Jr. The effects of male age on sperm analysis by motile sperm organelle morphology examination (MSOME). Reprod Biol Endocrinol 2012;10:19.
8. Costabile RA, Spevak M. "Characterization of patients presenting with male factor infertility in an equal access, no cost medical system". Urology 2001;58(6):1021–25.
9. Ahmet Gudeloglu and Sijo J Parekattil, Update in the evaluation of the azoospermic maleClinics (Sao Paulo). 2013 Feb; 68(Suppl 1): 27–34.
10. Matthias Schurich, Friedrich Aigner,Ferdinand Frauscher, Leo Pallwein. The role of ultrasound in assessment of male fertility, EJOG, vol 144, SUP 1:S192–8.
11. Andrea Ipak, Patrik Stani, Koraljka Uri, Tihana Serdar, Ernest Suchanek. Sperm morphology assessment according to WHO and strict criteria: method comparison and intra-laboratory variability. Biochemia Medica 2009;19(1):87–94.
12. Schiff JD1, Ramírez ML, Bar-Chama N. Medical and surgical management of male infertility. Endocrinol Metab Clin North Am. June 2007; 36(2):313–31.
13. Gual-Frau J, Abad C, Amengual MJ, Hannaoui N, Checa MA, Ribas-Maynou J, Lozano I, Nikolaou A, Benet J, García-Peiró A, Prats J. Oral antioxidant treatment partly improves integrity of human sperm DNA in infertile grade I varicocele patients. Hum Fertil (Camb) June 2015 19:1–5.
14. Cho KS, Seo JT.Effect of varicocelectomy on male infertility. Korean J Urol Nov 2014; 55(11):703–9.
15. Boomsma CM, Heineman MJ, Cohlen BJ, Farquhar C. Semen preparation techniques for intrauterine insemination. Cochrane Database Syst Rev 2007.
16. Herman Tournaye. Male factor infertility and ART. Sian J Androl Jan 2012;14(1):103–08.
17. Boulet SL, Mehta A, Kissin DM, Warner L, Kawwass JF, Jamieson DJ. Trends in use of and reproductive outcomes associated with intracyto-plasmic sperm injection. JAMA Jan 2015 20; 313(3):255–63.
18. Van Peperstraten A, Proctor ML, Johnson NP, Philipson G. Techniques for surgical retrieval of sperm prior to intracytoplasmic sperm injection (ICSI) for azoospermia.Cochrane Database Syst Rev Apr 2008;16;(2).

19

Female Infertility

• Renu Misra

Infertility is the inability of a couple to conceive after 12 months of regular unprotected intercourse, or after six months in women over the age of 35 years. On an average, 84% couples will achieve a pregnancy within one year and 92% in two years. The problem of infertility is rising globally. The overall incidence of infertility, which was 1 in 10 couples (10%) for a long time has increased to 15%. Increasing female age at planning pregnancy, obesity, and their consequences like endometriosis and fibroids being major contributors. The role of male partner in this increase is equally important; sperm counts have fallen worldwide by 50% over the last five decades.

NORMAL REPRODUCTIVE CYCLE

The chances of conception per cycle in a young healthy couple at best are 20–25%. To diagnose the reasons for infertility, it is important to first underst and the process of normal reproductive cycle. For pregnancy to occur in a cycle, the following prerequisites must be met.

- Maturation and release of an egg or ovulation from the ovary.
- Normal tubo-ovarian relation to ensure the egg is picked up by the tube when it is released.

- Normal semen analysis with adequate sperm count and motility.
- Normal tubal patency and function for the sperms to reach the site of the egg in the fallopian tube for fertilization and migration of the fertilized egg (embryo) from the tube to the uterine cavity.
- Receptive endometrium for implantation of the embryo.

Every month, hundreds of eggs are recruited from the dormant pool of eggs in the ovary to the active pool, which are now capable of growth and maturation. However, in a natural cycle, only one of these eggs will survive and grow, while the rest will degenerate. The growing egg which is contained in a fluid-filled sac called follicle, moves to the periphery of the ovary as it matures. Finally, the egg is extruded out of the ovary through a small surface rent on the ovary. This process is called ovulation. The residual follicular granulosa and theca cells form the corpus luteum and begin to secrete the hormone progesterone. If the embryo fails to implant, the corpus luteum degenerates in 14 days, the progesterone levels fall, and menses begin. In case a pregnancy occurs, the corpus luteum continues to produce progesterone to provide adequate uterine environment to maintain pregnancy.[1]

The fimbrial end of the fallopian tube spreads over the ovary at the time of ovulation and collects the egg. With peristaltic activity, the egg moves towards the midportion of the tube. The sperms which are deposited in the upper vagina at coitus swim up through the uterine cavity into the fallopian tube to meet the egg. One sperm can only penetrate the egg resulting in fertilization. The fertilized egg, now called an embryo slowly migrates from the tube to the endometrial cavity and implants resulting in pregnancy.

CAUSES OF INFERTILITY

The normal reproductive cycle can encounter problems at multiple places leading to infertility. The common causes of infertility in the female and male partner are as follows:

Female

1. Ovulatory dysfunction
2. Tubal block
3. Uterine pathology
4. Endometriosis

Male

1. Low sperm count (oligozoospermia) <15 million/ml
2. Low sperm motility (asthenozoospermia) <40%
3. Absent sperms (azoospermia)—no sperms seen
4. Abnormal morphology (teratozoospermia)—normal <4%.

Both male and female partners contribute to infertility equally. In 40% of infertile couples, the male partner is either the sole cause or a contributory factor to infertility.[2] 20–25% couples have unexplained infertility where no identifiable cause of infertility is detected on investigations.

If a woman has never conceived in her life, it is called primary infertility. Infertility following one or more conceptions, whether they end in miscarriage, ectopic pregnancy or viable birth (live or still), is called secondary infertility.

FEMALE INFERTILITY

The two major reasons for infertility in the female are ovulatory disorders and tubal pathology. Other causes are uterine abnormalities and endometriosis. The preliminary investigations should always start with a semen analysis to exclude male factor, followed by tests for ovulation detection and establishing tubal patency. Causes and management of female infertility will be discussed in detail in this chapter.

Ovulatory Disorders

Ovulatory dysfunction is the most common cause of infertility. Menstrual history can give a good insight into the ovulatory status of a patient. Women with irregular periods at intervals longer than 35 days are typically more likely to have ovulatory dysfunction, whereas regular menstrual cycles are usually ovulatory.[3] The incidence of ovulatory disorders also increases with age as the egg reserve is slowly depleted. The World Health Organization classifies ovulation disorders into three categories.

- *Group I:* Hypothalamic pituitary failure (hypogonadotrophic hypogonadism)
- *Group II:* Hypothalamic-pituitary-ovarian dysfunction (normogonadotrophic anovulation)
- *Group III:* Ovarian failure (hypergonadotrophic hypogonadism)

The hormone profile in different categories is shown in Table 19.1.

Table 19.1: Hormone profile indifferent categories

WHO group	FSH	LH	E2
I	Low	Low	Low
II	Low/ Normal	High/ Normal	High/ Normal
III	High	High	Low

WHO group I accounts for 5–10% of patients with anovulation. The defect lies at the level of hypothalamus or pituitary. The hormone profile shows low levels of follicle-stimulating hormone (FSH) and luteinizing hormone (LH), and low estradiol level as a consequence. This may be caused by primary pituitary disease resulting in primary amenorrhea as in Kallmann syndrome. Secondary causes of amenorrhea include suppression of hypothalamus (stress or exercise related amenorrhea, anorexia nervosa) or pituitary disease as in postpartum pituitary necrosis (Sheehans syndrome) or pituitary tumors (prolactinomas). These patients do not respond to oral ovulation inducing agents. To achieve pregnancy, administration of human menopausal gonadotropin which has both FSH and LH activity, or pulsatile GnRH, is required for follicular maturation and ovulation.

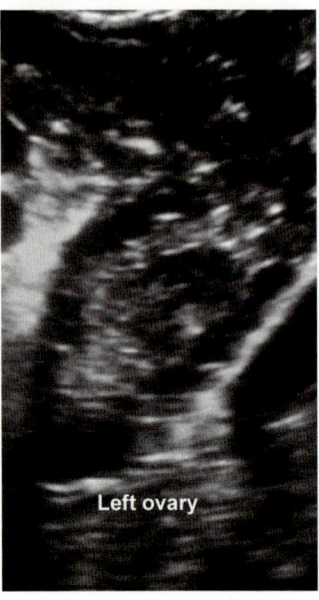

Fig. 19.1: Ultrasound showing polycystic ovary with peripherally arranged follicles

Hyperprolactinemia: High prolactin levels secreted by pituitary prolactinomas inhibit GnRH pulsatility causing secondary hypogonadotrophic hypogonadism. The treatment for these patients is to lower prolactin levels by dopamine agonist drugs like bromocriptine or cabergoline; surgery may be required in a minority of patients to treat macroprolactinoma.

WHO group II accounts for 75–90% of patients with anovulation, the vast majority are contributed by women with polycystic ovarian syndrome (PCOS). Their FSH and estradiol levels are normal. Classically, the LH level is elevated, at least twice that of the FSH level, but it may be normal in almost 50% women.[4] Ultrasound typically shows multiple small follicles arranged on the periphery giving a necklace appearance (Fig. 19.1). The pathophysiology of PCOS is poorly understood. It has a multifactorial origin with a genetic predisposition. The various pathways include abnormal gonadotropin secretion due to reduced hypothalamic feedback response to circulating sex steroids, disordered insulin action and androgen excess.[5] The end result is chronic anovulation. Menstrual cycles vary from oligomenorrhea to secondary amenorrhea.

Progestogen challenge test: Withdrawal bleeding almost always occurs in PCOS in response to progesterone because the endogenous estrogen levels are normal. This is an important clinical test which differentiates class II patients from class I and III, which are both hypo-estrogenic and do not get withdrawal to progestogen alone.

Women in this group who are obese, particularly BMI more than 30 should be counselled that losing weight may promote ovulation and improve the response to medication. Several studies have shown that even 5–10% reduction in weight can restore fertility.[6] These patients respond well to ovulation inducing agents, the commonest drug used is clomiphene citrate. It is given at a dose of 50 mg for five days starting any day between day 2 and 5 of the period. Follicle tracking is done by ultrasound to assess the response of treatment. An injection of HCG is not routinely required for follicular rupture and release of the egg, unless a procedure like intrauterine insemination (IUI) has to be timed. If there is no follicular growth or evidence of ovulation, the dose is increased to 100 mg in the next cycle, up to a maximum of 150 mg. If ovulation occurs, the same dose can be continued for a maximum of six cycles, provided other causes of infertility like tubal block has been excluded. In case of failed ovulation, metformin can be added to clomiphene. Metformin is given continuously in a dose of 1000–1500 mg per day in twice daily dosage. It should be emphasized that it should be taken after meals as it can cause gastrointestinal disturbances. Alternatively, if there is poor response to clomiphene, letrozole which is an aromatase inhibitor can be tried to induce ovulation. Currently however the drug is not approved by the Drug Controller of India to be used for fertility treatment in India.

Second line treatment for ovulation induction in women who fail to ovulate on first line drugs is either gonadotropin injections or laparoscopic ovarian drilling. Both have their pros and cons. Gonado-trophins are expensive, need to be given by injection, need greater monitoring as they carry a greater risk of multiple pregnancy compared to clomiphene (14% versus 8%). In comparison, laparoscopic ovarian drilling is an operative procedure with the inherent risks of anesthesia and surgery. However, laparoscopy has other advantages. It allows evaluation of the whole pelvis including patency of fallopian tubes, exclusion of endometriosis, adhesions, etc. It is a one-time procedure but the endocrinological effects may last for many years.[7] The rate of multiple pregnancy is also lower than gonadotropin injections.[8] When drilling fails to achieve pregnancy on its own, it makes the ovaries more responsive to ovulation inducing agents.

WHO group III patients include women with primary or secondary ovarian failure, and account for 5% women with ovulation problems. Hormone profile is characterized by high FSH and LH with low E_2 (estradiol) levels. Ovulation induction is futile as there are no eggs in the ovary, which can be stimulated. The only logical treatment is *in vitro* fertilization with donor eggs.

Tubal Pathology

Tubal patency is an essential requirement in the natural conception cycle. Tubal patency and function can be compromised either because of disease affecting the tubal lumen or exogenous obstruction due to adhesions, leading to tubal block. Mucosal disease is usually a result of pelvic inflammatory disease which is due to polymicrobial infection. Tuberculosis is also an important etiological factor in tubal disease in India. When the infection heals, it causes scarring and tubal obstruction. In the other scenario, a healthy tube may get entrapped and get obstructed in conditions associated with moderate to severe pelvic adhesions like endometriosis or previous pelvic surgery. Surgical procedures to restore tubal patency have better outcome in the latter group as the tubes have otherwise uncompromised function. Hysteroscopic tubal cannulation can be tried in proximal tubal block with successful recanalization in 60–70% patients.[9,10] Fimbrial phimosis and terminal block can be treated laparoscopically, although pregnancy rates depend on the condition of the tubal mucosa. Grossly distended tubes (hydrosalpinx) may be removed or clipped followed by IVF, which gives better chance of pregnancy than conservative surgery to create a new tubal ostium. Surgery has a limited role when tubes are diseased, as they tend to develop multiple blocks. *In vitro* fertilization is a better option to achieve pregnancy in these patients.

Uterine Pathology

Uterine abnormalities including endometrial polyps, submucous fibroids, uterine septum or intrauterine adhesions are identified in 10% to 15% of women seeking infertility treatment.[11] Presence of intrauterine pathology interferes with implantation and reduces the chances of pregnancy. Transvaginal ultrasound can detect uterine conditions like fibroids and adenomyosis which may have a negative impact on fertility. Intrauterine pathology like polyps or submucus fibroids may be picked up on ultrasound, although hysteroscopy is diagnostic. There is evidence to show that hysteroscopic surgery in these patients, particularly resection of a submucous fibroid or endometrial polyp, improves pregnancy rates.

Endometriosis

Endometriosis is a common condition in women which primarily manifests with pain and infertility. The incidence of endometriosis in general population is 6–10% but it is as high as 25–50% in infertile women.[13] It is a condition characterized by presence of ectopic endometrium outside the uterine cavity. This ectopic endometrium responds to ovarian hormones like the normally situated endometrium resulting in bleeding, local inflammation and scarring. Delay in planning pregnancy and continued menstruation increases the likelihood of developing endometriosis in genetically predisposed women.

Although there are many theories how endometriosis develops, Sampson's theory of retrograde menstruation seems to be most plausible as the common sites of endometriotic lesions correspond to areas which are likely to come in contact with the menstrual blood discharged from the tubes.[14] Thses include the ovaries, posterior cul-de-sac, uterosacral ligaments, and rectosigmoid colon. Ovaries are the commonest site. There may be lesions on the surface, but with more severe disease, cysts containing old blood form in the ovary, which are also called chocolate cysts.

Several mechanisms have been proposed to explain the association between endometriosis and infertility, which include:
- Distorted pelvic anatomy due to scarring and adhesions
- Altered peritoneal function
- Altered humoral and cellular immunity
- Endocrine and ovulatory abnormalities
- Impaired implantation

Laparoscopy is generally required to confirm the diagnosis. However, ovarian involvement in the form of endometriotic cysts can be diagnosed on imaging modalities like ultrasound and magnetic resonance (MR). They appear as cysts with echogenic contents due to the blood present in the cyst (Fig. 19.2). Since the disease has varied involvement of pelvic structures from a few millimeter peritoneal implants to large endometriomas, American Society for Reproductive Medicine has proposed a clinical staging based on laparoscopic findings (stages I to IV) for prognosis and treatment.

Although medical treatment to suppress endometriois can help resolve the symptoms of pain, it does not help in achieving pregnancy. On the contrary, it delays treatment of infertility and is therefore not recommended as primary treatment in infertile women. Laparoscopic ablation of endometriotic implants in stgaes I and II disease has been shown to significantly improve the live birth rates.[15,16] Women with stage III/IV have more severe disease and overall lower pregnancy

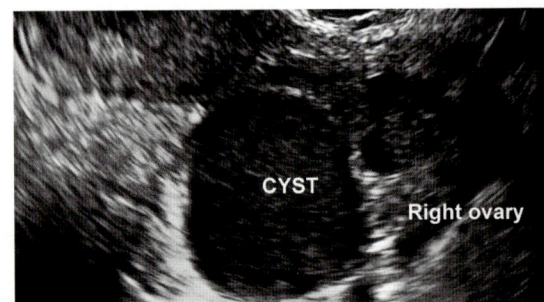

Fig. 19.2: Ultrasound showing endometriotic cyst in the right ovary

rates. Conservative surgery including ablation of peritoneal implants, excision of endometriotic cysts and releasing adhesions can increase the chances of conception. When spontaneous conception does not occur afte surgery, ovulation induction with intrauterine insemination (IUI) should be advised in early stage disease. In advance stages, *in vitro* fertilization (IVF) following surgery increases the chances of pregnancy. However, patients should be counselled that pregnancy rates with IVF are lower in women with endometriosis compared to those undergoing IVF for other indications.[17]

UNEXPLAINED INFERTILITY

When no detectable cause for infertility is found on investigation, it is categorized as unexplained infertility. Generally, the diagnosis is acceptable when basic tests for semen analysis, ovulation, tubal patency, and uterus are normal. If there is a suspicion of endometriosis on the basis of history, a diagnostic laparoscopy should also be performed. In this group of women who are already ovulating, giving clomiphene alone for ovulation induction is usually not very useful. Controlled ovarian stimulation should be combined with intrauterine insemination, and tried for 3–4 cycles in younger women. In women with long standing infertility or age more than 35 years, IVF is a better choice.[18]

WORK-UP OF AN INFERTILE COUPLE

History

A detailed history from both partners is important in ascertaining the cause of infertility and to plan treatment for the couple. History should include:

1. Age of both partners
2. Number of years married and cohabitation
3. Any contraception used and for how long
4. Previous partners if any and their reproductive history
5. Any pregnancy from current or previous partner and its outcome

6. Menstrual history
   - Menarche
   - No of days of bleeding
   - Interval between two periods (day 1 to day 1 of bleeding)
   - Associated dysmenorrhea
   - Last menstrual period
7. Past history
   - Medical disorders, e.g. diabetes, hypertension, hypothyroidism
   - History suggestive of PID, galactorrhea, tuberculosis
   - Known allergies
   - Any previous surgery
8. Family history of birth defects, developmental delay, early menopause, or reproductive problems
9. Coital history
   - Frequency of coitus
   - Any coital problem
   - Problem with erection/ejaculation
   - Dyspareunia
10. Details of investigations done
11. Details of previous treatments and their outcome
12. Use of tobacco, alcohol, or illicit drugs

Examination

The following must be documented:

1. Weight, body mass index
2. Blood pressure, pulse
3. Thyroid enlargement
4. Breast examination including checking for galactorrhea
5. Signs of androgen excess like hirsutism, acne
6. Abdominal examination for any abdominal or pelvic tenderness, any masses
7. Speculum examination for any vaginal or cervical abnormalities
8. Bimanual pelvic examination for
   - Uterine size, position and mobility
   - Adnexal mass or tenderness
   - Cul-de-sac masses, tenderness, nodularity

Investigations

Semen analysis: Basic investigations in an infertile couple should start with a semen test. Semen sample is produced by masturbation after 2–3 days of abstinence. Too short and too long period of abstinence, both affect semen quality. The reference values for semen parameters are given by World Health Organization.[19] The lower limit for the normal or the 5th percentiles is given in Table 19.2.

Table 19.2: Reference values for human semen by World Health Organization (2009)

Semen characteristics	5th percentile
Volume	1.5 ml
Concentration	15 million/ml
Total sperms/ejaculate	39 million
Vitality	58%
Progressive motility	32%
Total motility	40%
Morphology	4%

An abnormal semen report must be repeated before making a definite diagnosis. Tests for sperm antibodies or semen culture are not routinely recommended.

TESTS FOR OVULATION

Ovulatory disorders are found in 25–40% women who present with infertility. The integral endocrine events associated with ovulation include an LH surge followed by rise in progesterone level, which form the basis of a number of tests of ovulation.

Basal body temperature (BBT): Serial basal body temperature charting is an age-old method for ovulation detection. It is based on the principle that the basal body temperature increases after ovulation due to progesterone secretion. However, it is tedious and does not define the time of ovulation reliably, and therefore not routinely recommended.

Serum progesterone level measured one week before the onset of menses is a reliable method for ovulation detection. Progesterone level greater than 3 ng/ml indicates ovulation.

Urinary luteinizing hormone (LH): Kits are available commercially which can detect mid-cycle LH surge. Ovulation occurs one to two days following the LH surge.

Endometrial biopsy is done during the premenstrual phase or on the first day of period if the cycles are irregular. Histology showing secretory endometrium is considered diagnostic of ovulation in that cycle, as it is a sign of progesterone secretion which occurs only in ovulatory cycles. It has been considered as the gold standard for a long time to diagnose ovulation and luteal phase defect, but in modern practice, it is recommended only if there is a strong suspicion of endometritis or other endometrial pathology.

Transvaginal ultrasonography provides indirect evidence of ovulation as the growth and rupture of the follicle can be tracked by performing serial ultrasounds in a cycle.

TESTS FOR TUBAL PATENCY

Tubal disease is an important cause of infertility as it leads to tubal block. It is more often seen in women with secondary infertility than primary. Pelvic infection is the usual cause, but at times tubes may be blocked due to adhesions distorting normal pelvic anatomy. The standard tests for checking tubal patency are as follows:

Hysterosalpingogram (HSG): It is an out-patient procedure which does not require anesthesia. Water or lipid soluble contrast media is injected into the uterus using the Leisch Wilkinson cannula or a disposable plastic cannula via the cervix. The contrast opacifies the uterus, then the tubes and a peritoneal spill is seen if the tubes are patent. The test has a 94% negative predictive value and 38% positive predictive value,[20] which means that a test showing patent tubes is more likely to be correct than one showing tubal block. Figure 19.3 shows a normal HSG. Besides tubal patency, the test may demonstrate the site of the block, and intrauterine abnormalities.

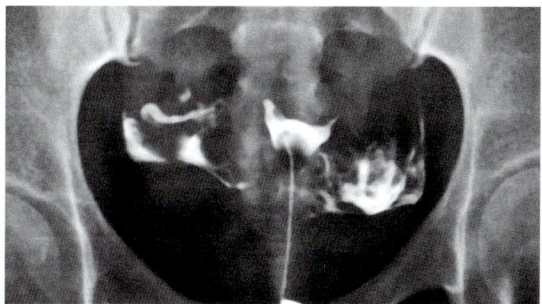

Fig. 19.3: Hysterosalpingogram showing bilateral tubal patency

Saline infusion sonography (SIS) is an ultrasound based procedure in which saline is injected via the cervix as in HSG and fluid is observed in the cul-de-sac. The test does not differentiate between unilateral and bilateral patency.[20]

Laparoscopy and chromotubation, also called lap and dye test involves demonstration of tubal patency on laparoscopy by introducing methylene blue or indigo carmine via the cervix. It can diagnose proximal or distal tubal block, and also correct fimbrial block or peritubal adhesions.

Uterine Pathology

Transvaginal ultrasound is a very useful investigation in infertility. It not only helps to suspect or diagnose uterine pathology but also shows the structure of ovaries to exclude polycystic ovaries or ovarian cysts, and any other pathology in the pelvis.

Hysteroscopy is the gold standard for diagnosing intracavitary uterine pathology like fibroids, polyps, adhesions, and developmental abnormalities like septate uterus. Figure 19.4 shows a hysteroscopic picture of an endometrial polyp. It also provides opportunity to correct these pathologies hysteroscopically at the same sitting or later.

Tests for Ovarian Reserve

Unlike men who produce sperms on an ongoing basis, women are born with the total number of oocytes or eggs they will ever have. According to estimates, the average number of eggs at birth is 500,000 to 1,000,000. This number decreases with increasing age as the oocytes undergo atresia. Moreover, not only the quantity but the quality of eggs also deteriorates, which correlates with the declining fertility with age.

Ovarian reserve implies the number and quality of remaining oocytes and therefore a marker of reproductive potential. It is usually not of concern in young women, but as the age increases beyond 30, it may become an important factor contributing to infertility. A number of tests for ovarian reserve are available which include biochemical tests and ultrasound imaging of the ovaries.

Biochemical tests include basal measurement of follicle-stimulating hormone (FSH), estradiol, inhibin B, and anti-mullerian hormone (AMH). As the number of follicles decline with age, inhibin B and AMH decline, whereas the basal (days 2, 3, or 4 of the cycle) FSH and estradiol rise.

Antral follicle count (AFC) is the measurement of the number of follicles on transvaginal ultrasound between 2 and 10 millimeters in diameter in both the ovaries. It is performed in the early follicular phase of the menstrual cycle, and correlates with the remaining follicular pool. Another ultrasound marker of ovarian reserve is the **ovarian volume,** which diminishes with falling ovarian reserve.

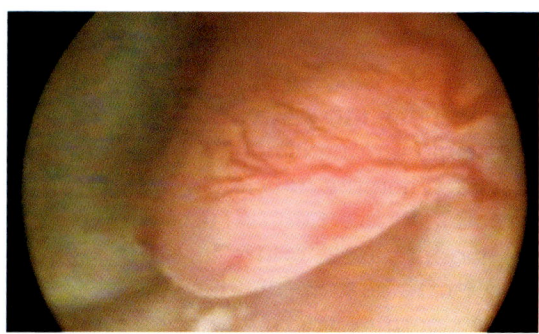

Fig. 19.4: Hysteroscopic view of endometrial polyp

The most commonly performed tests in clinical practice are basal FSH, AMH and AFC.

Treatment

Counseling is an important component of infertility treatment. Providing basic information about conception, fertile period, and above all giving hope to the couple who are often under a lot of stress can be of a great help in achieving pregnancy. Treatment for specific conditions leading to infertility has been discussed with the etiological factors. If such treatment fails to achieve conception, or in case of unexplained infertility, assisted reproductive techniques for conception should be offered.

Assisted Reproductive Technology (ART)

The greatest advancement in infertility treatment in the last two decades has been in the area of ART. Assisted reproductive technology includes all treatments which involve handling of sperms and oocytes. The most commonly used techniques are intrauterine insemination (IUI), *in vitro* fertilization (IVF) and intracytoplasmic sperm injection (ICSI).

Intrauterine insemination: This involves processing of a semen sample to improve the quality and quantity of sperms. The semen is washed and the sperms with good motility are separated, and injected into the uterus around the time of ovulation. This may be done in a natural cycle or a stimulated cycle with clomiphene or gonadotrophins. The success rate per cycle is usually 7–9% with clomiphene and 10–12% with gonadotrophins. Follicle monitoring is done to track follicular growth. When the follicle is mature (18 mm or more), an injection of HCG is given and IUI is done 36–40 hours later. The semen sample may be from the husband or in case of azoospermia, sperms are obtained from certified semen banks and donor IUI is done.

In vitro fertilization (IVF): It implies fertilization outside the body. In a typical IVF cycle, ovaries are stimulated with hormone injections (FSH and LH) for multiple follicular development. When the eggs are mature, HCG injection is given and eggs from the ovary are retrieved after 34–36 hours. The gametes are placed in an incubator and the fertilized embryos are replaced in the uterus after 2–5 days. The success rates vary depending on the age and ovarian reserve of the patients.

Intracytoplasmic sperm injection (ICSI): In conventional IVF, the oocytes and sperms are placed together in a dish and left in the incubator for the sperms to penetrate the eggs and fertilization to occur. In ICSI, the sperm is selected by the embryologist and introduced into the egg via a needle. ICSI is performed in couples to improve fertilization rates when the probability of fertilization by the natural process is lower, as in semen with low sperm count or motility.

Surgical sperm retrieval can be performed by aspiration or biopsy from the testis in azoospermic men. These sperms can then be used for IVF-ICSI.

Age is an important single factor which determines fertility in women. As age increases, the ovarian reserve falls, reducing the chances of conception and increasing the risk of abortion. Moreover, with increasing age, conditions like endometriosis and fibroids may develop which further reduce the chances of pregnancy. A proper evaluation of both partners should be undertaken to identify the cause if possible, and plan treatment accordingly. When the primary treatment targeted to the problem fails, or in case of unexplained infertility, ART gives hope of successful pregnancy. However, it should be resorted to early rather than late, as pregnancy and take home baby rates decline with age in ART as with other infertility treatments.

References

1. Niswender GD, Juengel JL, Silva PJ, Rollyson MK, McIntush EW. Mechanisms controlling the function and lifespan of the corpus luteum. Physiol Rev Jan 2000;80(1):1–29.

2. Fertility problems: assessment and treatment. NICE guidelines February 2013.

3. Baird DT. Amenorrhoea. Lancet 1997;350:275–9.

4. Anaszewska B, Spaczyñski RZ, Pelesz M, Pawelczyk L. Incidence of elevated LH/FSH ratio in polycystic ovary syndrome, Women with normo- and hyperinsulinemia. Rocz Akad Med Bialymst 2003;48:131–4.

5. Dumesic DA, Oberfield SE, Stener-Victorin E, Marshall JC, Laven JS, Legro RS. Scientific statement on the diagnostic criteria, epidemiology, pathophysiology, and molecular genetics of polycystic ovary syndrome. Endocr Rev. Oct 2015;36(5):487–525.

6. ESHRE Capri Workshop Group. Health and fertility in World Health Organization group 2 anovulatory women. Hum Reprod Update. Sep-Oct 2012 ;18(5):586–99.

7. Amer SA, Banu Z, Li TC, Cooke ID. Long-term follow-up of patients with polycystic ovary syndrome after laparoscopic ovarian drilling: endocrine and ultrasonographic outcomes. Hum Reprod. Nov 2002;17(11):2851–7.

8. Moazami Goudarzi Z, Fallahzadeh H, Aflatoonian A, Mirzaei M. Laparoscopic ovarian electrocautery versus gonadotropin therapy in infertile women with clomiphene citrate-resistant polycystic ovary syndrome: A systematic review and meta-analysis. Iran J Reprod Med. Aug 2014;12(8):531–8.

9. Chung JP, Haines CJ, Kong GW. Long-term reproductive outcome after hysteroscopic proximal tubal cannulation—an outcome analysis. Aust N Z J Obstet Gynaecol Oct 2012; 52(5):470–5.

10. Hou HY, Chen YQ, Li TC, Hu CX, Chen X, Yang ZH. Outcome of laparoscopy-guided hysteroscopic tubal catheterization for infertility due to proximal tubal obstruction. J Minim Invasive Gynecol Mar-Apr 2014;21(2):272–8.

11. Bosteels J, Kasius J, Weyers S, Broekmans FJ, Mol BW, D'Hooghe TM. Hysteroscopy for treating subfertility associated with suspected major uterine cavity abnormalities. Cochrane Database Syst Rev. 2015 Feb 21;2:CD009461.

12. Bosteels J, Weyers S, Puttemans P, Panayotidis C, Van Herendael B, Gomel V, Mol BW, Mathieu C, D'Hooghe T. The effectiveness of hysteroscopy in improving pregnancy rates in subfertile women without other gynaecological symptoms: a systematic review. Hum Reprod Update Jan-Feb 2010;16(1):1–11.

13. Bulletti C, Coccia ME, Battistoni S, Borini A. Endometriosis and infertility. Journal of Assisted Reproduction and Genetics. 2010;27(8):441–7. doi:10.1007/s10815-010-9436-1.

14. Burney RO, Giudice LC. Pathogenesis and Pathophysiology of Endometriosis. Fertility and sterility. 2012;98(3):10.

15. Marcoux S, Maheux R, Bérubé S. Laparoscopic surgery in infertile women with minimal or mild endometriosis. Canadian Collaborative Group on Endometriosis. N Engl J Med. 1997 Jul 24; 337(4):217–22.

16. Parazzini F. Ablation of lesions or no treatment in minimal—mild endometriosis in infertile women: a randomized trial. Gruppo Italiano per lo Studio dell'Endometriosi. Hum Reprod. May 1999;14(5):1332–4.

17. Practice Committee of the American Society for Reproductive Medicine. Endometriosis and infertility: a committee opinion. Fertil Steril. Sep 2012;98(3):591–8.

18. Sadeghi MR. Unexplained infertility, the controversial matter in management of infertile couples. J Reprod Infertil Jan-Mar 2015;16(1):1–2.

19. Cooper TG, Noonan E, von Eckardstein S, Auger J, Baker HW, Behre HM, Haugen TB, Kruger T, Wang C, Mbizvo MT, Vogelsong KM. World Health Organization reference values for human semen characteristics. Hum Reprod Update May-Jun 2010;16(3):231–45.

20. Practice Committee of American Society for Reproductive Medicine. Diagnostic evaluation of the infertile female: a committee opinion. Fertil Steril 2015;103:e44–50.

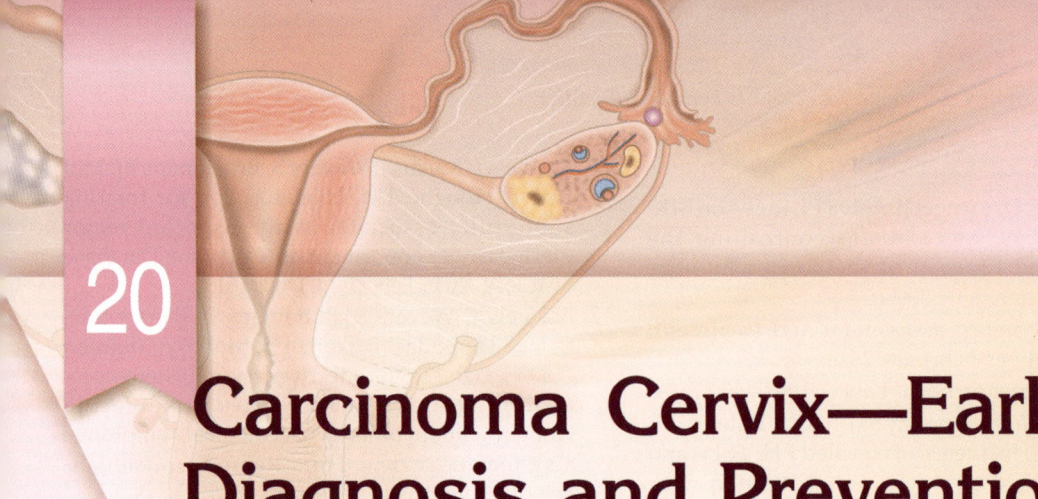

20

Carcinoma Cervix—Early Diagnosis and Prevention

• Sushma Rastogi

Let us make 'cancer' only a 'Zodiac' sign

Cancer cervix occupies the top rank among cancers in women in developing countries. The growing risk of cancer cervix in India (aged 0–64 years) is 2.4% compared to 1.3% for the world. India contributes 20% of the global burden of cervical cancer. Moreover, 70% of our patients come in the late stage because of lack of awareness among women and their relations about the significance of early symptoms. Unfortunately early symptoms are sometimes ignored by practitioners as well and medications are given without proper clinical examination and investigation.

Diagnosis

Women with early cancer cervix and pre-cancer have no symptoms. Symptoms do not begin until a pre-cancer becomes a true invasive cancer and grows into nearby tissue. When this happens the most common symptoms are:

1. Abnormal vaginal bleeding such as bleeding after coitus, bleeding after menopause, bleeding and spotting between periods and having longer or heavier menstrual periods than usual. Bleeding after douching or after a pelvic examination is a common symptom of cervical cancer but not pre-cancer.
2. An unusual discharge from the vagina— may contain some blood and may occur between periods or after menopause.
3. Pain during intercourse (screening is required).

Screening for cervical cancers: Cancer can ruin a beautiful life. Early detection can save one. There is as yet no organized screening program for the country. **American Cancer Society (ACS) Guidelines** for prevention and early detection of cervical cancer include:

- Screening should start at the age of 21 years or within 3 years of first sexual activity, whichever comes first; women aged 21 to 29 years should have a Pap test every 3 years. HPV testing should not be used in this age group unless it is needed after an abnormal Pap test result.
- Women between age 30 and 65 years should have a Pap test and HPV test (called **"co-testing"**) every 5 years or Pap test alone every 3 years.
- Women above 65 years and who had regular screening in the previous 10 years with normal results should not be tested for cervical cancer. Women with history of

serious cervical pre-cancer should continue to be tested for at least 20 years after that diagnosis.

- Women who had total hysterectomy for reasons not related to cervical cancer and who have no h/o cervical cancer should not be tested.
- A woman who has been vaccinated against HPV should still follow the screening recommendations for her age group .
- Some women because of their health history (HIV infection, DES exposure, organ transplantation) may need to have a different screening schedule for cervical cancer.

Since cervical cancer starts with *pre-cancer changes,* there are **two ways** to stop this disease from developing:

1. To find and treat pre-cancers in the first place.
2. To prevent the pre-cancers in the first place.

Finding cervical pre-cancers: A well proven way to prevent cervical cancer is to have testing (screening) to find pre-cancers before they can turn into invasive cancer. The **Pap test** (Pap smear) and the **HPV test** are used for this. If found, it can be treated, stopping cervical cancer before it really starts. Since no HPV vaccine provides complete protection against all of the HPV types that can cause cancer cervix, it cannot prevent all cases of cancer cervix. So screening should continue. Most invasive cancers are found in women who have not had regular screening.

Things to do, to prevent pre-cancer and cervical cancer

- Avoid contact with HPV
- Use condoms
- Do not smoke
- Get vaccinated—girls aged 11 to 12 years should routinely be vaccinated for HPV with the full series of 3 shots. Women aged 13–26 years who have not yet been vaccinated get "catch-up" vaccinations.

What Tests (or treatment) one needs, depends on the results of Pap test?

- **Atypical squamous cells** (ASC-US and ASC-H)— repeat the Pap test in 12 months or test for HPV.
  - 21–24 years old and HPV DNA positive– repeat Pap test in a year
  - 25 years old and HPV DNA positive– colposcopy to be done
- **If HPV not detected**—Pap test can be repeated in 3 years

  25 years old—Pap test +ve, HPV test to be done.

  If atypical squamous cells on Pap test, one cannot exclude high grade squamous intraepithelial lesion (ASC-H)—colposcopy is done
- **Squamous intraepithelial lesions**

  i. **Low grade (LSIL)**—further testing depends upon HPV testing
     - HPV negative—repeat Pap test and HPV in one year; HPV positive—colposcopy
     - No HPV test was done and the woman is 25 years—colposcopy to be done.

  ii. **High grade squamous intraepithelial lesion (HSIL)**—either colposcopy or a loop electrosurgical procedure is recommended for woman 25 years old or more.

     Under 25 years of age—colposcopy is advised.
- **Atypical glandular cells and adenocarcinoma in situ** (on a Pap test) but abnormal cells do not seem from endometrium— need coploscopy with endocervical curettage (scraping)

  If abnormal cells seen from endometrium— colposcopy with EB is done.
- **Abnormal Pap test results—work-up**

  Pap test is a screening test, not diagnostic, cannot reveal certainly that cancer is present, so other tests are required and also done to follow-up a positive HPV test results. One needs:
- Colposcopy

- Cervical biopsy—it may be:
  - Colposcopic
  - Endocervical curettage (scraping), and
  - Cone biopsy—electrosurgical procedure (LEEP or LLETZ) or knife cone biopsy. **Precancerous changes on a biopsy are called CIN (cervical intraepithelial neoplasia)** while on a Pap test they are called SIL (squamous intraepithelial lesion). CIN is graded on a scale of 1 to 3 depending upon how much of the cervical tissue looks abnormal when viewed under the microscope?
  - CIN1—not much tissue [least tissue] looks abnormal
  - CIN2—more tissue looks abnormal
  - CIN3—most of the tissue looks abnormal (most serious pre-cancer); term "Dysplasia" has also been used instead CIN in the past.

Prevention

Cervical cancer starts with pre-cancer changes, there are **two ways** to stop this disease from developing.

1. One way is to find and treat pre-cancer before it becomes true cancer, and
2. The other is to prevent the development of pre-cancers in the first place. Education, screening and vaccination are the most important pillars in the prevention of cervical cancer.

Primary Prevention

1. **HPV** infection—about 95% of women with invasive cervical cancer have evidence of HPV infection. HPV types 16 and 18 cause about 70% of cases of cancer cervix worldwide. Following measures can be undertaken to avoid HPV infection:
   i. Abstinence from sexual activity
   ii. Barrier protection and/or spermicidal gel during sexual intercourse
   iii. HPV vaccination
   iv. Avoid cigarette smoking

   v. Reproductive behaviour—high parity is associated with increased risk
   vi. Long-term use of oral contraceptives—women who use it for more than 5 years are likely to have approximately three times the incidence of cancer cervix.

HPV vaccine has been approved by FDA to prevent HPV infection. Routine vaccination is recommended for girls aged 10–12 years (before the onset of sexual activity). Three doses are given.

Finding cervical pre-cancer tests to be done include:

1. Pap test
2. HPV test

Full assessment by a gynecologist is necessary to treat infection, anemia, nutritional deficiency and follow-up: advise Pap test and manage accordingly; consider biopsy and treat accordingly; some cases seen as erosion after abortion or delivery may not require active treatment—just nip it in the bud.

1. *Pap smears* from ectocervix and endocervix. The Pap test (sometimes called a Pap smear or cervical cytology). Pap smear is most widely used method for screening of premalignant and malignant lesions of cervix. Sensitivity ranges from 55 to 80%. To avoid the sampling and preparation errors of Pap smear, newer methods like computer-assisted screening **(two systems-Auto Pap and Pap net (Pap sure)** are approved) and **liquid-based cytology (Thin prep) are** available. Pap stained cervical cell images, acquired through a CCD camera adapted to an optical microscope—Pap smear images of cervical region based on cell nuclei distribution and shape and size analysis (image processing tool box) has also been used.

2. *HPV testing*—HPV **DNA** testing by hybrid capture II (HC 2) is method most widely used. HPV genotyping for oncogenic HPVs is another method (most useful for primary screening). HPV vaccine (Gardasil-quadri-

valent vaccine against HPV types 16,18, at 0, 2, 6 months and cervarix—a bi-valent vaccine given at 0, 1 and 6 months). They provide efficient protection in non-exposed females; antibody titres are maintained for 4–5 years but further persistence is uncertain; have a high safety profile. **ACOG recommends that vaccination should be offered to all females aged 9–26 years who have not been previously vaccinated, along with regular cervical cytology screening**. Efficacy in older women is questionable.

3. *Colposcopy:* Though HPE (histopathological examination) is the gold standard test, the colposcope is unique in identifying the precursor lesions of cancer cervix. It is the most important tool for accurate diagnosis and its role cannot be overstressed. Even when the TZ line is not visualized making the view unsatisfactory, the identifying features of **abnormal vessels, intense acetowhite areas in affected cervix** strongly point to the nature of underlying disease and enabling the accuracy of selecting biopsy sites and provisional diagnosis. **Gynecologist** plays very important role in control of cervical cancer (assess the lesion—by colposcopy; enlighten and not to frighten the family); early lesions can be treated conservatively; perform cervical biopsy if necessary. The biopsy site may be cauterized with Monsel's paste or a silver nitrate stick; **endocervical curettage** if necessary (no abnormality on ectocervix, glandular lesion may be present, colposcopic examination–unsatisfactory). **Colposcopy is useful** to:

i. Confirm the presence of neoplasia

ii. Idendtify the grade of neoplasia, and

iii. Localize the lesion (cervical neoplasia—acetowhite area, keratosis, mosaic, punctuation and abnormal blood vessels).

A **biopsy** should be taken. Treatment depends upon the biopsy report—loop electro-surgical excision of the abnormal lesion, or cryotherapy. Use of magnascope instead of colposcope—low cost instrument has been found very useful. It has a built in light source and a fixed magnification of 5X.

4. *Cervicography:* A photograph is taken of the entire cervical os after applying 5% acetic acid to the cervix and sending it to the colposcopist for evaluation. A biopsy is taken from the appropriate site.

5. *Colposcopic directed biopsy:* Allows accurate localization of the abnormal tissue and reduces false negative findings.

6. *Cone biopsy:* Indications: (a) large area of abnormal lesion, (b) inner margin of the lesion has receded into the cervical canal, (c) SCZ is not completely visible during colposcopy, and (d) discrepancy is seen between the cytological report and colposcopic findings.

7. *HPV vaccines* are new hope as primary prevention. Let us say Good Bye to invasive cervical cancer. HPV testing and regular check-ups will make up a difference to the lives of women.

8. *Cervical cancer and STD* single sample system [one sample 4 tests—HPV DNA (high risk); Chlamydia DNA; Gonorrhoea DNA; HSV DNA—linear signal amplification (LSA) technology involving proprietary RNA probes and detection of full length RNA].

Screening of women in low resource setting includes

i. VIA (visual inspection of the cervix by 3–5% acetic acid) or VILI (visual inspection of the cervix by Lugol's iodine) or cervicoscopy.

ii. Use of magnascope instead of colposcope

iii. Single visit approach

iv. Cryosurgery for VIA +ve women

v. Education and counseling

vi. Increasing coverage by camp approach

vii. Low cost HPV tests, and

viii. HPV vaccines

Downstaging of cervical cancer: Downstaging is defined as a process of screening for cancer using clinical approaches for early detection of the disease. This is distinct from screening test and results in detection of the disease at a less advanced stage in the absence of screening. This approach is applicable in developing countries where cytological screening is not possible at present. In this method, paramedical staff trained for minimum period will be able to identify any abnormality including suspicious cervix and refer the case early to centres where facilities exist for treatment of premalignant and malignant lesions, including educating the women regarding risk factors, symptoms of disease and prophylaxis. This experimental methodology recommended by WHO for developing countries like India has to be evaluated by monitoring various ongoing projects where visual inspection screening method is used. The results are collected which include feasibility, compliance, costing, referral methodology, difficulties in implementation, specificity, sensitivity, positive predictive value and drawbacks. This methodology has been advocated as a means of improving survival and reducing mortality.

i. All the doctors, health workers need to be trained for early detection of cancer by Pap smear, on examination if any abnormality detected, and to refer the case for investigations.

ii. Society should be aware about predisposing factors, e.g. age of marriage, contraception, multiple sexual partners, general hygiene, use of barrier methods (STDs).

iii. Every woman married, multipara, >35 years of age—should have Pap smear.

iv. Proper treatment of pre-cancerous lesions to prevent development of invasive cervical cancer.

"Cervical cancer is, more than ever, a totally preventable cancer". "Better testing is cheaper than more visits".

Conclusion

All the doctors need to be trained for proper examination and early detection of carcinoma cervix. Paramedical staff should be able to identify any abnormality on the cervix and refer the case to the centre where facilities exist for the diagnosis of cancer cervix.

Society should be aware about predisposing factors so that proper care could be taken. All women who are married, above 35 years of age should have Pap smear. Women should be educated regarding risk factors, symptoms of disease and prophylaxis.

We should organise camps regularly in rural areas to educate women about cancer cervix, risk factors, contraceptive methods, HPV vaccine for girls, role of screening and its prevention.

Index

Outstanding Awards

- Awarded *"**Padmashri**" by the **President of India** in 1985.*
- FOGSI "**Late Prof. D Kutty Life Time Achievement Award**" in 2008.
- FOGSI "**Late RB Dr. SN Malhotra Award**"- 2012
- "**Dr. BC ROY National Award**" by the **President** of India in 1996.
- **World Record** of performing **611** Laparoscopic Ligation in 24 hrs at Aligarh in October 1982.
- "**Hari Om Ashram Alembic Research Award**" by the **President** of India in 1993.
- "**Indira Gandhi Priyadarshini Award**" in 1992.
- "**Rashtriya Rattan Award and Gold Medal**" in 2005.
- "**Jewel of India Award**" and a "**Certificate of Merit**" in 2005.

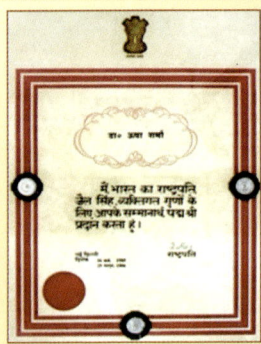

> **Awarded "Padmashri" by the President of India in 1985**

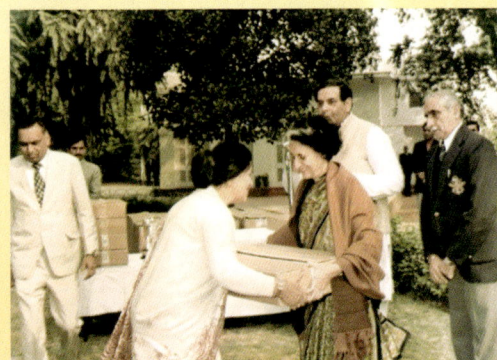

> **Awarded Laparoscope by Late Prime Minister Mrs Indira Gandhi for outstanding fieldwork in the country in 1982**

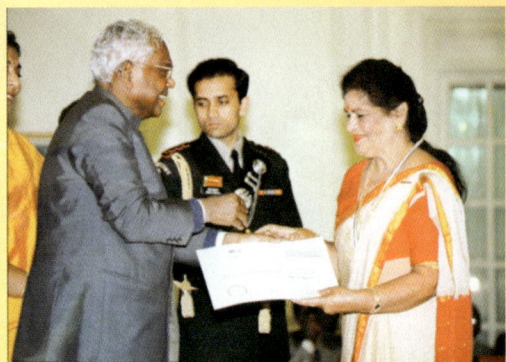

> **Hari Om Ashram Alembic Research Award by the President of India in 1993**

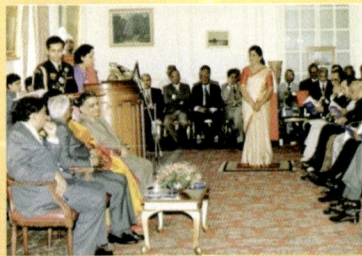

> **Dr. BC Roy National Award for Eminent Medical Teacher by the President of India in 1996**

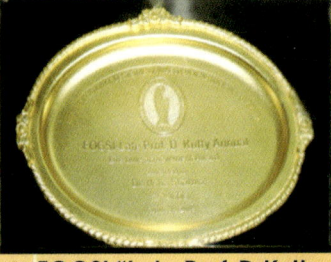

> **FOGSI "Late Prof. D Kutty Life Time Achievement Award" in 2008**

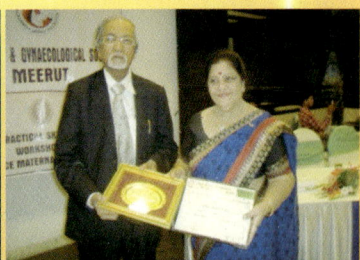

> **FOGSI "Late Prof. D Kutty Life Time Achievement Award" in 2008**